AORTIC DISEASES
Clinical Diagnostic Imaging Atlas

DVD Table of Contents

Chapter 1. Aortic Physiology and Function
- Animations (3 clips)

Chapter 2. Anatomic Variants of the Aorta
- Videos (2 clips)

Chapter 3. Examination and Imaging of the Aorta
- TTE (4 clips)
- TEE (4 clips)
- MRA (1 clip)

Chapter 4. Acute Aortic Dissection
- Animation (3 clips)
- Aortography (1 clip)
- Surgery (1 clip)
- TEE (11 clips)
- TTE (2 clips)
- Clinical cases (10 cases, 52 clips)

Chapter 5. Aortic Intramural Hematoma
- Videos (4 clips)
- Clinical cases (3 cases, 8 clips)

Chapter 6. Late Complications of Aortic Dissection
- Clinical cases (3 cases, 7 clips)

Chapter 7. Aortic Complications of Catheterization, Surgery, and Instrumentation
- Clinical cases (2 cases, 7 clips)

Chapter 8. Plaques, Debris, and Obstruction
- Video (1 clip)
- Clinical cases (4 cases, 9 clips)

Chapter 9. Thrombosis, Thromboembolism, and Atheroembolism
- Clinical cases (4 cases, 9 clips)

Chapter 10. Ulcers and Penetrating Aortic Ulcers
- Clinical cases (2 cases, 12 clips)

Chapter 11. Thoracic Aortic Aneurysms
- Clinical cases (3 cases, 8 clips)

Chapter 14. Diseases of the Aortic Root
- Videos (2 clips)
- Clinical cases (2 cases, 5 clips)

Chapter 15. Congenital Bicuspid Aortic Valve
- Clinical cases (5 cases, 11 clips)

Chapter 16. Coarctation and Atresia of the Aorta
- Videos (4 clips)
- Clinical cases (2 cases, 9 clips)

Chapter 17. Marfan Syndrome
- Clinical cases (4 cases, 15 clips)

Chapter 18. Traumatic Disruption of the Aorta
- Clinical cases (3 cases, 10 clips)

Chapter 19. Tumors of the Aorta
- Videos (2 clips)

Chapter 20. Infectious and Mycotic Aneurysms
- Videos (2 clips)

Chapter 21. Takayasu's Disease
- Videos (1 clip)

Aortic Diseases

CLINICAL DIAGNOSTIC IMAGING ATLAS

Aortic Diseases

CLINICAL DIAGNOSTIC IMAGING ATLAS

Stuart J. Hutchison

MD, FRCPC, FACC, FAHA, FASE, FSCMR, FSCCT

Clinical Associate Professor of Medicine

University of Calgary

Foothills Medical Center

Stephenson Cardiac Magnetic

Resonance Imaging Center

Libin Cardiovascular Institute of Alberta

Calgary, Canada

With contributions by Mark D. Peterson and Edward B. Diethrich

SAUNDERS

ELSEVIER

Original artwork and animations by
Gail Rudakewich, Myra Rudakewich, and **Stuart J. Hutchison**

SAUNDERS
ELSEVIER

1600 John F. Kennedy Blvd.
Ste 1800
Philadelphia, PA 19103-2899

AORTIC DISEASES: CLINICAL DIAGNOSTIC
IMAGING ATLAS

ISBN: 978-1-4160-5270-8

Notice

Knowledge and best practice in this field are constantly changing. As new research and experience broaden our knowledge, changes in practice, treatment, and drug therapy may become necessary or appropriate. Readers are advised to check the most current information provided (i) on procedures featured or (ii) by the manufacturer of each product to be administered, to verify the recommended dose or formula, the method and duration of administration, and contraindications. It is the responsibility of the practitioner, relying on his or her experience and knowledge of the patient, to make diagnoses, to determine dosages and the best treatment for each individual patient, and to take all appropriate safety precautions. To the fullest extent of the law, neither the Publisher nor the Author assumes any liability for any injury and/or damage to persons or property arising out of or related to any use of the material contained in this book.

The Publisher

Library of Congress Cataloging-in-Publication Data
Hutchison, Stuart J.
    Aortic diseases : clinical diagnostic imaging atlas with DVD / Stuart J. Hutchison.—1st ed.
        p. ; cm.—(Cardiovascular emergencies : atlas and multimedia series)
    Includes bibliographical references.
    ISBN 978-1-4160-5270-8
    1. Aorta—Diseases—Diagnosis—Atlases. 2. Aorta—Imaging—Atlases. I. Title. II. Series.
    [DNLM: 1. Aortic Diseases—diagnosis—Atlases. 2. Diagnostic Imaging—Atlases. WG 17 H978a 2009]
    RC691.6.I52H88 2009
    616.1'380754—dc22   2008018556

Executive Publisher: Natasha Andjelkovic
Publishing Services Manager: Frank Polizzano
Project Manager: Rachel Miller
Design Direction: Lou Forgione
Illustration Direction: Ceil Nuyianes
Multimedia Producer: Bruce Robison

Printed in China.

Last digit is the print number: 9 8 7 6 5 4 3 2 1

To Noel Keith and Cindy Hutchison, for the immeasurable gifts of love and time.

To Elizabeth Radley Hutchison (1931–1985) and G. B. Alec Hutchison (1927–2006)—*memor esto.*

To the many wonderfully dedicated cardiac and vascular surgery colleagues that I have been privileged to work with, especially those at St. Michael's Hospital, whose openness, honesty, insight, and abilities provided many of the best apertures through which aortic diseases may be understood.

Contributors

Kim A. Eagle, MD, FACC, FAHA
Albion Walter Hewlett Professor of Internal Medicine,
University of Michigan Medical School; Clinical Director,
University of Michigan Cardiovascular Center, Ann Arbor,
Michigan

Edward B. Diethrich, MD
Medical Director, Arizona Heart Institute and Foundation,
Phoenix, Arizona

Stuart J. Hutchison, MD, FRCPC, FACC, FAHA, FASE, FSCMR,
FSCCT
Clinical Associate Professor of Medicine, University of Calgary
Division of Cardiology, Foothills Medical Center; Department
of Cardiac Sciences, Libin Cardiovascular Institute of Alberta,
Calgary, Canada

Mark D. Peterson, MD, PhD, FRCSC
Assistant Professor of Surgery, University of Toronto; Cardiac
and Endovascular Surgery, Division of Cardiac Surgery, St.
Michael's Hospital, Toronto, Ontario, Canada

Foreword

Aortic Diseases: Clinical Diagnostic Imaging Atlas is indeed a tour de force in furthering our understanding of the normal aorta and the various disorders that affect it. Stuart Hutchison has done a masterful job in creating a compendium of chapters that take us from normal aortic physiology and function, to the understanding of various imaging modalities, to the myriad of conditions that can present with either acute or chronic aortic conditions. Most notably, the provision of key points at the beginning of each chapter as well as the marvelous images, figures, and tables make this a usable reference for bedside patient evaluation as well as furthering our knowledge of aortic diseases. In my opinion, this is the finest work of its type ever produced.

Kim A. Eagle, MD, FACC, FAHA
Albion Walter Hewlett Professor of Internal Medicine
Clinical Director, Cardiovascular Center
University of Michigan Health System
Ann Arbor, Michigan

Preface

Aortic diseases are clinical giants that do not fall easily. Many clinical services are involved in their management: emergency physicians, family physicians, cardiologists, cardiac surgeons, vascular surgeons, radiologists, interventional radiologists, and intensivists. In order to achieve optimal outcomes, coordination and collaboration among them are paramount. Delivering the current standard of care in the management of aortic diseases requires clinical prowess, but advancing the standard of care requires remarkable insight into disease, inspiration, perseverance, and dedication.

Many presentations of aortic diseases are frank emergencies that are greatly challenging to the clinician, often in several ways, and their optimal management requires a breadth of clinical proficiency—maintaining suspicion and a command of diagnostic testing is paramount. The paradigms and thresholds for treatment of aortic diseases are evolving, and increasing permutations of interservice cooperation are also developing.

The fundamental basis of management of aortic diseases is knowledge—that of the natural history of different diseases, of the imaging characteristics, and of the available and optimal interventions. This book and its companion DVD have been structured to provide separate chapters for each disease topic, and the accompanying 100 clinical cases were included to serve as real-life examples and broaden the reader's perception of specific aortic diseases.

In the last five years there have been unparalleled advances in the imaging of aortic diseases (particularly by CT and MR), the determination of the natural histories and the intervened histories of aortic diseases (particularly by the IRAD Registry), and the surgical and interventional procedures. The topic of aortic diseases is now firmly mainstream and rapidly moving forward, and it includes a broader and broader range of physicians.

This book and its companion DVD provide an approach that integrates our knowledge of aortic anatomy, pathophysiology, and imaging. The book includes 22 chapters and a reasonable breadth of cases per chapter that represent the variants of the disorder. The intent was to allow the reader to gain anatomy-based and evidence-based knowledge and also learn the practical aspects of aortic lesions. It is my hope that increased knowledge of aortic diseases will lead to the optimization of their management and that much effort will continue to be applied to advance their management and improve patient outcomes.

Stuart J. Hutchison, MD

Acknowledgments

My sincere appreciation goes to Inga Tomas; Natasha Andjelkovic, PhD; Jehangir Appoo, MD; Daniel Bonneau, MD; Vern Campbell, MD; Robert Chisholm, MD; the CCU, cardiac ward, cardiac OR, and CVICU nurses; Edward B. Diethrich, MD; Kim A. Eagle, MD; Lee Errett, MD; Quentin Forrest, MB; Matthias Friedrich, MD; Geoffrey Gardiner, MD; Kate Holmes, RVT; Robert J. Howard, MD; Majo Joseph, MD; David Latter, MD; Yves Leclerc, MD; Howard Leong-Poi, MD; Anne Lenehan; Alan Lossing, MD; Danny Marcuzzi, MD; David Mazer, MD; Rachel Miller; Juan-Carlos Monge; Mark Peterson, MD; Susan Pioli; Michael Regan; Gail Rudakewich; Myra Rudakewich; Trevor Robinson, MD; Nazmi Said, RVT; Bradley Strauss, MD; and Subodh Verma, MD.

Stuart J. Hutchison, MD

Abbreviations

AAA, abdominal aortic aneurysm
AAD, acute aortic dissection
ACB, aortocoronary bypass
ACE, angiotensin-converting enzyme
AI, aortic insufficiency
AVR, aortic valve replacement
BP, blood pressure
bpm, beats per minute
CAD, coronary artery disease
CCS, Canadian Cardiovascular Society
CCU, coronary care unit
CHF, congestive heart failure
CMR, cardiac magnetic resonance
COPD, chronic obstructive pulmonary disease
CPB, cardiopulmonary bypass
CT, computed tomography
CTA, computed tomographic aortography; computed tomographic angiography
ECG, electrocardiography; electrocardiogram
EVAR, endovascular aortic repair
[^{18}F]FDG-PET, [^{18}F]-fluorodeoxyglucose positron emission tomography
FTA-ABS, fluorescent treponemal antibody absorption test
HR, heart rate
IAB, intra-aortic balloon
ICD, implantable cardioverter-defibrillator
ICU, intensive care unit
IMH, intramural hematoma
INR, international normalized ratio
IV, intravenous
IVC, inferior vena cava
IVUS, intravascular ultrasonography
LCA, left coronary artery
LV, left ventricle; left ventricular
LVH, left ventricular hypertrophy
MDCT, multidetector computed tomography
MR, magnetic resonance
MRA, magnetic resonance angiography; magnetic resonance aortography
MRI, magnetic resonance imaging
NYHA, New York Heart Association
PET, positron emission tomography
PISA, proximal isovelocity surface area
RBBB, right bundle branch block
RCA, right coronary artery
RR, respiratory rate
RV, right ventricle; right ventricular
RVH, right ventricular hypertrophy
SBP, systolic blood pressure
SEM, systolic ejection murmur
SLE, systemic lupus erythematosus
SVC, superior vena cava
TDA, traumatic disruption of the aorta
TEE, transesophageal echocardiography
TEVAR, thoracic endovascular aortic repair
TIA, transient ischemic attack
TOF, time-of-flight
TTE, transthoracic echocardiography
US, ultrasonography
VDRL, Venereal Disease Research Laboratory
VSD, ventricular septal defect
VTI, velocity-time integral

Contents

1. Aortic Physiology and Function: Anatomic and Histologic Considerations 1

2. Anatomic Variants of the Aorta 17

3. Examination and Imaging of the Aorta 33

4. Acute Aortic Dissection 55

5. Aortic Intramural Hematoma 113

6. Late Complications of Aortic Dissection 131

7. Aortic Complications of Catheterization, Surgery, and Instrumentation 141

8. Aortic Atheromatous Disease: Plaques, Debris, and Obstruction 155

9. Aortic Atheromatous Disease: Thrombosis, Thromboembolism, and Atheroembolism 169

10. Aortic Atheromatous Disease: Ulcers and Penetrating Aortic Ulcers 181

11. Thoracic Aortic Aneurysms 195

12. Abdominal Aortic Aneurysms 215

13. Endovascular Therapy for Thoracic Aortic Pathology 237
Mark D. Peterson and Edward B. Diethrich

14. Diseases of the Aortic Root 251

15. Congenital Bicuspid Aortic Valve–Associated Aortopathy 259

16. Coarctation and Atresia of the Aorta 271

17. Marfan Syndrome 297

18. Traumatic Disruption of the Aorta 315

19. Tumors of the Aorta 333

20. Infectious and Mycotic Aneurysms 337

21. Noninfectious Aortitis: Takayasu's Disease 341

22. Noninfectious Aortitis: Giant Cell Aortitis, Systemic Lupus Erythematosus, and Other Aortitides 347

Index 351

Aortic Physiology and Function: Anatomic and Histologic Considerations

KEY POINTS

Normal Aorta

▶ Aortic histology underlies its functions.

▶ Disease processes involving components of the histology will result in predictable clinical syndromes.

▶ Different segments of the aorta are prone to different diseases.

▶ Aortic functions are (1) antiatherosclerotic and antithrombotic and (2) capacitor, conduit, and pump.

▶ Anatomic relations explain many aortic disease presentations and complications.

▶ Descriptions of arterial (aorta) pressure are overly simplified by systolic and diastolic as these two variables are the result of numerous other cardiovascular variables.

Hypertensive Aorta

▶ Hypertensive distention of the aorta places the aorta at the steeply rising portion of its pressure:volume relation, rendering the aorta stiffer (a less efficient capacitor) and a faster propagator of the pulse wave, thereby augmenting the systolic pressure.

▶ Hypertension begets histologic changes of the aorta that are variable and may

▶ Change its physiologic properties (reduced capacitance—stiffer aorta; faster propagation of the pulse wave)

▶ Change its structural integrity (accelerating medial degeneration—cystic medial necrosis, rendering it susceptible to dilation and dissection)

▶ Promote atherosclerosis

To understand aortic disease, it is important to understand the gross anatomy of the aorta and the anatomic variants. The different segments of the aorta are subject to different diseases, have different imaging characteristics, have different branch vessels of different relevance, are accessed surgically by different approaches, and serve different physiologic functions. The microscopic anatomy of the aorta provides the substrate for its physiologic functions and also its susceptibility to diseases.

ANATOMY OF THE AORTA

The gross anatomy of the aorta may be divided into the following segments: (1) the aortic root; (2) the sinotubular junction; (3) the ascending aorta; (4) the aortic arch; (5) the isthmus and descending (thoracic) aorta; and (6) the abdominal aorta (Figs. 1-1 and 1-2).

The Aortic Root

The aortic root is the segment of the aorta from the aortic valve annulus to the sinotubular junction, including principally the sinuses of Valsalva (Fig. 1-3). The aortic root is intrapericardial and consists of three rounded, pocket-like dilations (sinuses) at the aortic valve leaflet level that allow the aortic valve leaflets to open to 90 degrees. Normal diameter of the aortic root is 2.9 ± 0.4 cm, with variation appropriate for body size.

The most common consequence of disease of the aortic root is valve function; dilation of the root lessens coaptation, and an event like dissection reduces the suspension of leaflets and leads to prolapse. The right sinus straddles the tricuspid valve and thus abuts both the right atrium and the right ventricle. The left sinus abuts the left atrium. The noncoronary sinus straddles the interatrial septum and thus abuts both the left and right atria. Normally, the left coronary ostium arises from the superior left coronary sinus, and the right coronary ostium arises from the

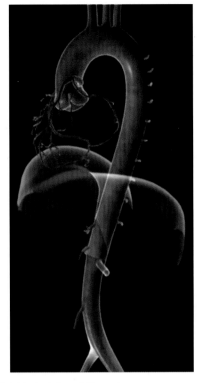

Figure 1-1. Graphic depiction of the aorta.

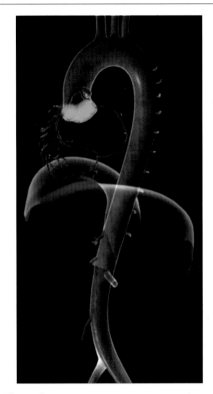

Figure 1-3. The aortic root.

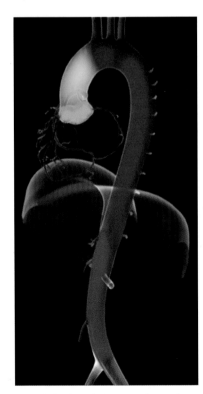

Figure 1-2. Segmental division of the aorta: the aortic root (LIGHT BLUE), the sinotubular junction (GREEN), the ascending aorta (YELLOW), the aortic arch (DARK BLUE), the isthmus and descending (thoracic) aorta (RED), and the abdominal aorta (PINK).

superior right coronary sinus. Some bicuspid aortic valves are associated with only two aortic root sinuses.

Branch vessels consist of the left coronary artery and right coronary artery. Anomalies and variations of coronary artery ostia and course are fairly common.

Disease Involvement

Disease involvement of the aortic root includes abscess extension from aortic valve endocarditis; dissection (most of the mortality of acute dissection is due to anatomic disruption of the aorta at the root level by rupture into the pericardial space, dehiscence of the aortic valve, or coronary ostial disruption); intramural hematoma; aneurysm (isolated to a sinus of Valsalva or generalized to involve the root and ascending aorta); sinus of Valsalva fistula; false aneurysms; noninfectious and infectious aortitis; traumatic disruption; and atherosclerosis. Congenital variants may occur in association with bicuspid aortic valves and present as two sinuses or dilation and aneurysm.

Imaging Considerations

The motion of the aortic root—about 1.5 cm per cardiac cycle—confers motion artifact to nongated imaging with low temporal resolution. High-resolution imaging of the ascending aorta requires either high temporal resolution (e.g., multidetector computed tomography [MDCT]) or electrocardiography (ECG) gating.

Computed Tomography High-attenuation streak artifacts from concentrated contrast dye in the adjacent superior vena cava (SVC) are common and clinically important problems because these streak artifacts can contaminate the depiction of the aortic root. Pacemaker leads in the SVC may also project artifacts across the aortic root. Mechanical aortic valves may also project artifacts into the aortic root.

Cardiac Magnetic Resonance Mechanical aortic valves may cause susceptibility artifacts within the aortic root.

Echocardiography The aortic root is usually well seen by transthoracic echocardiography, although artifacts may in some cases be prominent. Mechanical aortic valves and bioprosthetic aortic valves with thick wire stents produce posterior aortic root reverberation and shadowing artifact by transthoracic echocardiography and anterior aortic root reverberation and shadowing artifact by TEE. Transesophageal echocardiography (TEE) affords superior detail in most cases. Echocardiography is the best means to identify the presence and severity of functional complications of diseases of the aortic root, such as aortic insufficiency, myocardial ischemia, and tamponade.

Aortic Root and Its Anatomy: Clinical Relevance
- The aortic root is a frequently diseased site of the aorta.
- Its anatomy establishes the support and therefore integrity of the aortic valve.
- Disruption of the aortic root, as by dissection, usually results in prolapse of aortic valve leaflets and aortic insufficiency.
- Dilation of the root (particularly of the sinotubular junction) results in malcoaptation of the aortic valve leaflets centrally and central aortic insufficiency.
- Surgical approach is by median (midline) sternotomy; surgery requires cardiopulmonary bypass.
- Surgical root replacement (Bentall composite grafting) requires coronary artery reimplantation.
- Rupture of the root, as with type A aortic dissection or intramural hematoma, occurs into the pericardial sac, producing tamponade.
- Coronary anomalies confer technical challenge to angiographers and interventionalists.
- Some coronary anomalies are clinically symptomatic.
- Bicuspid aortic valves are common and associated with other aortic developmental anomalies and their complications.

The Sinotubular Junction

The sinotubular junction is normally a well-defined site at which the rounded and wider sinuses of Valsalva join the narrower tubule-shaped ascending aorta (Fig. 1-4). Effacement (erasing or blurring) of the usually well defined sinotubular junction suggests annuloaortic ectasia, an often marfanoid type of pathology. However, degrees of effacement may be seen in other clinical contexts, such as bicuspid aortic valves. Disease that involves the aorta proximal to this risks compromise of the suspension of the aortic valve commissures and also the coronary arteries whose ostia are within the sinuses. Normally, the sinotubular junction has the same dimension as the aortic annulus and constitutes a critical support to the superior aspect of the aortic valve commissures. Normal diameter of the sinotubular junction is 2.6 ± 0.3 cm, with variation appropriate for body size.

Loss of support of the commissure leads to leaflet prolapse. Dilation of the sinotubular junction confounds the correct spatial arrangement of the commissures and typically results in central malcoaptation and aortic insufficiency. Replacement of an aneurysmal ascending aorta and sinotubular junction with a tube graft of correct diameter often corrects aortic insufficiency by reestablishing the correct spatial suspension of the aortic valve. Similarly, reestablishing integrity of a dissected sinotubular junction by sewing the dissected root components to a tube graft that supplies support to the repaired sinotubular junction may also

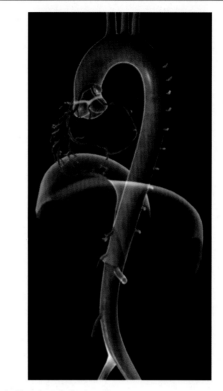

Figure 1-4. The sinotubular junction.

correct aortic insufficiency from an aortic dissection. Surgical tube graft replacement of the ascending aorta may be anastomosed to the root at the sinotubular junction, sparing aortic valve replacement and coronary implantation and their potential complications.

Imaging Considerations
Imaging issues are the same as for imaging of the aortic root.

Disease Involvement
Diseases involving this segment of the aorta include all of those listed for the aortic root. Particularly relevant diseases include annuloaortic ectasia (Marfan-like ballooning of the root and ascending aorta with loss of the "waist" imparted by the sinotubular junction) and dissection (cleavage of proximal dissection down to the sinotubular junction may compromise coronary ostial and aortic valve integrity). Surgical access is achieved through median (midline) sternotomy.

Sinotubular Junction and Its Anatomy: Clinical Relevance
- The sinotubular junction confers suspension to the aortic valve.
- Marked dilation (effacement) of the sinotubular junction is often associated with Marfan syndrome.

The Ascending Aorta

The ascending aorta is the segment of the aorta from the sinotubular junction to the first great arch vessel (Fig. 1-5). Although it is conceptually a simple definition, as the normal arch vessels arise only from the outer curvature, identifying the distinction of the ascending aorta from the arch on the outside curvature is

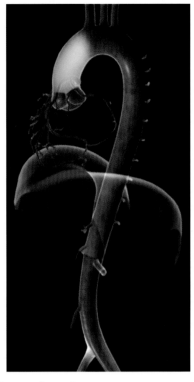

Figure 1-5. The ascending aorta.

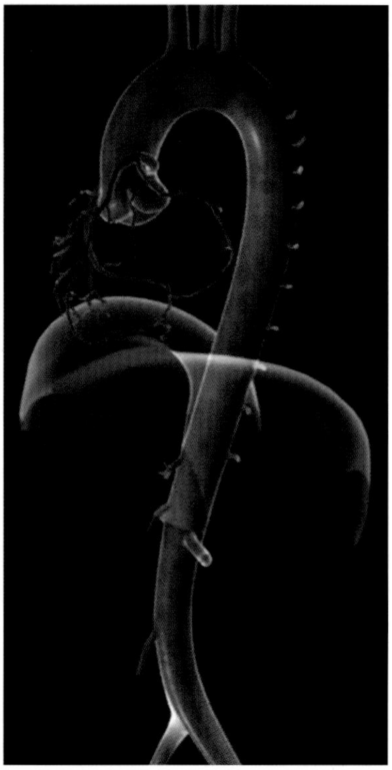

Figure 1-6. The aortic arch.

easier than it is on the inside curvature. This segment of the aorta is frequently involved in dissections and aneurysms. Surgical manipulation of the aorta is greatest here, as both the cross-clamp and the afferent bypass cannula insertion sites are within the ascending aorta. The ascending aorta is intrapericardial, as the pericardium reflects distally at the first branch vessel. Normal diameter of the ascending aorta is 2.6 ± 0.3 cm, with variation appropriate for body size.

The posterior inferior relations of the ascending aorta are the right pulmonary artery, the left mainstem bronchus, the left recurrent laryngeal nerve, and the roof of the left atrium. The anterior relation is the pulmonary artery. The right relation is the SVC, hence streak artifacts from contrast dye and pacer wires.

Imaging Considerations

The ascending aorta is subject to motion artifact on nongated imaging with low temporal resolution. High-resolution imaging of the ascending aorta requires either high temporal resolution (e.g., MDCT) or ECG gating.

Computed Tomography High-attenuation streak artifacts from concentrated contrast dye in the adjacent SVC are common and clinically important problems because these streak artifacts can contaminate the depiction of the ascending aorta. Pacemaker leads in the SVC may also project artifacts across the ascending aorta.

Echocardiography The ascending aorta is less well seen by transthoracic echocardiography, and the best depiction of it usually requires higher parasternal views and often high right parasternal views. Artifacts over this segment of the aorta are a usual problem for transthoracic echocardiography. TEE affords superior detail in almost all cases but often generates artifacts over this segment of the aorta. It visualizes a variable amount of the ascending aorta, depending on the course of the esophagus and the trachea and right mainstem bronchus.

Disease Involvement

Disease involvement of this segment of the aorta includes aneurysms (aneurysms associated with congenitally bicuspid aortic valves commonly involve predominantly or entirely the ascending portion of the aorta, sparing the root), dissection, false aneurysms, aortitis, syphilitic aortitis, traumatic disruption, atherosclerosis, plaques, ulcers, thrombi, and penetrating ulcers.

The Ascending Aorta and Its Anatomy: Clinical Relevance

- The ascending aorta is a frequently diseased segment of the aorta and gives rise to most dissections and intramural hematomas of the aorta.
- The most common cause of death due to dissection and intramural hematoma is rupture of the ascending aorta and aortic root into the pericardial space.
- High-attenuation streak artifacts on CT scanning from the SVC are common and clinically important because these streak artifacts can contaminate the depiction of the ascending aorta. The heart confers substantial motion to the ascending aorta and therefore confers motion artifact to nongated imaging with low temporal resolution. High-resolution imaging of the ascending aorta requires either high temporal resolution or ECG gating.
- Cardiac surgery is performed with extensive manipulation of the ascending aorta.
- Surgical access is achieved through median (midline) sternotomy.

The Aortic Arch

The aortic arch is the transverse portion of the aorta from the first arch vessel to the left subclavian artery ostium (Fig. 1-6). The aortic arch is mostly extrapericardial. Normal diameter of the aortic arch is 2.5 ± 0.2 cm, with variation appropriate for body size.

The arch arcs over the right pulmonary artery, the left mainstem bronchus, the left recurrent laryngeal nerve, and the roof of the left atrium. The esophagus lies to the left posterior aspect of the arch, and the trachea lies to the right posterior aspect. From the TEE (posterior) perspective, the tracheal air column often obscures the right part (anterior arch, upper ascending).

Branch vessels include right brachiocephalic artery (right subclavian artery and right common carotid artery), left carotid artery, and left subclavian artery (aortic arch branch variations are common).

Imaging Considerations
The aortic arch is subject to lesser motion artifact.
Computed Tomography High-attenuation streak artifacts from concentrated contrast dye in the adjacent brachiocephalic vein may occur, as they may from pacemaker leads in the brachiocephalic vein.
Echocardiography The aortic arch is not well seen by transthoracic echocardiography. Suprasternal views or supraclavicular views afford the best depiction. The left subclavian and left common carotid artery takeoffs may be seen, but imaging of the innominate takeoff is unlikely. Artifacts over the aortic arch are essentially inevitable for transthoracic echocardiography. TEE affords superior detail in almost all cases but is blinded over some portion of the arch by the tracheal air column.

Disease Involvement
Disease involvement of this segment of the aorta includes aneurysms, dissection, intramural hematoma, aortitis (especially giant cell arteritis and Takayasu's arteritis), atherosclerosis, plaques, ulcers, thrombi, and penetrating ulcers. Congenital variants include an arch branch vessel variant (incidence 1:3) and right-sided arches.

The Aortic Arch and Its Anatomy: Clinical Relevance
- Surgery on the cranial portion of the aortic arch entails interruption of blood flow to the arch vessels; thus, potential neurocognitive risks are particularly significant from surgery on this portion of the aorta.
- Surgery may be performed on the more proximal lower portion of the arch without interruption of blood flow to the arch vessels by clamping along the length of the arch.
- Surgical access is achieved by median (midline) sternotomy.
- Dissection of the aortic arch does not lend itself easily to standard classification.

The Isthmus and Descending Thoracic Aorta

The isthmus is the short portion of the aorta after the left subclavian artery to the present or former ductus arteriosus. It garnered its name from the in utero observation that the aorta is slightly narrower in this segment, as the aorta proximal to it is larger due to inflow of blood from the aortic valve (but which then diminishes as it outflows via the arch vessels), and the aorta distal to it is larger due to inflow of blood from the patent ductus arteriosus. The descending aorta is the vertically oriented portion of the aorta continuing from the isthmus to the level of the diaphragm

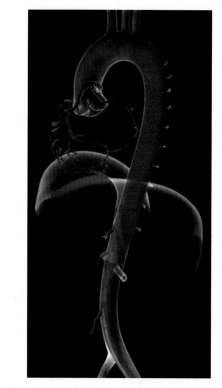

Figure 1-7. The isthmus and the descending aorta.

(Fig. 1-7). The esophagus runs alongside (within 0.5 cm) the descending aorta.

Normal diameter of the descending proximal aorta is <3.0 cm (mean ± 2 SD). At the eleventh rib level, it is <2.3 cm (mean ± 2 SD).

Branch vessels of the isthmus include the ductus arteriosus. Branch vessels of the descending aorta include intercostal arteries, spinal arteries including the artery of Adamkiewicz, and bronchial arteries.

Imaging Considerations
The descending aorta is subject to little motion artifact.
Computed Tomography CT is subject to few artifacts through the descending aorta, except from spinal prostheses (e.g., Harrington rods).
Echocardiography In infants and children, the isthmus region and very proximal descending aorta are well imaged and hence ductal flow and location are well depicted. In older children and most adults, the descending aorta is very poorly imaged by transthoracic echocardiography. The retrocardiac aorta is seen in cross section on the parasternal long-axis view and in long axis on some apical 2- or 3-chamber views. A left pleural effusion affords some means to image the descending aorta in lateral or posterior chest views. Although the proximity of the esophagus to the descending aorta greatly facilitates TEE imaging of this segment of the aorta, TEE generates near-field artifacts in some cases, and intimal calcification can generate misleading reverberation artifacts.

Disease Involvement
Disease involvement of this segment of the aorta includes coarctation, atresia, patent ductus arteriosus, atherosclerosis, plaques, ulcers, thrombi, penetrating ulcers, aneurysms, dissection, intramural hematoma, false aneurysms, traumatic disruption, aortitis,

and late complications of coarctation surgery or angioplasty. Congenital variations of the isthmus and descending aorta include right-sided aorta, aberrant right subclavian artery origin and course, and ductal diverticulum.

Surgical access is achieved through left thoracotomy. Importantly, the left pleural space abuts the descending aorta; hence, surgical access is usually through the left pleural space, and good pulmonary function, particularly of the right lung, is particularly important.

The Isthmus and Its Anatomy: Clinical Relevance

- The isthmus is a frequently diseased and malformed segment of the aorta.
- The awkwardness of surgery on the descending aorta with its greater comorbidity has been a significant factor driving the development of interventional procedures on this segment of the aorta.
- Rupture of the descending aorta is either into the mediastinum or into the large left pleural cavity, which is catastrophic.

The Abdominal Aorta

The abdominal aorta is the infradiaphragmatic aorta down to the aortic bifurcation (Fig. 1-8). Branch vessels include inferior phrenic arteries, celiac artery branches (hepatic artery, gastroepiploic artery, and splenic artery), renal arteries, superior mesenteric artery, inferior mesenteric artery, lumbar and spinal arteries, and iliac arteries (internal iliac artery: anterior division [obturator artery, inferior gluteal artery, internal pudendal artery, and visceral branches] and posterior division [superior gluteal artery, iliolumbar artery, and lateral sacral arteries]; and external iliac artery).

Normal diameter of the suprarenal abdominal aorta is 2.0 cm (mean ± 2 SD), and normal diameter of the infrarenal

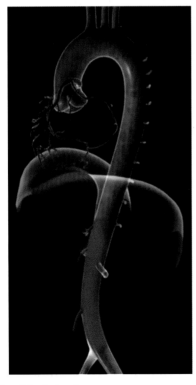

Figure 1-8. The abdominal aorta.

abdominal aorta is <2.0 cm (mean ± 2 SD). The venerable and beside "rule of thumb" is that the abdominal aorta is the size of the patient's thumb.

Imaging Considerations

The abdominal aorta is subject to little motion artifact.

Computed Tomography CT is subject to few artifacts over the descending aorta.

Echocardiography Transthoracic echocardiography can approximately depict the diameter and flow of the abdominal aorta in many cases but less well than dedicated broad ultrasound probes. Ultrasound imaging of the abdominal aorta by any form struggles against midline gas and obesity. Ultrasound is not a reliable means to identify leakage of the abdominal aorta.

Disease Involvement

Disease involvement of this segment of the aorta includes aneurysms (abdominal aortic aneurysm is one of the most common aortic aneurysms; thoracoabdominal aneurysms may extend down from the chest), atherosclerosis, plaques, ulcers, thrombi, penetrating ulcers, and aortitis.

Disease of the abdominal aorta is dominated by atherosclerosis and aneurysms. The abdominal aorta is the most frequently aneurysmal site of the aorta. Identification of abdominal aortic aneurysm (AAA) is increasingly difficult without imaging in an era of rampant obesity that has diminished the chance of recognition by physical examination alone. Rupture of an AAA or of a repaired AAA may occur into the retroperitoneal space, the peritoneal space, the overlying duodenum (aortoenteric fistula), or the inferior vena cava (aortocaval fistula).

The relation of an AAA to the renal arteries is so clinically important that AAAs are categorized as either infrarenal (95%) or suprarenal (5%). The level of surgical clamping of the aorta is similarly important and categorized by the level of the branch (and therefore its difficulty, and what it renders ischemic) as infrarenal, suprarenal or infraceliac, and supraceliac.

Surgical access is achieved through midline abdominal incision, laparotomy, or retroperitoneal dissection.

The Abdominal Aorta: Anatomic Relations

- The abdominal aorta equals the infradiaphragmatic aorta down to the aortic bifurcation.
- The bifurcation of the abdominal aorta occurs at L4-5 (the level of the bifurcation is variable). In older persons, the bifurcation is frequently lower because of elongation of the aorta from hypertension or other disease.
- The duodenum overlies the abdominal aorta.
- The inferior vena cava lies to the right side of the aorta.
- A horseshoe kidney wraps around the aorta and may be lost in operating on an AAA.

HISTOLOGY OF THE AORTA

The basic components of the aorta are the intima, media, and adventitia (Table 1-1; Figs. 1-9 and 1-10).

The Intima

The basic structure of the intima is the endothelial monolayer and the subendothelial "space." If it is normally functioning and

Table 1-1. Aortic Layers in Health and Disease

Layer	Function in Health	Loss of Function Consequences in Disease
Intima	Antithrombotic Antiatherosclerotic	Atherosclerotic plaques, stenoses, ulcers, thrombi
Media	Elastic tissue layers enable accommodation of the stroke volume at physiologic pulse pressure and store energy to be released passively in diastole, passively propelling blood forward. Fibrous tissue layers resist overdistention of the aorta and rupture.	Sclerosis, atherosclerosis, and overdistention (hypertension) result in excessive stiffness, increasing the pulse pressure. Weakness leads to aneurysm, dissection, intramural hemorrhage, and rupture. Concentric layering of the wall elements enables propagation of dissection proximally and distally.
Adventitia	Wrap (nutritive) layer	Rupture, disease invasion

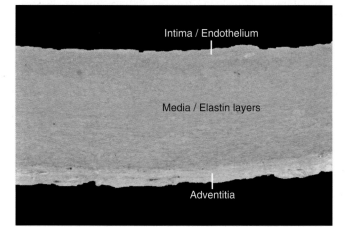

Figure 1-9. The media is the thickest layer of the aorta, principally containing layers of concentric elastic sheets joined by elastin fibers. Thus, the dominant property of the aorta is compliance, capacitance, and dynamic compression supplied by the large quantity of elastic material. The intima (endothelium and subintimal space) is extremely thin compared with the media. The outer layer, the adventitia, contains small blood vessels to sustain the metabolic needs of the aorta and collagen to supply strength and noncompliance to limit overdistention.

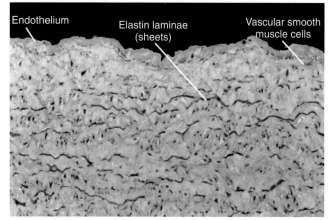

Figure 1-10. Reticulin stain for elastin. The elastin sheets are apparent. Their wavy configuration is due to the nonpressurized state of the histologic preparation. A few endothelial cells are apparent.

without trauma or disease, the intima resists atherosclerosis and thrombosis. If it is diseased by risk factors (hypertension, smoking, dyslipidemia, diabetes) or traumatized, the intima is prone to development of atherosclerotic plaques, ulcers, and thrombi.

The Media

The basic structure of the media consists of concentric layers of elastic sheets joined by elastin fibrils and collagen sheets, interposed with ground substance and a few smooth muscle cells. The aorta is notable for a thick media dominated by layers of elastin sheets (or lamellae). Peripheral arteries have different architecture with elastin at an internal layer and external layer and muscle in between. Elastin:collagen ratio is 70:30 in proximal aorta (hence, it is the most cushioning segment of the aorta), 50:50 in distal aorta, and 30:70 in peripheral arteries. This histologic structure results in the following properties of the media: (1) accommodation of the stroke volume at physiologic pressures (cushioning function); (2) storage of energy once it is distended (capacitor function) and release to passively pump blood (Windkessel phe-

nomenon); (3) maintenance of the integrity of the vessel; and (4) provision of a conduit to branch vessels.

If the media is defective because of a congenital or hereditary disorder (e.g., bicuspid aortic valve, Marfan syndrome, Ehlers-Danlos syndrome) or diseased from an acquired disorder (hypertension, atherosclerosis) or trauma, it is prone to (1) overdistention and stiffening, which may result in inability to receive the stroke volume at physiologic pressures, resulting in systolic hypertension, and acceleration of the pulse wave velocity, also resulting in systolic hypertension; (2) weakening and dilation, resulting in aneurysms or spontaneous or traumatic cleavage between layers, leading to dissection or intramural hematoma (the basic structure of the aorta, with such distinct lamellae with slight adhesion between them, is permissive of dissection more than in any other artery); and (3) invasion by atherosclerotic plaques, resulting in further stiffening, penetration, intramural hematoma, or rupture.

The Adventitia

The adventitia is a thin external layer mainly composed of collagen and the vasa vasorum—the fine blood supply to the aorta. The adventitia therefore supports the metabolic needs of the aorta and acts as a final barrier to rupture. In disease, it appears to supply the route of invasion of syphilitic treponemes. Also, the areas of the aorta with lesser vasa vasorum appear to have greater chance for development of atherosclerosis (e.g., the abdominal aorta).

PHYSIOLOGY OF THE AORTA

The length of the aorta averages about 1.2 m in adults. Over this length, there are temporal delays in the transmission of the pressure and flow down the aorta. The temporal delay in transmission of pressure between the proximal and distal aorta is 0.8 second; the temporal delay in transmission of volume is 3 seconds (heart rate dependent).

As long as there is a competent aortic valve and no other means of retrograde runoff, the blood will be pumped by the aorta distally as a result of its proximal capacitor function. The conversion of pulsatile flow proximally in the aorta (cyclic introduction of stroke volume into the aorta) into continuous flow in the more distal aorta occurs through the capacitor function and Windkessel effect. The cushioning function of the aorta and the capacitor function and Windkessel effect both result from the high elastin content of the proximal aorta, which confers elasticity, absorbing the systolic volume load, retaining potential energy in systole and releasing it in diastole, converting the energy to kinetic energy that moves blood distally in diastole. The degree of cushioning and capacitance is proportional to the amount of elastin in the aorta (Table 1-2).

Table 1-2. The Degree of Cushioning and Capacitance Is Proportional to the Amount of Elastin in the Aorta

	Cushioning and Capacitance	Percentage Elastin
Proximal aorta	Highest	70%
Abdominal aorta	Lower	40%
Peripheral arteries	Least	30%

The term *Windkessel* arose in a German translation of Stephen Hales' treatise on aortic pressure to exemplify the passive pump function of the aorta. The Windkessel was a component (the pressurized air bladder) of a manual fire engine pump. A manually powered piston pushed water into a reservoir, which, by storing potential energy (pressure) in the air bladder, converted the intermittent inflow into more continuous flow by maintaining pressure on the water reservoir such that even between strokes of the piston, there was some pressure (stored potential energy in the reservoir transformable to kinetic energy) to drive water out of the reservoir and to maintain flow (Fig. 1-11).

The aorta, like every chamber, has a passive pressure:volume relationship that reflects the interaction of volume and the capacitance or stiffness of the aorta. The greater the volume within the aorta, the higher the pressure. One of the best examples of this is intra-aortic balloon (IAB) counterpulsation: with diastolic inflation of the 40-mL IAB, the diastolic pressure in the aorta rises—the pressure augmentation effect.

The aortic pressure:volume relationship is nonlinear. As the aorta is distended further, the elastic reserve of the wall is exhausted and the pressure begins to rise more rapidly. When the aorta is overdistended by pressure, there is no further elastic reserve, and any further increase results in a nearly vertical rise in pressure as the pressure response is now determined only by the collagenous properties of the wall. The pressure:volume relation changes with age and with disease and remodeling of the aorta. Unfortunately, hypertension begets hypertension, as a more distended aorta has less elastic reserve and compliance. Sclerosis of the aorta and atherosclerosis increase aortic stiffness. Chronic aortic insufficiency results in remodeling of the aorta, and other vessels, to accommodate the hugely increased stroke volume at only slightly increased systolic pressure (Fig. 1-12).

Blood Pressure Descriptions

Because blood pressure is ubiquitously measured as systolic (highest) and diastolic (lowest), it is common practice to describe blood pressure as such; however, there are limitations to this practice. Such a simplistic description has engendered a wide-

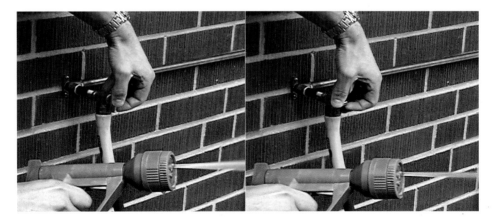

Figure 1-11. The Windkessel effect can be seen in the conversion of intermittent flow into the garden hose (valve switched on and off) into continuous flow. The tap is alternately turned on and off, intermittently introducing water into the hose. The flow of water, though, is continuous out of the low resistance of the nozzle. LEFT, Valve opened. RIGHT, Valve closed. Analogous to the heart and the aorta, the hose is converting phasic flow into continuous flow by the Windkessel effect of cushioning (capacitance) and passive conversion of stored potential energy into kinetic energy.

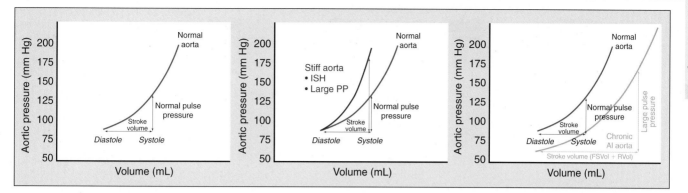

Figure 1-12. LEFT, Aortic pressure:volume relationship is a nonlinear relationship. The normal aorta accepts the normal stroke volume index (35 mL/m²) at about 1 mm Hg/mL/m² of (40 mm Hg) pulse pressure at normal pressure ranges. MIDDLE, The stiff aorta accepts the normal stroke volume at higher (hypertensive, nonphysiologic) pressures. RIGHT, The volume-overloaded aorta (e.g., chronic aortic insufficiency, patent ductus arteriosus) remodels to accept a larger stroke volume at less than expected pressures. AI, aortic insufficiency; FSVol, forward stroke volume; ISH, isolated systolic hypertension; PP, pulse pressure; RVol, regurgitant volume.

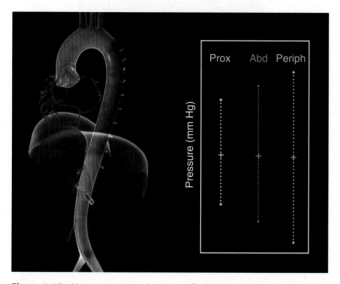

Figure 1-13. Mean pressure and pressure fluctuations. Mean pressure changes are determined by resistance, inertia, and viscosity. As these are minor factors along the aorta, the mean pressure decreases only slightly. Fluctuations around the mean are determined by the stiffness of the vessel. As the arterial vasculature has relatively less elastin distally, it is relatively stiffer and acquires greater pressure fluctuations, influencing the systolic and diastolic pressures.

spread outlook that the two variables sufficiently represent distinct and unrelated phenomena, for example, that systolic pressure describes predominantly cardiac function and diastolic pressure describes resistance alone. The ubiquity of measuring the aortic pressure as such has reduced general understanding of the multiple phenomena that contribute to arterial pressure. The expression of pressure by these two easily measurable variables places practicality over insight.

A more physiologic approach is to describe blood pressure as having a mean pressure and fluctuations about the mean. The mean pressure falls little along the aorta as it is an excellent conduit. The pressure fluctuations (or oscillations) increase distally as distal vessels are less elastic and are closer to reflected waves. Proximal fluctuations are usually 30% of the mean pressure; distal fluctuations are usually 40% of mean pressure. This generally adds 10 to 15 mm Hg and often up to 25 mm Hg of pressure (Fig. 1-13).

Different physiologic and pathologic factors influence the mean and the fluctuations. Mean pressure changes are determined by resistance, inertia, and viscosity. As these are minor factors along the aorta, the mean pressure decreases only slightly. Fluctuations around the mean are determined by the stiffness of the vessel. As the arterial vasculature has relatively less elastin distally, it is relatively stiffer and acquires greater pressure fluctuations, influencing the systolic and diastolic pressures (Fig. 1-14). Pressure fluctuations in the proximal aorta are 100 ± 20 mm Hg; in the abdominal aorta, 98 ± 22 mm Hg; and in the peripheral arteries, 95 ± 25 mm Hg.

Arterial Pressure:Age Relationship

With age, there is both a rise in the mean pressure due mainly to a rise in overall peripheral resistance (preponderant tissues are less vascular) and an increase in fluctuations about the mean as vessels stiffen and cushion less well (Fig. 1-15). There is also a remarkable near doubling of blood pressure between the first and the seventh decades of life.

The Aortic Pulse Wave

The aortic pulse and pressure wave emanates at high speed outward from the heart as the aortic valve opens (Fig. 1-16). It propagates increasingly rapidly as it moves peripherally, as the velocity of propagation is inversely proportional to the compliance of the aorta, and the more proximal aorta is more compliant because it contains more elastin, as its structure relates to its function to receive distention from injection of the stroke volume of the left ventricle, at tolerable pressure. Reflections of the pulse wave occur at all peripheral arteriole narrowings, with the largest reflections being clinically relevant and produced at the enormous resistance bed of the leg muscles. Pulse wave velocity of propagation is 4 m/s in the proximal aorta, 6 m/s in the abdominal aorta, and 12 m/s in the peripheral arteries.

The aortic pulse wave moves at 4 to 6 m/s in a healthy aorta, whereas the blood flows at 1 m/s; therefore, it is usually far ahead of the stroke volume specific to that cardiac cycle. The pulse wave, moving at 4 to 6 m/s, runs the length of the aorta and major peripheral arteries within a fraction of a second, reflects off of

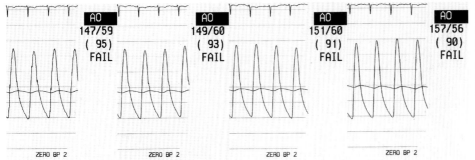

Figure 1-14. Pressure tracings from (LEFT TO RIGHT) the ascending aorta, the proximal descending aorta, the abdominal aorta, and the femoral artery of the same patient. The mean pressure varies little, but the fluctuation about the mean is increasing peripherally as the aorta and arteries are increasingly stiffer peripherally.

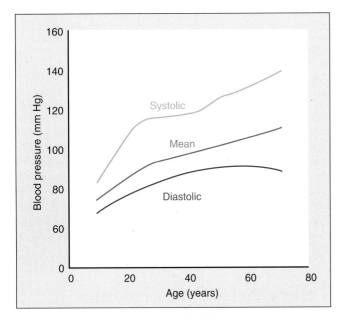

Figure 1-15. Arterial pressure:age relationship. With increasing age, there is both a rise in the mean pressure due mainly to a rise in overall peripheral resistance (preponderant tissues are less vascular) and an increase in fluctuations about the mean as vessels stiffen and cushion less well. Note also the near doubling of pressure between the first and the seventh decades of life.

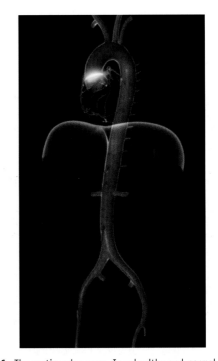

Figure 1-16. The aortic pulse wave. In a healthy and normal aorta, with aortic valve opening, the pulse wave propagates outward at high speed, accelerates as it travels, reflects off of large arteriole beds, and returns toward the heart. A healthy and compliant aorta propagates the pulse wave at a speed that although fast is not so fast that it returns during systole (ejection), but rather later, after the aortic valve closes.

peripheral arterioles, and returns to the heart in less than a second.

If the aorta is healthy, compliant, and a slow conductor of the pulse wave, the reflected wave returns after the completion of systole, in diastole. This is revealed in some patients by the presence of a diastolic pressure wave—the reflected pressure wave.

Reflected Pressure Waves in the Aorta

The aortic and arterial pulse wave transmits easily to the peripheral vasculature. It is prone to reflecting off of (1) arterial bifurcations, as a wave would reflect back off of any structure it encountered, and (2) resistance vessels. The reflected waves return backward, at speeds similar to outgoing velocities of propagation. The outbound pulse wave velocity and the returning pulse wave velocities are fast (4 to 13 m/s); hence, they return within a cardiac cycle and render the pressure wave at any point the sum of the outbound and returning (reflected) pressure waves (Table 1-3). They arrive within the systolic wave in the more peripheral vessels. They arrive later and spread either within systole and diastole or

Table 1-3. Pulse Wave Velocity in Different Arterial Segments

Arterial Segment	Pulse Wave Velocity
Ascending aorta	4-5 m/s
Descending aorta	4-7 m/s
Abdominal aorta	5-8 m/s
Iliac artery	7-8 m/s
Femoral artery	8-13 m/s

within diastole in the proximal aorta (in health). When they arrive in diastole, they contribute to diastolic pressure; and when they arrive in systole, they will summate with the systolic wave (Fig. 1-17).

In disease, when the aorta becomes stiffer and transmits the pulse wave faster, the reflected waves return sooner (within

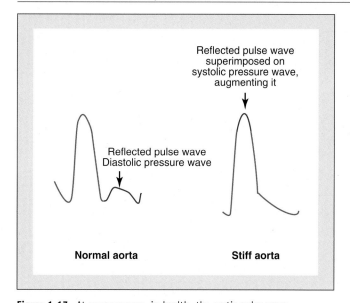

Figure 1-17. At younger ages, in health, the aortic pulse wave propagates and returns slowly, therefore later—and arrives in diastole in the proximal aorta (LEFT TRACING). With a stiff aorta, the pulse wave emanates and returns rapidly, therefore earlier, and arrives in systole, summating with the systolic pressure and augmenting systolic pressure—hence, the self-perpetuation of systolic hypertension by stiffening of the aorta.

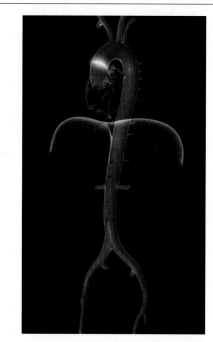

Figure 1-18. A hypertensive aorta is less compliant and therefore a faster propagator of the pulse wave. Unlike the healthy and compliant aorta, the hypertensive aorta conducts the outbound and returning pulse waves so quickly that they return in systole, summating with the aortic pressure to increase it.

systole) and will summate with the systolic waves, altering the waveforms, not only their amplitude (blood pressure).

Pulse wave velocity increases with age (increased intrinsic stiffness and increased stiffness due to higher distending pressure) and diseases such as hypertension (after elastic stretch from elastin is exhausted, tensile strength from collagen predominates and the aorta stiffens under high pressure), atherosclerosis (the process of atherosclerosis leads to disruption of elastin and loss of elasticity), and arteriosclerosis.

Aortic Pulse Wave and Hypertension

As the aorta stiffens (e.g., with hypertension), the pulse wave travels at least one third faster. If the aorta is stiff because of hypertension, atherosclerosis, or other disease and is a fast conductor of the pulse wave, the reflected wave returns *before* the completion of systole, thereby increasing systolic pressure, impedance to left ventricular ejection, and myocardial work (MVo_2) (Fig. 1-18). Thus, self-perpetuation and a vicious circle of hypertension occur: hypertension leads to a stiff aorta, which leads to overdistention and elevation of systolic pressure due to loss of compliance, early return of the pulse wave to superimpose its pressure on systolic pressure, early return of the pulse wave, increased myocardial work, and less efficient cardiac ejection.

The Aortic Pulse Pressure Contour

The aortic pulse pressure contour has four components: (1) the upslope, (2) the dome/peak, (3) the dicrotic notch (incisura), and (4) the pressure decay (Figs. 1-19 and 1-20). The aortic pulse pressure magnitude and contour is the summation of *multiple*

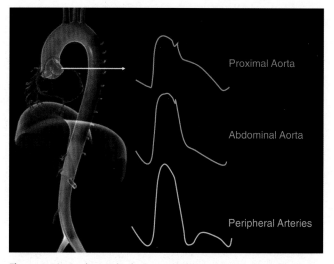

Figure 1-19. In the proximal aorta, systolic waveform is dome-like. Dicrotic notch is present due to aortic valve closure. Diastolic waveform is present, has a shallow dome or linear descent, and may include reflected pressure waves. In the abdominal aorta, systolic waveform is taller while still rounded and slightly delayed compared with proximal aorta. Dicrotic notch is no longer present. Diastolic waveform is present and has a smaller, linear descent. In the peripheral arteries, systolic waveform is taller, steeper, triangular, and not rounded. It is even further delayed compared with proximal aorta and usually includes reflected waves. Diastolic waveform shows a small secondary wave.

effects and the site of sampling. The effects that influence the aortic pulse pressure magnitude and contour are volume ejected into aorta, rate of ejection into aorta, compliance (capacitance or cushioning effect), Venturi effect, timing of reflected waves, magnitude of reflected waves, and peripheral resistance.

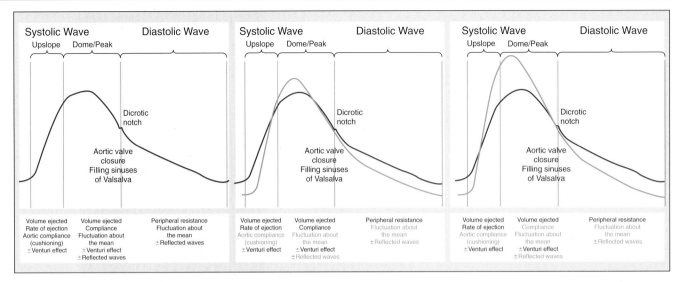

Figure 1-20. LEFT, Aortic pressure tracing. MIDDLE, Peripheral aortic pressure tracing is characterized by (1) more rapid upstroke; (2) higher peak pressure, due to slightly lesser compliance and cushioning, greater systolic pressure fluctuation, and summation of pressure waves in systole (that occurred nearby and therefore returned earlier); and (3) lower diastolic pressure, due to greater fluctuation about the mean and reflected waves no longer present in diastole (returned in systole). RIGHT, Aortic pressure tracing in stiff aorta. In addition to more rapid upstroke, higher peak pressure, and lower diastolic pressure, there is also more triangular systolic wave.

Aortic Pressure Waveform

The upslope is the interaction of the volume entering the aorta, and the stiffness or elasticity of the local vessel determines the rate of pressure rise. The stiffer the vessel, the more rapid the upslope, and the larger the volume, the more rapid the upslope. In health, vessels become stiffer toward the periphery; in disease, they may become very stiff. The rate of left ventricular pressure rise (dP/dt) and presence or absence of a local Venturi effect (aortic stenosis, aortic stenosis–aortic insufficiency) that would reduce pressure and thereby pressure rise are also determinants of aortic pressure waveform. Waveform considerations in proximal aorta, abdominal aorta, and peripheral arteries are illustrated in Figures 1-21 to 1-23.

Height of systolic pressure is determined by the interaction of the volume entering the aorta, and the stiffness or elasticity of the local vessel also determines the rate of pressure rise and presence or absence of reflected pressure waves superimposing on the systolic pressure. In health, this does not happen significantly in the proximal aorta. Shape of the systolic pressure wave is determined by upstroke:stroke volume (compliance ± Venturi effect) and reflected pressure waves if they are returning in systole (summate with incident pressure wave). Dicrotic notch is due to aortic valve closure and is seen well only in the proximal aorta. Diastolic pressure wave is due to peripheral resistance, rate of distal or proximal runoff (e.g., aortic insufficiency), and reflected pressure waves if they are arriving in diastole.

As blood pressure is recorded more distally, there is a very slight progressive fall in mean pressure (Table 1-4), increase in pressure fluctuations about the mean, increasing phase delay in the systolic pressure rise, and loss of the dicrotic notch in the abdominal and femoral artery pressure tracings.

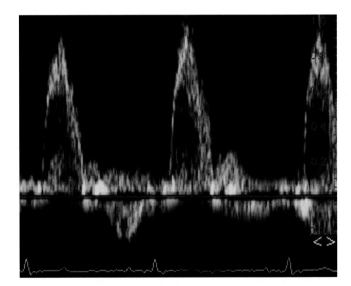

Figure 1-21. Flow in the proximal aorta. There is a small amount of diastolic flow reversal normally, due to flow into the coronary arteries.

Table 1-4. Differences Between Mean Pressure Proximally to Distally

	Blood Pressure (mm Hg)	Mean (mm Hg)
Ascending	147/59	95
Descending	149/60	93
Abdominal	151/60	91
Femoral	157/56	90

Table 1-5. Functions of the Aorta

Function		Proximal Aorta	Abdominal Aorta	Peripheral Arteries
Antiatherogenic		Yes	Yes	Yes
Antithrombotic		Yes	Yes	Yes
Conduit function	To carry blood from the heart to branch vessels, without loss of energy through turbulence or resistance.	Yes	Yes	Yes
Cushion function	To accept the ejected blood volume into the aorta and to accommodate this volume at a physiologically tolerable pressure increase. Normally, the aorta distends about 4% with systole as a measure and a means of accommodation.	Significant	Some	Some
Capacitor function	To harness the energy (as potential energy) used in stretching of the aorta by systolic distention	Significant	Slight	Little
Pump function	To release the potential energy stored within the wall (by systolic distention) through recoil of the conduit function. All segments of the aorta are low-resistance conduits to more distal vasculature that permit flow distally without turbulence and loss of energy. There is only very slight (mean) pressure drop along the aorta.	Significant	Slight	Little

Table 1-6. Structure and Function of the Aorta

	Proximal Aorta	Abdominal Aorta	Peripheral Arteries
	The first ~20 cm of the aorta receives the stroke volume each cardiac cycle.		
Structure	The most prominent structural feature is the multiple layers of elastin sheets to provide cushion and capacitance. To a lesser extent, there are collagen fibrils within the media and the adventitia to arrest maximal distention and thereby to avoid aortic disruption. There is relatively little smooth muscle to confer contractile properties.	Mixture of layers of elastin sheets and collagen fibrils within the media and the adventitia to arrest maximal distention, to avoid disruption. Relatively little smooth muscle to confer contractile properties	Balanced mixture of elastin for compliance, collagen for strength and ability to resist excessive distention, and smooth muscle to confer vasoconstrictor ability. 30% elastin only
Function	The proximal aorta has the greatest cushioning and capacitor function of all blood vessels.		
Cushion and capacitor	Cushion function: prominent cushion function to accommodate the stroke volume at physiologically tolerable pressure. Capacitor function: prominent capacitor function to store potential energy in the elastin fibrils during distention in systole and to release energy in diastole, driving blood forward	Cushion function: some Capacitor function: some	Cushion function: little Capacitor function: little
Conduit	To its branch vessels and the more distal aorta	The principal function is as a conduit to the branch vessels.	The principal function is as a conduit to the peripheral branch vessels.
Pulse wave velocity	4 m/s As the proximal aorta has the greatest elastin content and elasticity of any artery, it is the least stiff and therefore the slowest conducting blood vessel.	7-8 m/s Higher than in the proximal aorta: as the abdominal aorta contains less elastin and is relatively stiffer than the ascending proximal aorta, it is a faster pulse wave conductor.	12 m/s Higher than in the aorta because of the low content of elastin and thereby lesser compliance and relatively greater stiffness and faster conduction properties

Table 1-6. Structure and Function of the Aorta—cont'd

	Proximal Aorta	Abdominal Aorta	Peripheral Arteries
Pressure	Age dependent	Age dependent	Age dependent
Mean	100 mm Hg The mean pressure in the proximal aorta is usually the diastolic $+^1/_2$ pulse pressure due to rounded systolic waveform.	100 mm Hg The mean pressure is usually the diastolic $+^1/_3$ pulse pressure due to now taller, peaking systolic waveform.	Slightly less than the central aorta (<5 mm Hg difference) The mean pressure is usually the diastolic $+^1/_3$ pulse pressure due to more narrow and peaked systolic waveform.
Fluctuations	±20 mm Hg Pulse pressure only 40 mm Hg due to efficient cushion function	±20 mm Hg Pulse pressure only 40 mm Hg due to cushion function	± Those of the central aorta + An additional 10 mm Hg
Waveform			
Systolic	Steep vertical upstroke Rounded dome, full shaped	Steep vertical upstroke Taller Dome is still rounded, full shaped Slightly delayed vs. proximal aorta	Taller, steeper Triangular, not rounded Further delayed vs. proximal aorta Usually includes reflected waves: reflected waves are local and return rapidly in systole, augmenting systolic pressure
Dicrotic notch	Usually obvious, due to closure of aortic valve	Diminished or no longer present	No longer present
Diastolic	Present, shallow dome or slightly convex upward or linear descent May include reflected pressure wave returning from peripheral arteries	Present, smaller, linear descent Slightly convex upward, may include reflected pressure waves back from peripheral arteries	Small secondary wave
Blood flow			
Velocity	Systolic: anterograde flow 0.8-1.2 m/s Diastolic: brief retrograde flow	Systolic: anterograde flow 0.6-0.8 m/s Diastolic: brief retrograde flow	Systolic: anterograde flow 0.6-0.9 m/s Diastolic: brief retrograde flow
Waveform	Very brief accentuated diastolic retrograde due to closing of the aortic valve and the filling of the sinuses of Valsalva Mid and late diastolic flows are competing: distal runoff from Windkessel effect, and proximal (root) runoff due to flow into coronary arteries Overall, there is little net forward or backward flow.	Flow in proximal abdominal aorta: systolic and diastolic anterograde due to the Windkessel effect of proximal aorta and low resistance to runoff in renal arteries allowing diastolic anterograde flow Flow in distal abdominal aorta: triphasic or biphasic (high-resistance) pattern due to generally high arteriolar resistance of distal tissue beds (predominantly muscle) in their resting state	High-resistance pattern: biphasic or triphasic pattern Systolic anterograde Early diastolic reversal Short anterograde diastolic flow Low-resistance pattern (when vascular bed, usually muscular, is vasodilated): • Systolic anterograde • Diastolic anterograde

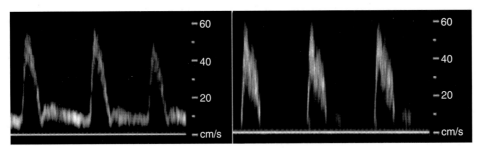

Figure 1-22. Flow in the abdominal aorta. LEFT, Above the renal arteries, there is both anterograde systolic and diastolic flow because of the low resistance within the renal arteries (that allows renal anterograde flow in diastole) distal to the site of sampling. RIGHT, Lower abdominal aorta. The flow pattern is systolic only—a high-resistance pattern due to the high resistance of the more distal branch vessels.

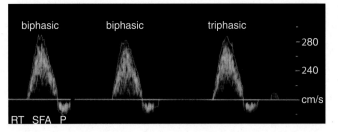

Figure 1-23. Flow in the superficial femoral artery (SFA). The pattern is high resistance with a brief diastolic reversal due to the locally reflecting pressure waves.

Arterial Pressure and Arterial Flow

There is too high a degree of variation of arterial pressure and flow for aortic pressure to be a trustworthy surrogate for aortic flow, cardiac output, and tissue perfusion. Peripheral resistance (an enormously wide-ranging variable, especially in younger patients and in older hypertensive patients), distal stenoses, and occlusions render proximal pressure of little correlation with respect to flow to distal organs. There are two major exceptions to correlation of aortic pressure and forward flow: (1) an occluded artery or aorta typically has higher than normal pressure as the reflected pulse wave is greater; and (2) in aortic insufficiency, flow will reverse in the aorta in diastole.

Therefore, arterial blood pressure is a tenuous clinical surrogate for arterial flow. The correlation of arterial blood pressure and cardiac output, in disease states and under pharmacologic influence, is much worse than is generally believed (Fig. 1-24).

INTEGRATING THE ANATOMY, HISTOLOGY, AND PHYSIOLOGY OF THE AORTA

Tables 1-5 and 1-6 present an integrated summary of aortic function based on anatomic, histologic, and physiologic considerations.

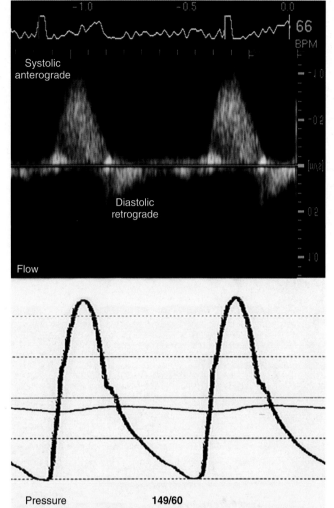

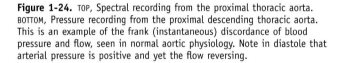

Figure 1-24. TOP, Spectral recording from the proximal thoracic aorta. BOTTOM, Pressure recording from the proximal descending thoracic aorta. This is an example of the frank (instantaneous) discordance of blood pressure and flow, seen in normal aortic physiology. Note in diastole that arterial pressure is positive and yet the flow reversing.

CHAPTER 2

Anatomic Variants of the Aorta

KEY POINTS

▸ The anatomic relations of the aorta are frequently important in terms of
  ▸ Disease manifestations
  ▸ Surgical access
  ▸ Surgical complications

▸ Anatomic variants of most segments of the aorta are
  ▸ Relatively common
  ▸ Important for diagnosis
  ▸ Important for surgery and intervention

This chapter focuses on the anatomic variants of the aorta and its branches. Anatomic variants are reviewed per segment of the aorta with use of the terminology established in Chapter 1.

EMBRYOGENESIS OF THE AORTA

In earliest embryogenesis, vessels throughout the body are plexiform. With growth, they become confluent, but early on, arteries and veins are indistinguishable endothelial cell–lined tubes. As the fetal size develops, vessels assume their recognizable conduit character. The adult aorta and aortic arch system result from the regression and fusion of components of the six pairs of aortic arches that evolve the design from six symmetric arches into the asymmetric final pattern (Fig. 2-1). The arches develop serially, that is, the first and second arches first, then the third and fourth, then the fifth and sixth. Initially, there are six aortic arches and two dorsal aortas. The eventual outcome of aortic arch evolution is as follows:

1. The proximal ascending aorta derives from the truncus arteriosus, as does the proximal pulmonary artery.
2. The distal ascending aorta, the aortic arch until the left common carotid artery, and the brachiocephalic trunk derive from the aortic sac.
3. The right subclavian artery derives from the fourth aortic arch, the right dorsal aorta, and the right intersegmental artery.
4. The common carotid arteries derive from the third aortic arch.
5. The aortic arch between the left common carotid artery and the left subclavian artery isthmus portion of the aorta derives from the fourth aortic arch.

6. The left subclavian artery derives from the left intersegmental artery.
7. The ductus arteriosus derives from the sixth aortic arch.
8. The descending aorta derives from the left dorsal aorta.

From this very basic description, it can be understood that many of the observed congenital malformations of the aorta result from maldevelopment of a segment, persistence of a segment, or misconnection.

VARIANT ANATOMY OF THE AORTIC ROOT

Variant Anatomy of the Sinuses

Congenital variations of the aortic valve are responsible for differences in the number of aortic root sinuses. Bicuspid aortic valve malformation, seen in 1% to 2% of males and less than 0.5% of females, may result in two sinuses, whose orientations and sizes are different from those of usual tricuspid valves. Quadricuspid valves (0.01% incidence) result in four sinuses, often of differing sizes. A bicuspid aortic valve is a significant lesion because of its risk of dysfunction and also because of its association with other aortic defects and diseases and other cardiac anomalies.

Significant aortic associations of bicuspid aortic valves and two sinuses include aortic developmental abnormalities (ascending aneurysms, coarctation), aortic dissection, and other vascular (e.g., patent ductus arteriosus) and cardiac anomalies. Bicuspid aortic valves are one of the principal reasons of aortic dissection in patients younger than 45 years (10 times more common than Marfan syndrome as a cause of aortic dissection).

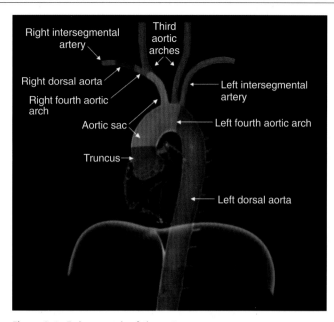

Figure 2-1. Embryogenesis of the aorta.

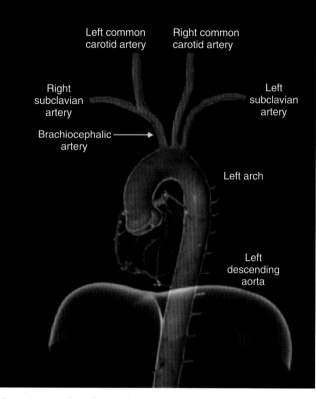

Figure 2-2. Aortic arch: normal branch vessel anatomy.

Congenital variation of the size of sinuses does occur such that the sizes are unequal. Congenital fistula, usually into a right-sided heart chamber, may also occur.

Branch Variant Anatomy: Anomalies of Coronary Arteries

Anomalies of the coronary arteries may affect dominance, number, ostia, course, and termination.

Anomalies of Coronary Artery Dominance Coronary artery dominance is determined on the basis of supply of the posterior descending coronary artery. In 80% of individuals (normal), it is supplied from the right coronary artery (right dominance). Variants include 10% from the left circumflex artery (left dominance) and 10% from both the right coronary artery and the left circumflex artery (codominance).

Anomalies of Coronary Artery Number Normal is two separate coronary arteries. Variants include separate ostia of the left anterior descending and left circumflex arteries; a solitary coronary artery may occur, or an accessory fourth coronary artery may occur.

Anomalies of Coronary Artery Ostia Anomalies of coronary artery ostia include high ostium (above sinotubular junction) and ostium arising from opposite sinus.

Anomalies of Coronary Artery Course Anomalies of coronary artery course are classified as follows:

type A, *a*nterior to the pulmonary artery;
type B, *b*etween the pulmonary artery and aorta (intra-arterial);
type C, through the *c*rista supraventricularis of the septum; and
type D, *d*orsal to the aorta (retroaortic).

Intramyocardial course (bridging) is very common, especially of the left anterior descending coronary artery.

Anomalies of Coronary Artery Termination Anomalies of coronary artery termination include fistulas.

Clinical Relevance of Variant Anatomy of the Aortic Root

Bicuspid aortic valves are common and may be associated with aneurysms of the ascending aorta and coarctation of the aorta as well as other malformations. Bicuspid valves and their associations may result in aortic dissection, particularly in younger patients. Coronary artery anomalies, although they can be clinically symptomatic, increase the technical challenge of coronary angiography and interventional procedures.

VARIANT ANATOMY OF THE ASCENDING AORTA

There are few variations to the anatomy of the ascending aorta. The orientation may be abnormal in several congenital cardiac anomalies, but the ascending aorta itself is generally normal.

VARIANT ANATOMY OF THE AORTIC ARCH

Regression of the right dorsal aortic root arch results in the normal left aortic arch (Fig. 2-2). The left aortic arch, left descending aorta, three-arch vessel pattern is present in only 70% of

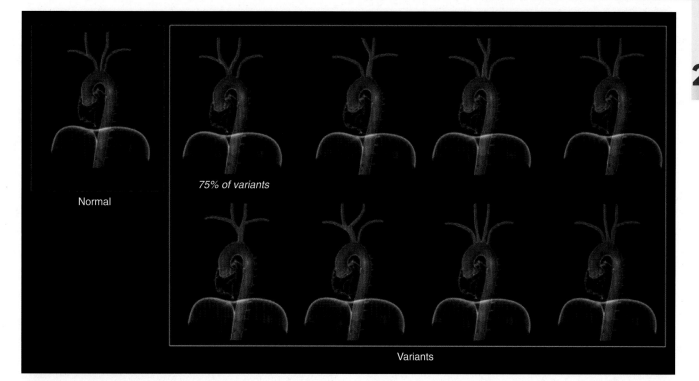

Figure 2-3. Aortic arch: variant anatomy.

individuals. Branch vessel anomalies are common, and right-sided aortic arches occur.

Usual Branch Anatomy Arising from the Aortic Arch

Brachiocephalic artery (usually 3 or 4 cm in length) branches into right subclavian artery (thyrocervical trunk, vertebral artery, and right internal mammary artery) and right common carotid artery (right internal carotid artery and right external carotid artery). Left carotid artery branches into left internal carotid artery and left external carotid artery. Left subclavian artery branches into left thyrocervical trunk, left vertebral artery, and left internal mammary artery.

Variant Anatomy of the Aortic Arch

Approximately 70% of individuals have what is considered normal branch vessel anatomy. Branch vessel variants of the aortic arch are present in approximately one third (30% to 35%) of individuals (Fig. 2-3). The most common arch vessel variant (20% of individuals) is the common origin of the brachiocephalic and left common carotid arteries (Figs. 2-4 and 2-5). Other variants are uncommon and include left vertebral artery arising from the arch (5% of individuals) and thyroid origin of the internal mammary artery (5% of individuals). See Table 2-1 for a classification of the aortic arch.

   Aberrant right subclavian artery (Figs. 2-6 and 2-7) occurs in 1% of individuals. It is mainly an isolated anomaly but may be associated with other lesions. It is believed to be due to involution of the right fourth arch and persistence of the right dorsal aorta. Its typical course is behind the esophagus (80%), and anomalies

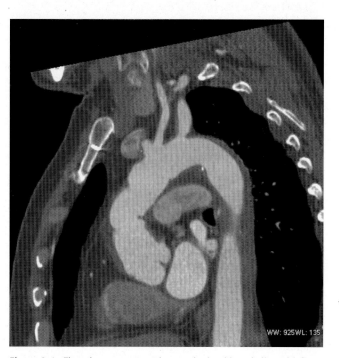

Figure 2-4. There is a common ostium to the brachiocephalic and left carotid arteries. The ascending aorta was previously repaired with a Dacron tube graft.

include course between the esophagus and trachea (15%) and anterior to the trachea (5%).

   In a patient with a left aortic arch, an aneurysm of the first portion of an aberrant left subclavian artery is referred to as Kommerell's diverticulum. The lesion can be seen combined with other malformations (Fig. 2-8).

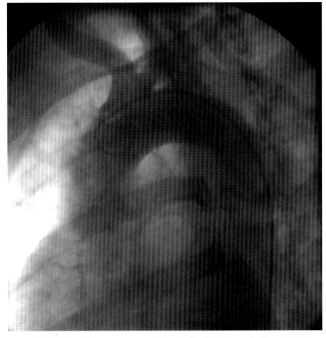

Figure 2-5. There is a common ostium to the brachiocephalic and left carotid arteries.

Table 2-1. Aortic Arch Classification
Normal left aortic arch
Left arch anomalies
Retro-esophageal subclavian artery
Left arch, right descending aorta
Right aortic arch anomalies
Mirror image right aortic arch
Right aortic arch with retro-esophageal left subclavian artery
Double aortic arch
Dominant right aortic arch
Equal-sized arches
Dominant left aortic arch
Persistent fifth aortic arch
From Weinberg, PM: Aortic arch anomalies. J Cardiovasc Magn Reson 2006;8:633-643.

Aberrant right brachiocephalic artery is a rare occurrence.

The sidedness of the arch is with respect to the tracheal air column.

Right-Sided Aortic Arch

A right-sided aortic arch (Fig. 2-9) is most commonly associated with an aberrant left subclavian artery and is seldom associated with congenital heart disease. Its branches include the left common carotid artery, the right common carotid artery, the right subclavian artery, and an aberrant left subclavian artery. The mirror-image type of aortic arch is often associated with congenital heart disease (usually cyanotic). Its branches include the left

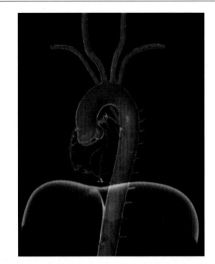

Figure 2-6. Aberrant right subclavian artery running posterior to the arch.

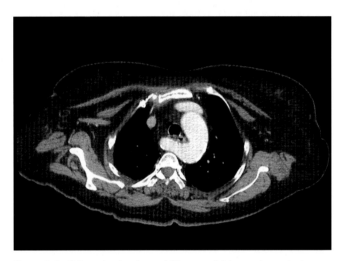

Figure 2-7. This contrast-enhanced CT scan axial image demonstrates an aberrant right subclavian artery origin (distal to the left subclavian artery) and course (posterior to the esophagus and trachea).

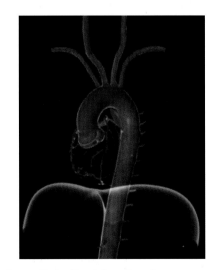

Figure 2-8. In a patient with a left aortic arch, an aneurysm of the first portion of an aberrant left subclavian artery is referred to as Kommerell's diverticulum.

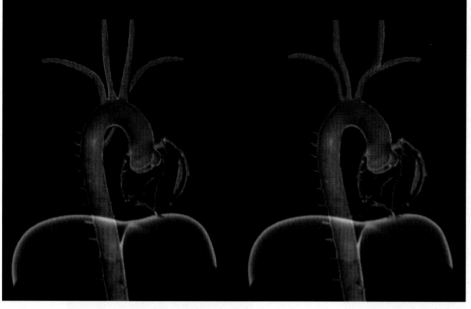

Figure 2-9. Right-sided aortic arches. LEFT, With associated aberrant left subclavian artery. RIGHT, Mirror-image type.

brachiocephalic artery, right common carotid artery, and right subclavian artery.

Double Aortic Arch

In cases of double aortic arch, the two arches are usually not equal in size, with the right arch tending to be larger. The descending aorta is usually on the left side but may be on the right side. The common carotid and subclavian arteries arise from the ipsilateral arch. The ductus arteriosus is usually on the left side. Double aortic arch is believed to be due to disappearance of the right sixth distal aortic arch.

As the esophagus and trachea are contained within a ring between the arches, symptoms, when present, are usually respiratory.

Cervical Aortic Arch

A cervical aortic arch is a rare anomaly that occurs because of atresia of the fourth primitive aortic arch. Arch branch vessel and cervical vessel anomalies may be associated (Fig. 2-10).

Clinical Relevance of Variant Anatomy of the Aortic Arch

One in three persons has an arch branch vessel variant. Right-sided arch may occur either with an aberrant left subclavian artery or with the mirror-image configuration that is frequently associated with severe congenital heart lesions.

VARIANT ANATOMY OF THE DESCENDING AORTA

The descending thoracic aorta gives rise to a large number of branch vessels that may be anomalous. The blood supply to the clinically and surgically very important anterior spinal artery occurs at multiple levels, which include the descending thoracic aorta. The ductal diverticulum at the isthmus of the proximal descending aorta is a common source of confusion.

Intercostal and Subcostal Arteries

Anterior intercostal arteries arise from the internal mammary artery. Posterior intercostal arteries arise from the superior inter-costal artery from the costocervical trunk of the subclavian artery (first to third) and from the descending thoracic aorta (fourth to twelfth).

Spinal Arteries

The anterior 80% of the spinal cord is perfused by the anterior spinal arteries; the posterior 20%, by the posterior (paired) spinal arteries. The anterior spinal artery arises near the vertebrobasilar junction and receives branches at a number of levels. The important artery of Adamkiewicz (arteria radicularis magna) arises on the left side between T5 and L2; but in 75% of individuals, it arises from T9-12. This important feeder vessel to the anterior spinal artery may arise within surgically accessed areas; therefore, anterior spinal ischemia may occur with surgery (Fig. 2-11).

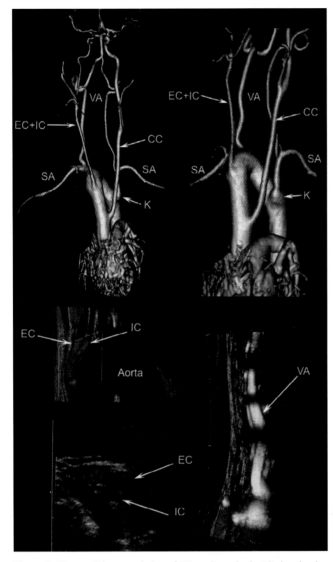

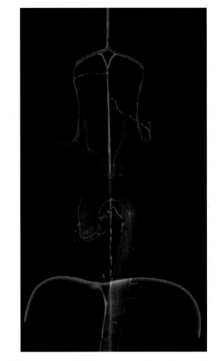

Figure 2-11. The anterior spinal artery supplies the anterior spinal cord and is fed by branches at several levels, one of which (the artery of Adamkiewicz) originates from the posterior proximal descending aorta.

Figure 2-10. TOP, Volume rendering of MR angiography in AP view (LEFT) and left lateral oblique view (RIGHT). BOTTOM, Doppler ultrasound of the carotid arteries (LEFT) and power Doppler ultrasound of the vertebral artery. (From Poellinger A, Lembcke AE, Elgeti T, et al: The Cervical Aortic Arch: A Rare Vascular Anomaly. Circulation 2008;117:2716-2717, with permission.)

Ductus Diverticulum

The ductus diverticulum is the residuum of the distal right fourth aortic arch. It has a variable appearance—generally a tapered or fusiform bulging of the ventromedial aspect of the proximal descending aorta (Fig. 2-12).

Clinical Relevance of Variant Anatomy of the Descending Thoracic Aorta

Loss, by disease or more likely by surgery, of the arteria radicularis magna (artery of Adamkiewicz) risks paraplegia, a dreaded complication of surgery of the descending aorta. The size of the artery and clinical significance of losing the artery of Adamkiewicz are almost impossible to predict. Another important clinical consideration that may arise is the confusion over the nature of the ductus diverticulum, particularly in cases of possible traumatic aortic disruption.

Bronchial Arteries

Bronchial arteries originate from the third to seventh intercostal arteries. Variants of bronchial arteries are common. Single or multiple (two to four) bronchial arteries per side are typical. Sixty percent of individuals have a single right bronchial artery.

Esophageal Arteries

Esophageal arteries originate from cervical, thoracic, and abdominal arteries (from the phrenic artery).

VARIANT ANATOMY OF THE ABDOMINAL AORTA

There are few anatomic variants of the abdominal aorta.

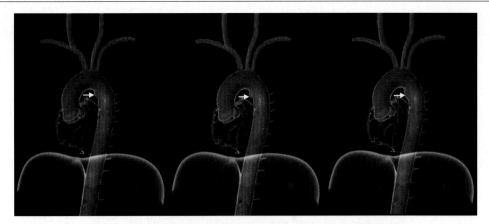

Figure 2-12. Ductus diverticulum is a tapered or fusiform bulge on the ventromedial aspect of the proximal descending aorta that is a residual of the distal right fourth aortic arch. It has a variable appearance. The most common appearance is a short and slightly rounded bulge (LEFT), but less rounded bulges (MIDDLE) and longer bulges (RIGHT) also occur.

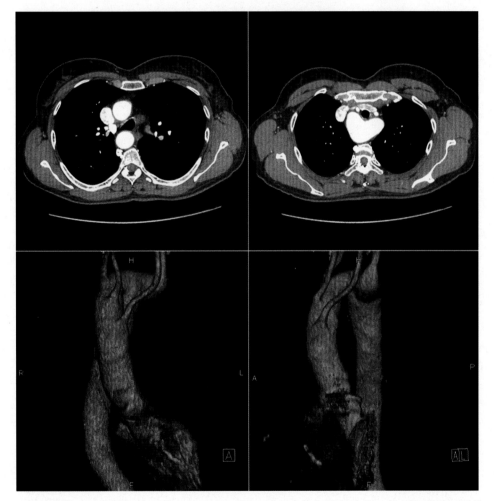

Figure 2-13. Contrast-enhanced CT scan. Multiple anomalies are present: The aortic arch is right-sided, there is a diverticulum of Kommerell from which arises the left subclavian artery, and the left common carotid artery arises as the first branch vessel from the posterior wall of the ascending aorta/proximal aortic arch. (Courtesy of Jehangir Appoo, MD, Calgary, Canada.)

CASE 1

Normal Anatomy

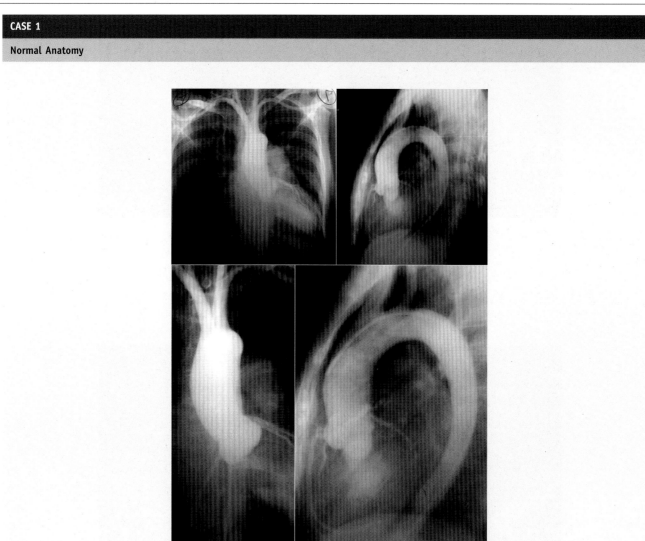

Figure 2-14. Aortographic appearance of the normal aorta. The arch and descending aorta are left sided. The arch vessel anatomy is normal. The separate ostia and course of the left common carotid artery and left subclavian artery are appreciated on the lateral view; on the posteroanterior view, they are superimposed, giving the false impression of a left brachiocephalic–innominate artery. (Courtesy of Andrew Common, MD, Toronto, Canada.)

CASE 2

Asymptomatic Aberrant Right Subclavian Artery

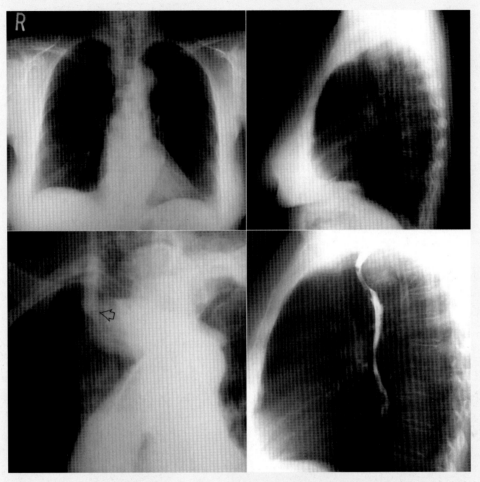

Figure 2-15. TOP, Chest radiographs demonstrating a left-sided aortic arch and an abnormal indentation on the posterior wall of the trachea seen on the lateral chest radiograph. Aortography (BOTTOM LEFT) demonstrates an aberrant right subclavian artery with an aneurysmal first portion (diverticulum of Kommerell). A barium swallow study (BOTTOM RIGHT) demonstrates that the esophagus is identically displaced by a rounded structure. (Courtesy of Andrew Common, MD, Toronto, Canada.)

CASE 3

Asymptomatic Aberrant Right Subclavian Artery

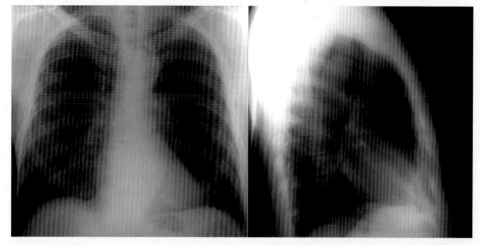

Figure 2-16. Left-sided aortic arch and left descending aorta. (Courtesy of Andrew Common, MD, Toronto, Canada.)

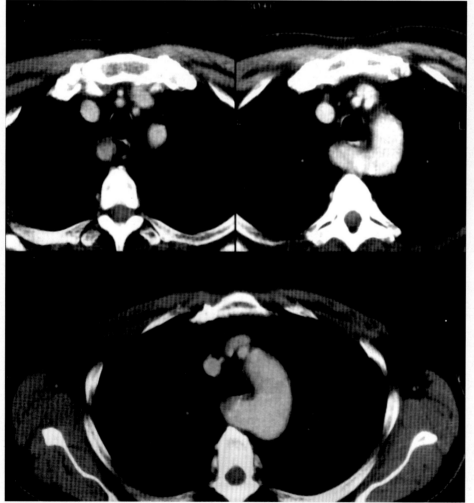

Figure 2-17. Contrast-enhanced CT scans. TOP LEFT, View of the arch branch vessels. The right subclavian artery is posterior to the trachea and immediately lateral to the esophagus and has a normal diameter at this level. TOP RIGHT, View of the dilated first portion of the aberrant right subclavian artery, which courses posterior to the esophagus and trachea. BOTTOM, View of the widest portion of the aneurysm of the aberrant right subclavian artery revealing that its size is identical to the aortic arch. (Courtesy of Andrew Common, MD, Toronto, Canada.)

2

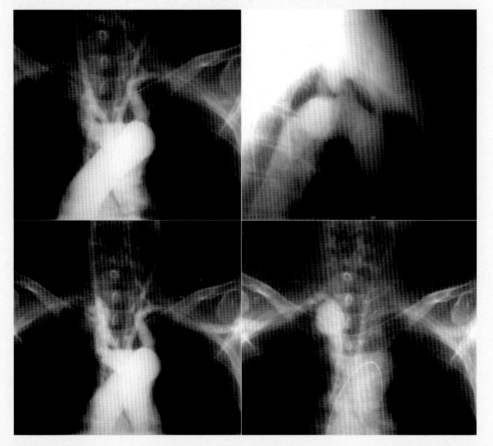

Figure 2-18. Aortography. Posteroanterior view (TOP LEFT) reveals the left-sided arch, the common carotid arteries arising from the left-sided arch, and an aberrant right subclavian artery with an aneurysmal first portion (diverticulum of Kommerell). Lateral view (TOP RIGHT) reveals the aneurysmal portion of the right subclavian end as a round lesion on the diameter of the aorta. BOTTOM, Aortography at different phases revealing an aneurysm of the right subclavian artery proper at and above the level of the right clavicle. (Courtesy of Andrew Common, MD, Toronto, Canada.)

CASE 4

Asymptomatic Aberrant Right Subclavian Artery

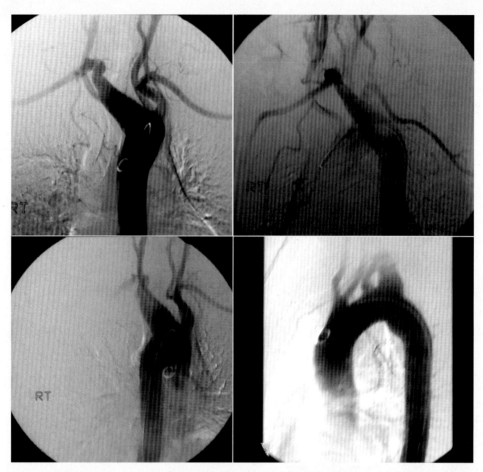

Figure 2-19. Aortography in different views revealing a left-sided aortic arch and descending aorta and an aneurysmal first portion of an aberrant right subclavian artery (diverticulum of Kommerell). The lateral view (BOTTOM RIGHT) reveals a ductal diverticulum of the inside curvature of the aorta in the proximal descending portion. (Courtesy of Andrew Common, MD, Toronto, Canada.)

2

CASE 5

Double Aortic Arch

▸ Progressive chronic cough and wheeze
▸ No dysphagia
▸ Patient was aware of pulsation in the throat area
▸ Never operated on

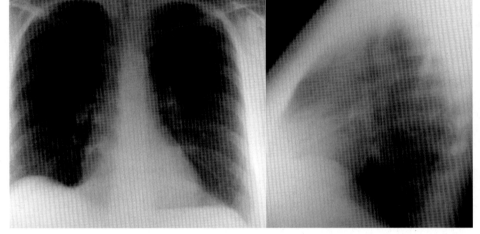

Figure 2-20. Chest radiographs revealing a double arch, with greater prominence of the right arch. Left descending aorta. (Courtesy of Andrew Common, MD, Toronto, Canada.)

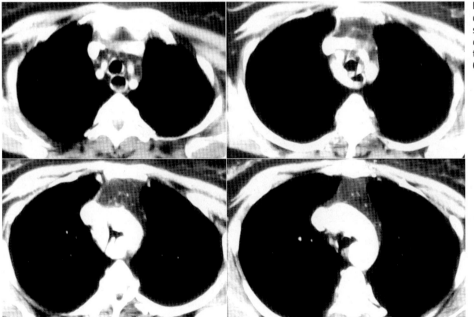

Figure 2-21. Contrast-enhanced CT scans demonstrating two aortic arches and a left-sided descending aorta. The common carotid and subclavian branches arise from the ipsilateral arches. (Courtesy of Andrew Common, MD, Toronto, Canada.)

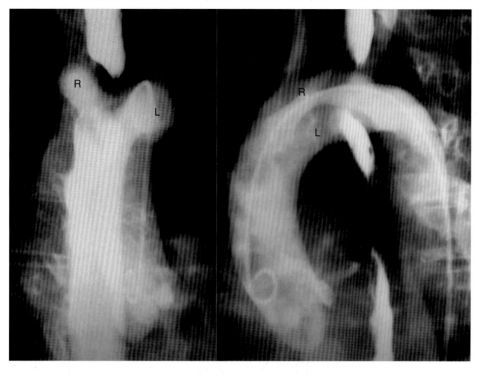

Figure 2-22. Aortography reveals that the left arch, although less prominent on the plain chest radiograph, is the larger one. (Courtesy of Andrew Common, MD, Toronto, Canada.)

CASE 6

Right-Sided Aortic Arch and Descending Aorta

▸ The patient had asymmetric upper extremity pulses.

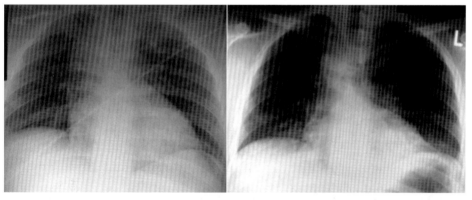

Figure 2-23. Chest radiographs with lesser (LEFT) and greater (RIGHT) penetration show a right-sided aortic arch and descending aorta. (Courtesy of Andrew Common, MD, Toronto, Canada.)

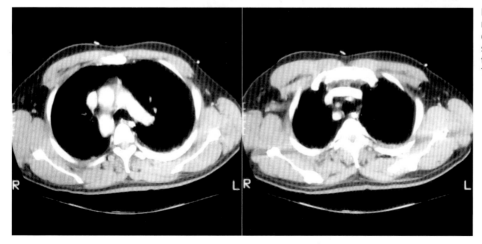

Figure 2-24. Contrast-enhanced CT scans. LEFT, Right-sided aortic arch and descending aorta. RIGHT, The aberrant left subclavian artery is posterior to the trachea. (Courtesy of Andrew Common, MD, Toronto, Canada.)

CASE 7

Asymptomatic Right-Sided Aortic Arch and Descending Aorta

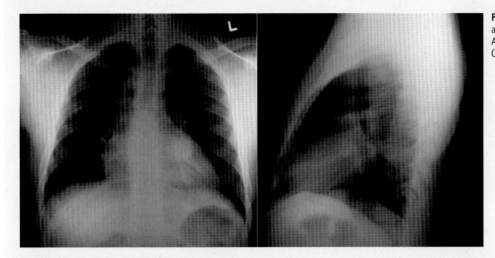

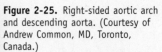

Figure 2-25. Right-sided aortic arch and descending aorta. (Courtesy of Andrew Common, MD, Toronto, Canada.)

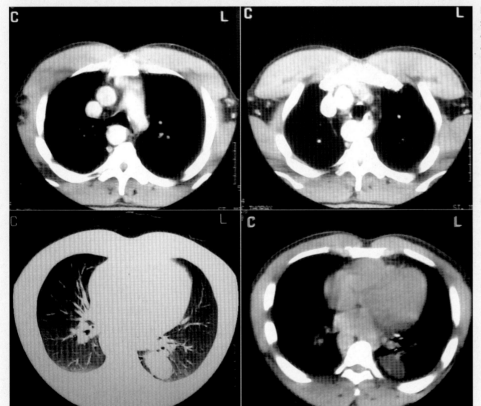

Figure 2-26. Contrast-enhanced CT scans. TOP LEFT, Right-sided aortic arch and descending aorta. TOP RIGHT, The aberrant left subclavian artery is posterior to the trachea. BOTTOM, A bronchogenic cyst (needle aspiration proven) is present in the left lower lobe. (Courtesy of Andrew Common, MD, Toronto, Canada.)

2

CASE 8

Symptomatic Right-Sided Aortic Arch and Descending Aorta

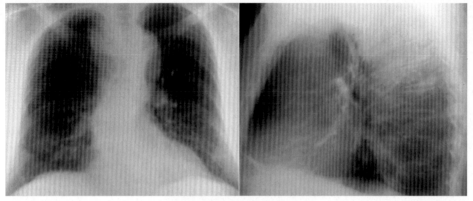

Figure 2-27. Right-sided aortic arch and left-sided descending aorta. (Courtesy of Andrew Common, MD, Toronto, Canada.)

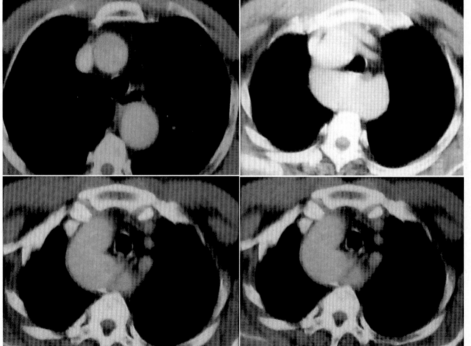

Figure 2-28. Contrast-enhanced CT scans. The aortic arch is right sided and the descending aorta is left sided. The origin of the aberrant left subclavian artery is seen as the last branch vessel of the arch. (Courtesy of Andrew Common, MD, Toronto, Canada.)

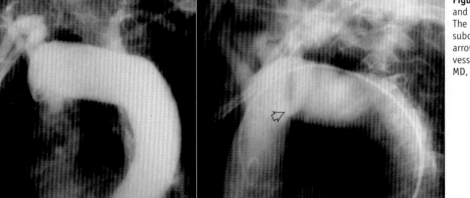

Figure 2-29. Right-sided aortic arch and a left-sided descending aorta. The origin of the aberrant left subclavian artery is indicated by the arrow and is the last arch branch vessel. (Courtesy of Andrew Common, MD, Toronto, Canada.)

CHAPTER 3

Examination and Imaging of the Aorta

- ▸ Clinical suspicion, acumen, and versatility with imaging modalities are all crucial to the assessment of the diseased aorta.
- ▸ CT scanning is the principal imaging modality for thoracic and abdominal aortic diseases, offering excellent anatomic depiction even in acutely ill patients.
- ▸ Echocardiography is useful for assessing related cardiac complications of aortic diseases, such as cardiac functional disturbances, and it is a good test for aortic dissection but much less useful for assessment of other

aortic diseases. It is an excellent test for acutely ill patients with disease of the ascending aorta.
- ▸ Ultrasonography is a suitable screening test for abdominal aneurysms.
- ▸ Cardiac MR is an alternative to CT scanning and is useful for avoiding radiation exposure in young patients or contrast toxicity in patients with renal insufficiency. It is not a very suitable test for acutely ill patients.

HISTORY AND PHYSICAL EXAMINATION

Elements of the history and careful physical examination are useful in the assessment of the aorta; both are often overlooked.

Medical History

Pain is the cardinal feature of acute aortic disease and immediately alters and escalates the evaluation and management. Dissection, intramural hematoma, and rupture pain is usually abrupt and maximal at the onset and may migrate. Although there is some correlation of location of pain with location of aortic dissection and rupture, the correlation is imperfect. Some distal (posterior) dissections also have pain anteriorly, and some anterior dissections have pain posteriorly. Pain due to enlargement of the aorta (and compression of adjacent structures) is usually a deep unrelenting ache.

Family History

The review of family history is useful in consideration of familial disorders with strong predilection for aortic abnormalities, such as Marfan syndrome, Ehlers-Danlos syndrome, familial thoracic

aneurysm/dissection syndrome, and familial abdominal aortic aneurysm syndrome.

Review of Systems

The review of systems is useful for considerations such as risk factors for aortic diseases (hypertension, atherosclerosis), trauma, infections (staphylococci, syphilis), and inflammatory diseases (giant cell arteritis, Takayasu's arteritis, systemic lupus erythematosus, rheumatoid arthritis) and for complications of aortic diseases such as heart failure from aortic insufficiency.

Physical Examination

Useful elements of physical examination include the following:

- Aortic insufficiency murmur (potentially indicating distortion or disruption of the root of the aorta) is a useful sign, but it is neither specific nor sensitive for aortic diseases.
- Pericardial rub (potentially signaling leakage of the ascending aorta into the pericardium) is an important sign, but it is neither specific nor sensitive for aortic diseases.
- Signs of tamponade (potentially signaling leakage of the ascending aorta into the pericardium) are important, but they also are neither specific nor sensitive for aortic diseases.

Table 3-1. Sensitivity of Physical Diagnosis for Detection of Abdominal Aortic Aneurysm

Parameter	Sensitivity
AAA diameter 3.0-3.9 cm	61%
AAA diameter 4.0-4.9 cm	69%
AAA diameter >5.0 cm	82%
Waist circumference <100 cm	91%
Waist circumference ≥100 cm	53%

AAA, abdominal aortic aneurysm.
From Fink HA, Lederle FA, Roth CS, et al: The accuracy of physical examination to detect abdominal aortic aneurysm. Arch Intern Med 2000;160:833-836.

- Tracheal tug is a rare sign of an aneurysm of the ascending aorta or arch.
- Pulsatile sternum may indicate a retrosternal aortic aneurysm.
- Pulsatile abdominal aorta

Physical Diagnosis of Abdominal Aortic Aneurysms

In slender patients, an expansile epigastric mass fairly reliably indicates an abdominal aortic aneurysm (AAA). It is usually located to the left of the midline. However, in obese patients, few AAAs can be detected by palpation. As obesity becomes more prevalent in the industrialized world, the challenge to clinically detect AAAs will only increase. Literature reviews of detection of AAA by physical diagnosis suggest limited sufficient accuracy: sensitivity, 33% to 100%; specificity, 75% to 100%; positive predictive value, 14% to 100%.[1] Only about half of AAAs are detected clinically; of 198 patients with AAA presenting during a 3-year period, 48% were detected clinically, 37% were detected radiographically, and 15% were detected at laparotomy. The average diameter of a palpable AAA was 6.42 ± 1.24 cm, and the average diameter of nonpalpable AAAs was 4.86 ± 1.38 cm.[2] Table 3-1 summarizes the sensitivity of physical diagnosis based on the diameter of the AAA and waist circumference.[3]

PLAIN RADIOGRAPHY

Chest Radiograph

Intimal calcification is a marker of atherosclerosis, and intimal displacement into the lumen is a marker of pathologic wall thickening (dissection or intramural hematoma). The anteroposterior and posteroanterior chest radiographs can depict aortic intimal atherosclerosis. Calcification is assumed to be intimal, but it may extend into the wall. Before 65 years of age, radiographically evident calcification is associated with a twofold increase in cardiovascular mortality; but as the incidence increases with age, beyond 65 years it is so common as to not be as prominent a marker of increased risk (Fig. 3-1).

When there is more than 0.5 or 1.0 cm of distance from the intimal calcification to the outside wall of the aorta, there is said to be intimal displacement, which is consistent with pathologic wall thickening such as may be seen with acute aortic dissection or intramural hematoma. Intimal displacement is not a sensitive sign for acute aortic dissection; also, it is not specific because a tortuous arch can mimic the sign (Fig. 3-2).

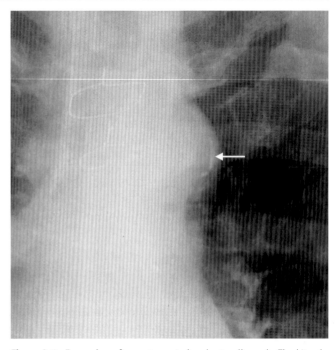

Figure 3-1. Zoom view of a posteroanterior chest radiograph. The lateral aspect of the aortic knob (distal arch)–proximal descending aorta clearly has extensive intimal calcification (from atherosclerosis). Extensive aortic atherosclerosis is nearly invariably associated with coronary artery disease. The sternotomy wires are from a prior aortocoronary bypass. The intimal location of the calcification establishes that the wall thickness is normal (no dissection or intramural hematoma that thickens the wall in this anatomic segment).

A left pleural effusion is a potentially ominous and urgent sign in the context of acute aortic disease as inflammation with exudation or leakage or frank rupture may occur into the left pleural cavity. Centesis can establish the nature of the fluid.

Aortic dissection is associated with an abnormal chest radiograph in most but not all cases. About 10% to 20% of dissections do not have aortic abnormalities that can be visible on a chest radiograph (such as enlargement, abnormal contour, or intimal displacement).

Utility of Chest Radiography for Detecting Specific Aortic Diseases

Aortic dilation or aneurysm is usually evident on the chest radiograph, but the sensitivity for detection of dilation relates to the extent of dilation (Fig. 3-3). The posteroanterior chest radiograph is far better at depicting aortic abnormalities than the anteroposterior chest radiograph is. Isolated dilation of the aortic root may not be seen unless it is frankly aneurysmal, as the root overlies the shadow of the heart, obscuring it on the chest radiograph. As the ascending aorta dilates, it lies over the right hilum and accordingly the hilar vessels are obscured—the hilar overlay sign on the posteroanterior chest radiograph. Dilation or aneurysm of the aortic arch is usually evident on a posteroanterior chest radiograph as a mediastinal widening. Rotation may create a false-positive to this sign. Dilation or aneurysm of the descending aorta may be difficult to distinguish from mere tortuosity. The basic problem is that the medial wall of the aorta cannot be determined on the chest radiograph; leftward position of the left margin of the aorta may occur from dilation (aneurysm or dissection) or from tortuosity.

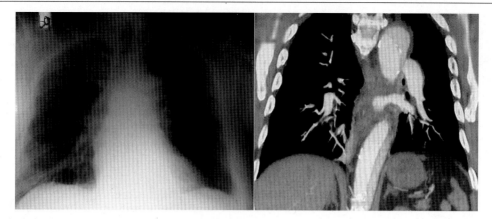

Figure 3-2. Intimal displacement. Displacement of intimal atherosclerotic calcification is a useful sign to denote the presence of a false lumen within the wall of the aorta. The anteroposterior chest radiograph on the left vaguely depicts calcification along the distal aortic arch. The contrast-enhanced CT scan coronal image on the right reveals the underlying dissection that resulted in the false lumen that widened the wall of the aorta and displaced the calcium within the intimal plaques. The aortic contour is abnormal on the chest film; intimal calcification is a more specific radiographic sign of acute aortic dissection, although insensitive.

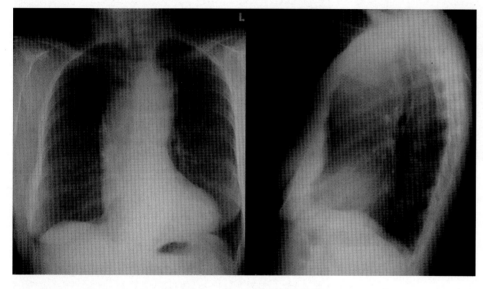

Figure 3-3. These plain anteroposterior and lateral chest radiographs do not show findings specific for a particular aortic disease but do show a dilated ascending aorta. The patient had an aneurysm limited to the ascending aorta, without dissection. The cardiopericardial silhouette is normal. There is a pectus excavatum.

Abdominal Radiograph

The lateral shoot-through plain abdominal film is able to depict prelumbar calcification of the anterior aortic wall, which is increasingly common with aging and reflects the calcification associated with the predilection of atherosclerosis for this segment of the aorta. The anterior wall of an AAA is usually (in 80% of cases) obvious on a plain lateral film because of its calcification (Fig. 3-4).

Plain Radiography for Evaluation of the Aorta: Clinical Summary

Advanced imaging has supplanted plain radiography for the assessment of aortic diseases, but current lack of familiarity with aortic abnormalities on plain film imaging is regrettable, as awareness of plain film manifestations of aortic diseases may assist in the recognition of disease and lead to more

specific advanced imaging. Important findings to be aware of are

1. *enlargement of the aortic contour,* suggesting dissection, aneurysm, or intramural hematoma or even coarctation;
2. *calcification of the aorta,* delineating its size;
3. *intimal displacement,* consistent with the presence of a dissection; and
4. *left pleural effusion.* Although a left pleural effusion is nonspecific toward the presence of thoracic aortic diseases, it is a potentially worrisome sign in the context of thoracic aortic disease, as it may denote leakage.

ECHOCARDIOGRAPHY

Transthoracic Echocardiography

Transthoracic echocardiography (TTE) is a modality that is significantly limited in its ability to depict the aorta. It is able to

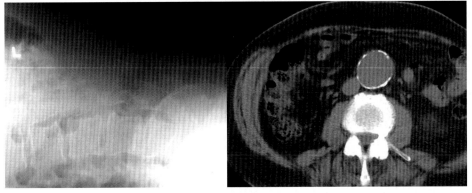

Figure 3-4. The lateral shoot-through radiograph on the left reveals an AAA by projecting the prelumbar anterior calcification (and posterior calcification) of the AAA away from the spine. The non–contrast-enhanced CT scan image on the right is from the same patient. The maximal diameter was nearly identical by radiography and CT scanning.

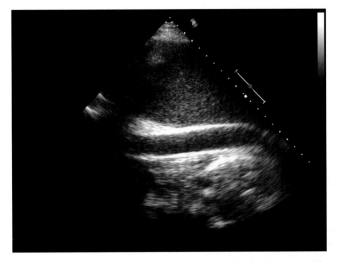

Figure 3-5. Vertically oriented transthoracic image obtained from the left lateral mid chest. The long tubular structure deep to the pleural effusion is the descending aorta, which is seen in fair detail.

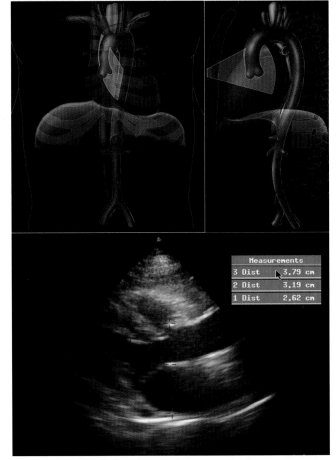

Figure 3-6. TTE parasternal views can image a variable amount of the aortic root and ascending aorta. Often, imaging from one rib interspace higher than for the standard parasternal long-axis view or from high right parasternal sites offers a depiction of a longer length of the aorta. The still-frame image on the left shows the aortic valve (open), the aortic root, and several centimeters of the ascending aorta. Although the image is fairly clear, there are multiple artifacts. Recognition of artifact is an important aspect of all forms of imaging.

visualize only the first several centimeters of the aorta in most individuals—usually the root and a few variable centimeters of the ascending aorta and, in half of individuals, the mid arch as well. This leaves large areas of the aorta poorly seen or not seen at all. Artifacts are regularly encountered by transthoracic imaging of the aorta.

Thus, in other than a few individuals, TTE is very limited in its ability to see the aorta, let alone resolve details of pathology other than intimal flaps. However, when a dissection is simply obvious by TTE, subsequent testing is often redundant and time-consuming. On occasion, a left pleural effusion will allow extensive visualization of the descending portion of the thoracic aorta (Fig. 3-5).

The key role of TTE in regard to the evaluation of aortic diseases is its ability to rapidly and accurately assess cardiac complications of aortic diseases (especially dissection), such as aortic insufficiency from root involvement, pericardial fluid from root or ascending involvement, wall motion abnormalities from coronary involvement, and left pleural fluid collection from descending aortic leakage.

The most useful TTE views to assess the aorta are (1) standard parasternal long-axis views for the aortic valve, root, and lower ascending aorta (Fig. 3-6); (2) high left or right parasternal views for the ascending aorta; (3) suprasternal views for the arch (Fig. 3-7); and (4) subcostal views for the abdominal aorta (Fig.

3-8). Other TTE views of potential utility are left posterior thoracic view through the chest wall; left posterior thoracic view through a pleural effusion; parasternal long-axis views, which offer usually at least the size of the aorta but rarely clearly show a dissection flap and which are virtually unable to show intramural hematoma; and apical 2-chamber or 3-chamber views that show the retrocardiac descending aorta.

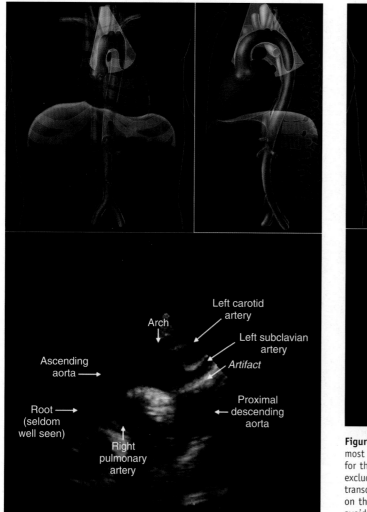

Figure 3-7. TTE suprasternal views are obtained by placing the transducer in the midline behind the suprasternal notch or the left supraclavicular space. Variable amounts of the aortic arch, ascending aorta, and descending aorta are imaged. The right pulmonary artery is seen conspicuously in cross section under the aortic arch. A view of the aortic arch by TTE usually entails a prominent artifact of the descending aorta. Often the very proximal portions of the arch vessels are seen. The right pulmonary artery is seen under the arch. Artifacts commonly overlie the proximal descending aorta. The plane of the view emerges out the side of the wall of the proximal descending aorta.

The brachiocephalic (innominate) vein runs over and parallel to the aortic arch. Suprasternal views often detect it. The thin wall between the two should not be mistaken for an intimal flap. Doppler sampling can resolve the differences in flow direction and pattern that would eliminate this potential false-positive (Fig. 3-9).

Ultrasonography of the Abdominal Aorta

Ultrasonography of the abdominal aorta is a useful technique to identify and to screen for AAA, to observe AAA for diameter changes, and to assess for abdominal branch complications of aortic disease or associated diseases, such as atherosclerotic occlusive disease of the iliacs or splanchnic vessels (Fig. 3-10).

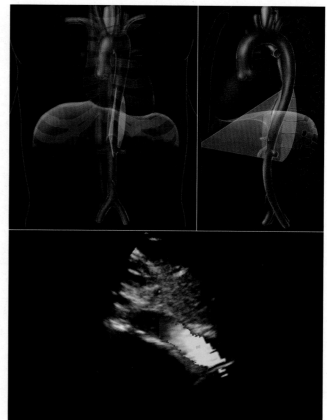

Figure 3-8. Subcostal TTE can garner views of the abdominal aorta in most individuals but struggles with less than optimal transducer design for the task and against rampant obesity. Images may be adequate to exclude aneurysm or dissection of the abdominal aorta. With the transducer oriented superiorly, the proximal abdominal aorta is displayed on the right. Superior orientation angles the sector through the liver, avoiding midline abdominal gas.

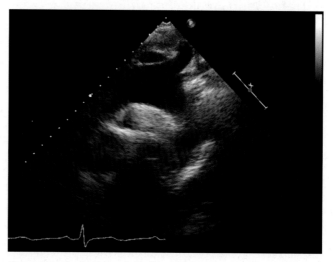

Figure 3-9. The brachiocephalic (innominate) vein is seen over the aortic arch, mimicking an intimal flap, with true and false lumens.

Vascular ultrasonography is readily available at the bedside, allowing rapid examination. Lack of radiation and contrast risk is also a positive feature. Inability to image in detail, especially in an unprepared patient, and some difficulty in determining branch involvement are regularly negative features.

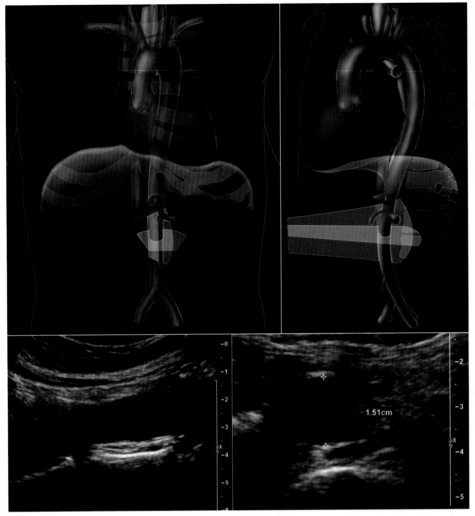

Figure 3-10. Vascular ultrasonography of the abdominal aorta can image longer lengths of the aorta, and lower segments of the aorta, as well as the celiac, superior mesenteric, and renal artery takeoffs. In this single view, the aorta is seen in long axis through the majority of its abdominal course. The ability of ultrasonography to screen for abdominal aneurysms is evident. By convention, the abdominal aortic diameter is measured on a short-axis view to ensure determination of the maximal diameter.

Transesophageal Echocardiography

Transesophageal echocardiography (TEE) is far better suited for imaging of the thoracic aorta than is TTE (Fig. 3-11), and it is also a superb test to define or to exclude cardiac involvement. In most individuals, the root and most of the ascending aorta are well imaged (Fig. 3-12), as well as the distal arch (Fig. 3-13) and the length of the descending thoracic aorta (Fig. 3-14). A full examination can be performed in 10 minutes at the beside. The most common uses of TEE for aortic diseases are as the second-line diagnostic test for aortic dissection or suspected dissection cases (potential intramural hematomas, penetrating ulcers) and for evaluation of cardiac complications of aortic diseases, such as the mechanism of aortic insufficiency and the potential reparability of the valve.

Problem areas for interrogation by TEE regularly include the mid and upper ascending aorta and the proximal arch (in both cases because of interposed tracheal air between the esophagus and these anatomic regions). Another potential problem is heavy calcification of the aorta that obscures imaging; therefore, in patients with severe atheromatous disease, the aorta cannot be well imaged. The narrowness of the near field of the sector limits depiction of near-field findings and potentially of their recognition. Availability of 24-hour TEE expertise is a limitation.

Because TEE probes have transducers that can be rotated to any degree, there are an infinite number of potential views of the aorta. The standard views that enable a systematic interrogation of the different aortic segments are reduced to short- and long-axis views of three segments of the aorta (Table 3-2).

COMPUTED TOMOGRAPHIC IMAGING OF THE AORTA

Computed tomographic aortography (CTA) is a superb modality to assess diseases of the aorta and has essentially established itself as the principal advanced diagnostic test for diseases of the aorta. CTA has advanced enormously in the last 5 years because of increases in the numbers of detectors and slices (currently 64 and 256) and the supporting software. This has yielded superb spatial resolution (better than magnetic resonance aortography), excellent temporal resolution, very fast scanning times (15 to 20 seconds), and numerous means to display images by post-processing software. Critically ill patients can be scanned by CTA because they are fairly readily monitored throughout, and door-to-door time is 15 minutes. Actual scanning time is 20 seconds. Risks include potential contrast nephropathy and allergy; radiation risks are on the order of one coronary angiogram.

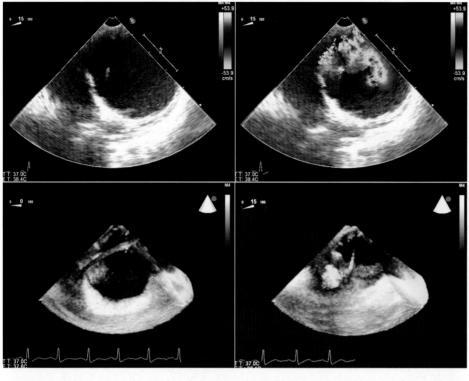

Figure 3-11. TEE imaging of the aorta. TOP, Standard 2D imaging in diastole (LEFT) and in systole (RIGHT) revealing an intimal flap with a large false lumen into which a jet enters in systole only. BOTTOM, Real-time 3D imaging showing the intimal flap, true (smaller) and false (larger) lumens (LEFT), and the intimal tear (defect in the intimal flap, RIGHT).

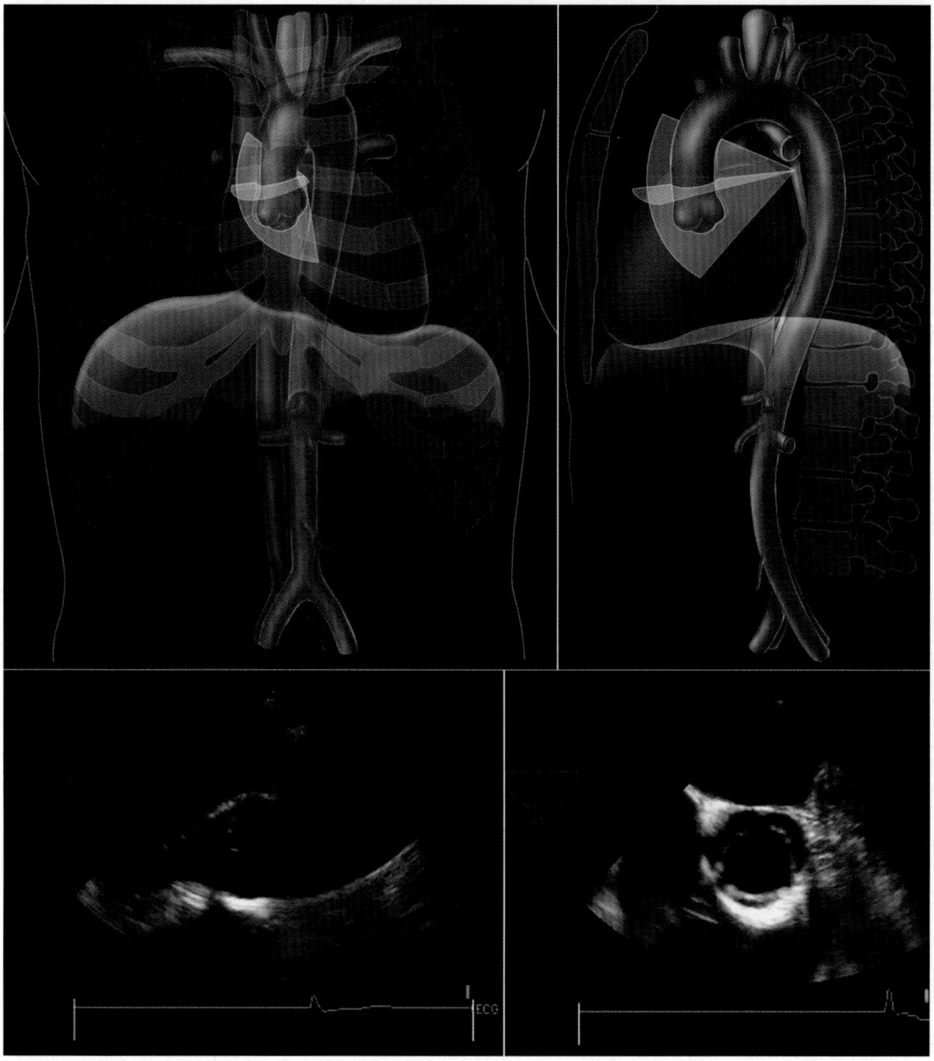

Figure 3-12. TEE view of the aortic valve, root, and ascending aorta. Acquired from the mid esophagus, transverse (short-axis, 30 to 40 degrees) and longitudinal (long-axis, 110 to 130 degrees) views. Short- and long-axis views are orthogonal to each other (different by 90 degrees). The competence of the aortic valve is easily determined by color Doppler flow mapping.

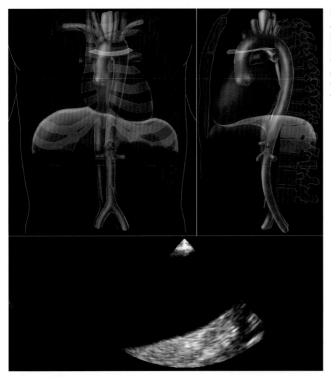

Figure 3-13. TEE views of the aortic arch. Horizontal-longitudinal view is acquired from the upper esophagus (0 degrees), avoiding the tracheal and left bronchial air columns, usually by acquiring the image from above them; a horizontal view looking obliquely along the arch of the aorta can be obtained in most people. A horizontal view looking along the arch of the aorta displays the distal portion on the right, the anterior wall opposite the transducer, and the proximal part of the arch the farthest away from the transducer on the left.

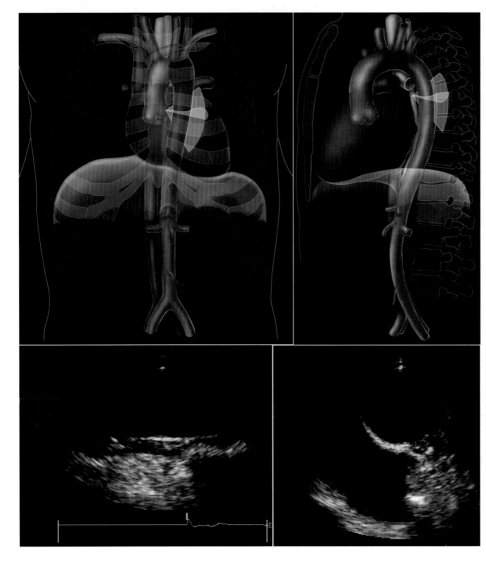

Figure 3-14. TEE views of the descending aorta. Acquired from the mid esophagus, transverse (short-axis, 0 degrees) and longitudinal (long-axis, 90 degrees) views are obtained at multiple levels. Short- and long-axis views are orthogonal to each other (different by 90 degrees). Imaging the entirety of an enlarged aorta may be difficult if its diameter is greater than the sector of imaging can encompass. This is most problematic for near-field imaging, where the sector is narrowest.

Table 3-2. Standard Transesophageal Echocardiographic Views for Systematic Inspection of Different Segments of the Aorta

Aortic Segment and View	Position of Probe Tip	Angle of Rotation
Aortic valve, root, ascending aorta		
Short-axis view: 30-40 degrees	Mid esophagus	30-40 degrees
Long-axis view: 110-130 degrees	Mid esophagus	120-140 degrees
Aortic arch		
Short-axis view	Upper esophagus	0 degrees
Long-axis view	Upper esophagus	90 degrees
Descending aorta		
Short-axis view	Mid esophagus, multiple levels	0 degrees
Long-axis view	Mid esophagus, multiple levels	90 degrees

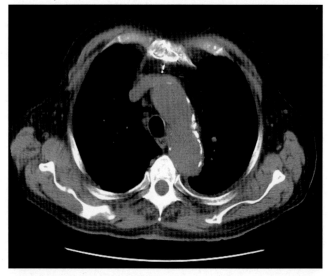

Figure 3-15. This non–contrast-enhanced axial CT image shows extensive intimal calcification. Intimal calcification is less readily appreciated in the presence of luminal contrast enhancement, as both have similar brightness (attenuation coefficients).

Technique and Modalities

For CTA, the field of view is verified by a pre-scan (surview or topograph). The delineation of the field of view determines the data volume acquired, which can subsequently be reconstructed and displayed according to the available software.

Non–Contrast-Enhanced Scan

- Breath-hold 15 to 20 seconds
- Initial scanning is done without the administration of contrast material to delineate calcification, wall thickening, and other details that are more clearly understood in the absence of contrast dye.

For example, intramural hematoma (if it is fresh) has a high signal density (60 to 70 Hounsfield units) that is best apparent on non–contrast-enhanced images (Figs. 3-15 and 3-16).

Contrast Scan

- Breath-hold 15 to 20 seconds
- Injection of 1 or 2 mL/kg (80 to 150 mL) of nonionic contrast material by power injector at 3 to 5 mL/s achieves homogeneous contrast.

The acquisition of images is initiated either by a sensing technique that identifies that the contrast material has arrived in the aorta or by having timed a test bolus of saline (Figs. 3-17 to 3-19).

Transaxial images from above the arch to the femoral arteries are reconstructed at 0.5-cm intervals. Axial images can be reformatted to yield 2-dimensional (2D) images along any plane and 3-dimensional (3D) images (Figs. 3-20 and 3-21).

Image Reformatting and Post-Processing

Reformatting and post-processing modalities that are commonly and easily preformed are reformatted 2D images, multiplanar image reformatting to display along nonaxial planes (e.g., sagittal

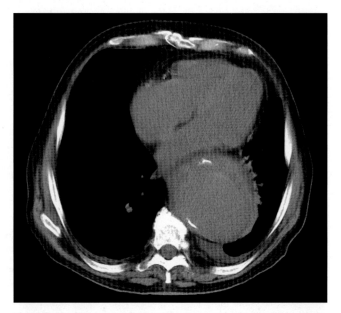

Figure 3-16. This non–contrast-enhanced transaxial CT view in a patient with renal insufficiency shows a large thoracic aortic aneurysm. There is calcification marking the position of the intima and the vague delineation of lumen from mural thrombus.

or any other plane or planes that image the aorta and its branches well), and maximum intensity projection, which enhances the maximum signal on any image slice. Reformatted 3D images can be obtained by shaded-surface display and volume rendering (Figs. 3-22 and 3-23).

Some newer workstations have vascular-specific software that can extract the vessel (aorta or other) and display it as a straightened structure, facilitating measurement or other analysis (Figs. 3-24 to 3-28). Most diagnoses are based on axial images; some post-processing images do assist with display but may introduce inaccuracies.

Text continued on p. 49.

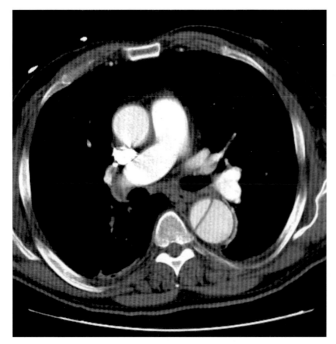

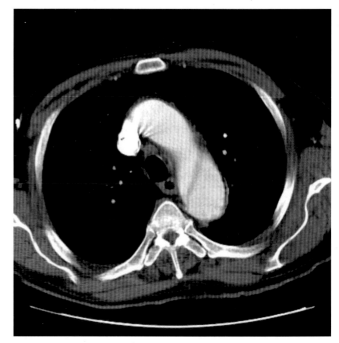

Figure 3-17. This contrast-enhanced axial CT image shows an intimal flap within the descending aorta and none in the aortic root, suggesting a type B dissection. There is an extremely common high-attenuation artifact streaking out from the residual dye in the superior vena cava into the ascending aorta, potentially misleading that there is an intimal flap in the ascending aorta.

Figure 3-18. This contrast-enhanced axial CT image of the aortic arch shows an intimal flap in the mid arch–descending aorta. On this older scanner, the resolution is not sufficient to clearly delineate the mobile flap. Again, there are streak artifacts from residual dye in the superior vena cava.

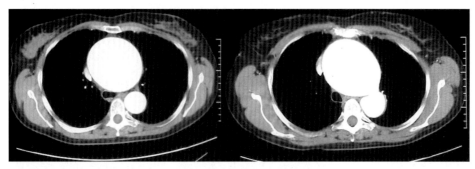

Figure 3-19. These contrast-enhanced axial CT images of the thoracic aorta depict an aneurysm of the ascending aorta. The diameter of the descending portion is normal. The right slice is at the level of the floor of the arch and shows a fold of the floor—pseudocoarctation.

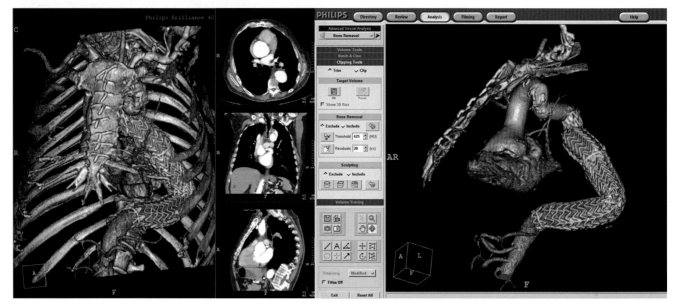

Figure 3-20. Contrast-enhanced 3D volume-rendered CT images. The reformatted image on the left reveals sternal wires, the thoracic cage, the heart cavities, and the stented thoracic aorta. The image on the right was obtained by rotating the image, use of bone removal software, and editing. The aorta is now more directly seen: the detail of the overlapping stents, the calcification of the arch of the aorta, and the markedly tortuous course of the arch portion.

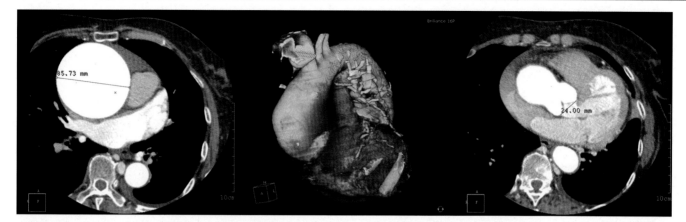

Figure 3-21. CT aortography of an ascending aortic aneurysm: axial and volume-rendered images. LEFT, This axial image depicts the maximal diameter of the aneurysm; it allowed measurement and demonstrated the absence of a flap. MIDDLE, The volume-rendered image depicts the exterior detail of the aorta, the distribution of the aneurysm, and patches of calcification. RIGHT, This axial image is another example of measurement function; here, a 24-mm composite graft would be suitable.

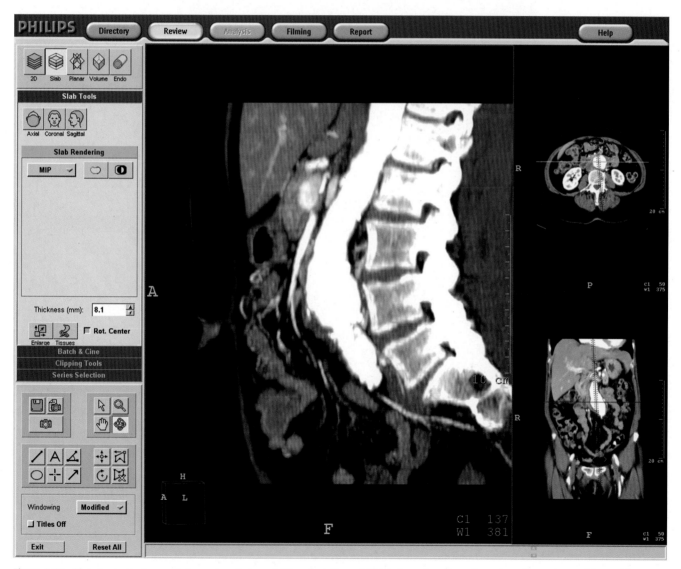

Figure 3-22. CT aortography: image display and analysis modalities. An infrarenal AAA is imaged on these three views. The main panel is an oblique sagittal view. The reference planes are depicted on the corresponding orthogonal views by the solid blue lines (the dotted blue lines describe the slice thickness, as is also depicted on the left-hand toolbar). The dataset can be reviewed by moving side to side on the sagittal view, up and down on the axial view, or front to back on the coronal view or by swiveling on any of them. There is irregular mural thrombus within the AAA.

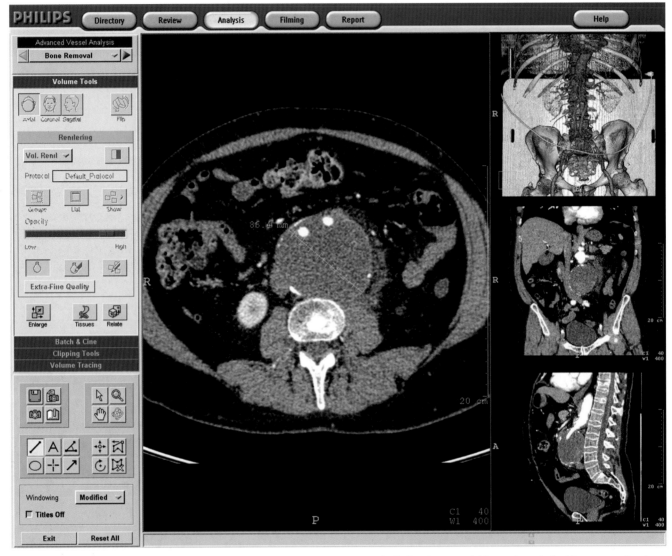

Figure 3-23. CT aortography: image display and analysis modalities. This stented AAA is displayed on an axial image (CENTER), by 3D reconstruction (TOP RIGHT), on a coronal image (MIDDLE RIGHT), and on a sagittal view (BOTTOM RIGHT). The axial image demonstrates the large AAA (measurement possible with calipers), with thrombosis around the graft limbs and with scattered calcification on all sides. The 3D volume-rendered view shows only the contrast-filled aorta, that is, only the lumen of the nonaneurysmal aorta and the graft.

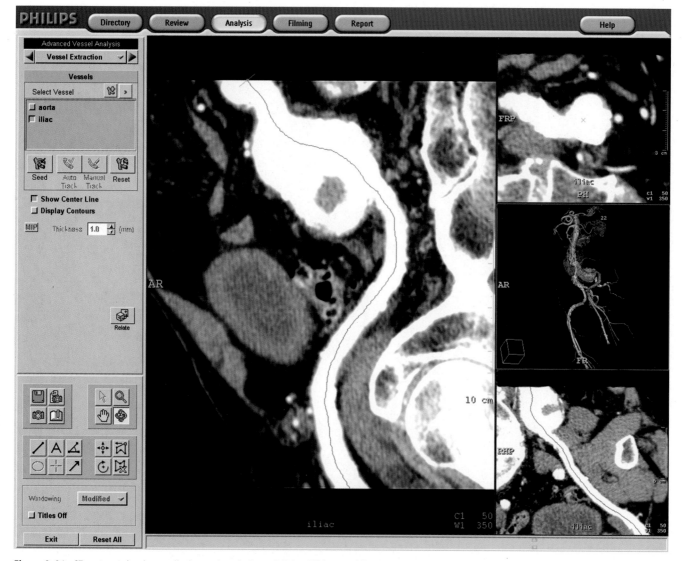

Figure 3-24. CT aortography: image display and analysis modalities. With use of features such as Advanced Vessel Analysis, this curved multiplanar reconstruction (CENTER) depicts an aneurysm not of the aorta but of the right iliac artery, which has been extracted by use of seed markers placed on the aorta proximal and distal to the site of interest on previous images. Thrombus is protruding into the lumen at the plane of imaging, as can be best seen on the straightened view (BOTTOM RIGHT). TOP RIGHT AND MIDDLE RIGHT, Orthogonal axial and sagittal images.

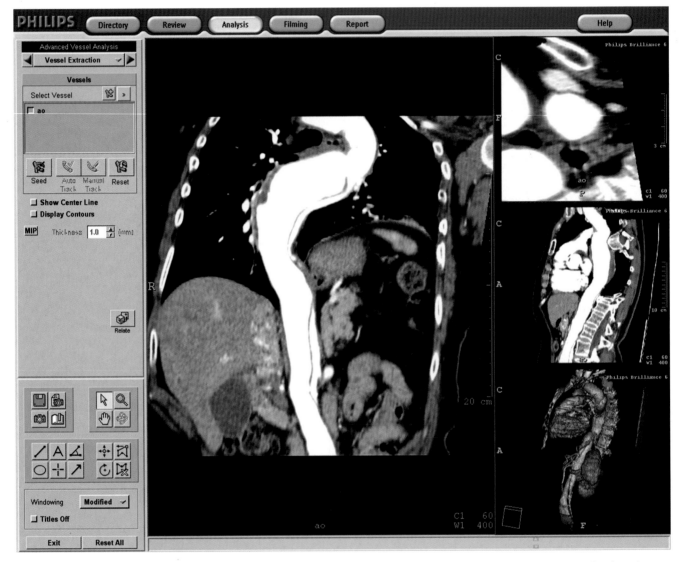

Figure 3-25. CT aortography: image display and analysis modalities. With Advanced Vessel Analysis, this curved multiplanar reconstruction (CENTER) depicts a dissection of the descending aorta, which has been extracted by use of seed markers placed on the aorta proximal and distal to the site of interest on previous images. The flap, entry, and re-entry tears are imaged. TOP RIGHT AND MIDDLE RIGHT, Orthogonal axial and sagittal images. The volume rendering function (BOTTOM RIGHT) is less suited to depiction of dissections than of aneurysms.

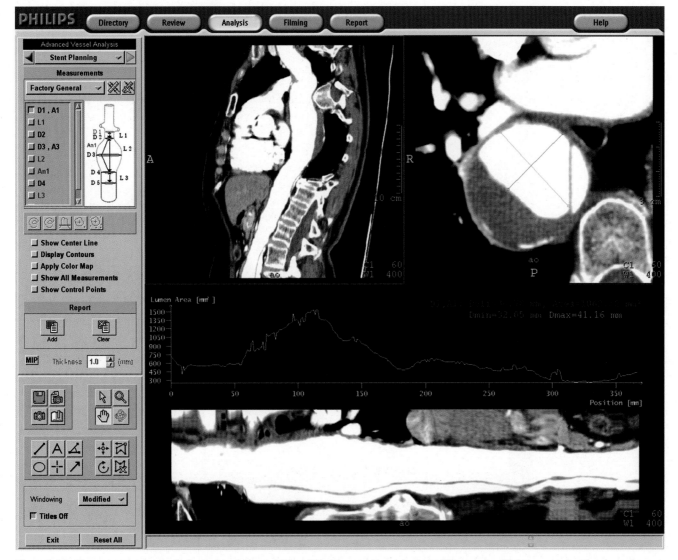

Figure 3-26. CT aortography: image display and analysis modalities. With Advanced Vessel Analysis, this curved multiplanar reconstruction (CENTER) depicts the dissection of the descending aorta, which has been extracted by use of seed markers placed on the aorta proximal and distal to the site of interest on previous images. For stent planning purposes, the software has automatically traced the area of the lumen along the length of the aorta depicted and plotted this. The lumen is characterized automatically by its area and maximum and minimum diameters.

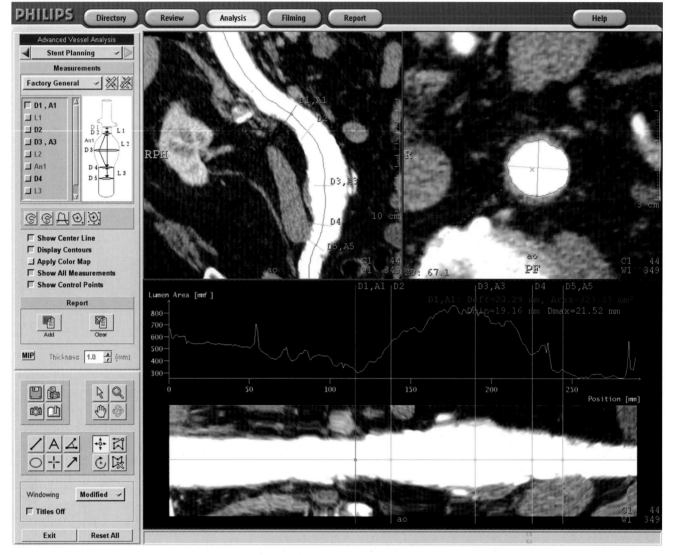

Figure 3-27. CT aortography: image display and analysis modalities. With Advanced Vessel Analysis, this curved multiplanar reconstruction (MAIN PANEL) depicts again the dissection of the descending aorta, which has been extracted by use of seed markers placed on the aorta proximal and distal to the site of interest on previous images. For stent planning purposes, the software has automatically traced the area of the lumen along the length of the aorta depicted and plotted this. The lumen is characterized automatically by its area and maximum and minimum diameters. The lower panel is a straightened depiction of the aorta and shows the entry tear, flap, and exit tear. Markers have been placed at the conventional positions of the upper and lower necks of the AAA, the landing positions, and the maximal diameter. At each site, the vessel areas and diameters are analyzed. The plot and matching straightened image of the aorta below depict the diameters along the aorta and the location of the markers.

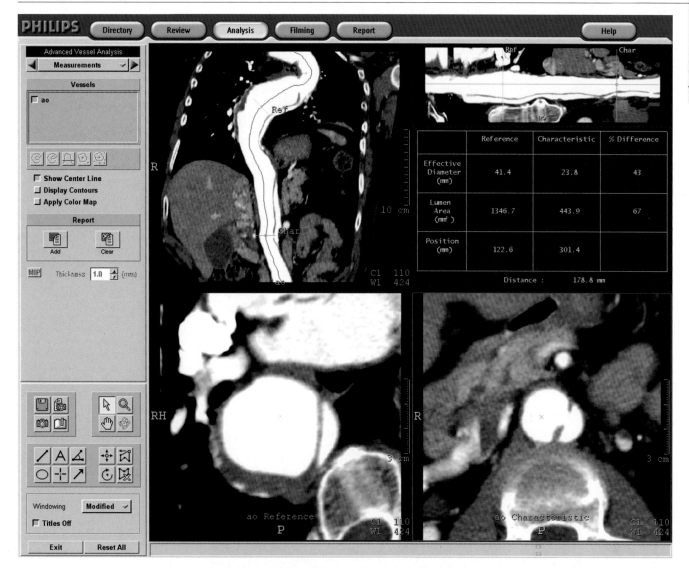

Figure 3-28. CT aortography: image display and analysis modalities. With use of vessel extraction software, a reference site and a series of characteristic sites can be depicted, along with automated analysis of diameter, luminal area, and distance between the sites. TOP LEFT, This panes displays the extracted multiplanar image of the aorta and allows placement of the reference and characteristic markers. BOTTOM LEFT, Image of the aorta at the reference site, automatically projected in short axis. BOTTOM RIGHT, The characteristic site, in this case at the exit tear, also automatically projected in short axis. TOP RIGHT, The automated analysis calculations of the two sites.

MAGNETIC RESONANCE IMAGING OF THE AORTA

Magnetic resonance aortography (MRA) and 64-slice helical CTA are essentially equivalent tests for the evaluation of the aorta in terms of diagnostic yield, but they differ in terms of logistics. The only advantages of MRA over CTA for diagnosis of aortic diseases are the absence of radiation risk and minimal contrast risk. Potential problems and limitations with MRA include lack of access at some centers, longer duration of scanning time, lesser suitability for scanning unstable and critically ill patients, artifacts due to respiratory motion in patients unable to breath-hold for sufficient time, claustrophobia occurring within the magnet, and lesser ability to identify calcification compared with CTA.

Common uses of MRA for assessment of aortic diseases vary considerably at many centers. They often include Marfan syndrome cases, chronic aortic dissection follow-up, occasional acute dissection evaluation, intramural hematoma (some ability to assess wall thickening and to identify blood in the wall), giant cell aortitis, Takayasu's or other aortitis (ability to see wall thickening as well as luminal narrowing), inflammatory aneurysms, and associated peripheral artery disease (Fig. 3-29). MRA provides an alternative to CT in patients with renal insufficiency (Fig. 3-30).

Techniques and Modalities

Spin Echo Images
T1 versus T2 weighting (longitudinal relaxation versus transverse or spin-spin relaxation) may be useful in characterization of aortic wall thickening, such as intramural hematoma. On T1-weighted images, intramural hematoma appearance equals wall

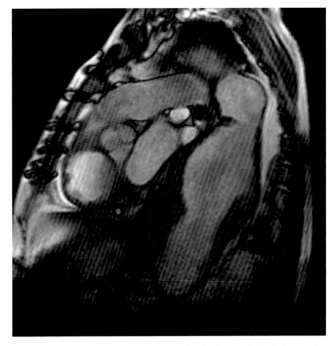

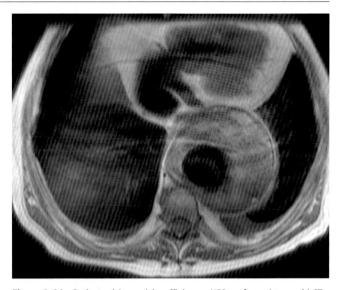

Figure 3-30. Patient with renal insufficiency, MRI performed to avoid CT contrast-related nephrotoxicity. Black blood technique reveals a very large thoracoabdominal aneurysm located behind the heart. Most of the aneurysm consists of mural thrombus—the lumen is but a fraction of the cross-sectional area. The black blood technique is prone to low-flow artifact.

Figure 3-29. MRA. The saccular nature of this thoracoabdominal aorta is evident, as is the varying amount of mural thrombus and the elongation of the aorta, leading to kinking. In this case, the folding and slight kinking of the aorta produce a pseudocoarctation appearance.

Figure 3-31. Black blood sequence (LEFT) and bright blood sequence (RIGHT) of a patient with an abdominal aortic aneurysm with a large crescentic mural thrombus.

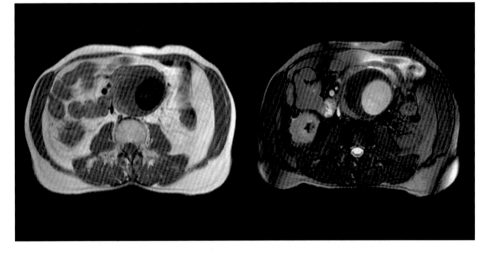

appearance; on T2-weighted images, fresh blood has high signal intensity, whereas 1- to 5-day-old blood has low signal intensity.

Black Blood Imaging

Signal from blood is suppressed, which works well for rapidly moving blood. This technique is slow and quite susceptible to artifacts, especially in longitudinal views, where the challenge is to distinguish black blood from other dark-appearing entities, such as calcification and air (Fig. 3-31).

Blood Pool Depiction

Gadolinium contrast–enhanced MRA is the principal modality for blood pool depiction (Figs. 3-32 to 3-34). Gadolinium shortens T1 relaxation and accentuates intravascular signal, yielding aortogram-like images in terms of narrowings, branches, and col-

laterals. It allows rapid acquisition of a large field of view; correct timing is critical. Like contrast aortography, it is best suited to aneurysm depiction, but it likewise suffers from inability to image thrombus (except by void) or the wall. It may show "phantomish" depiction of tissue and has been shown to depict inflammatory aneurysm changes.

Time-of-flight (TOF) imaging suppresses background to enhance inflowing blood, which appears bright. The primary use is in detection of aortic dissection and aneurysms. This modality allows delineation of the blood pool without use of contrast dye. TOF imaging, though, is subject to artifacts, such as high signal from fat or blood mimicking flow. Two-dimensional TOF technique allows rapid acquisition but is susceptible to motion artifact. Three-dimensional TOF allows high spatial resolution; it is sensitive to medium and high flow but insensitive to low flow.

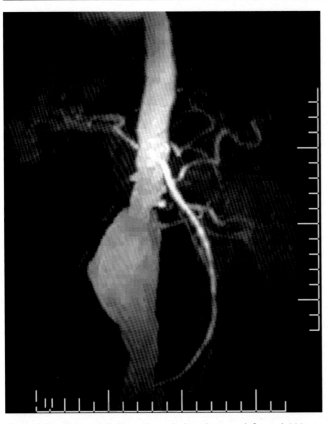

Figure 3-32. This gadolinium-enhanced view shows an infrarenal AAA. The lumen of the AAA is well depicted by the gadolinium enhancement, as is its relation to the branch vessels of the abdominal aorta. The depiction of mural thrombus, though, is phantomish and ambiguous.

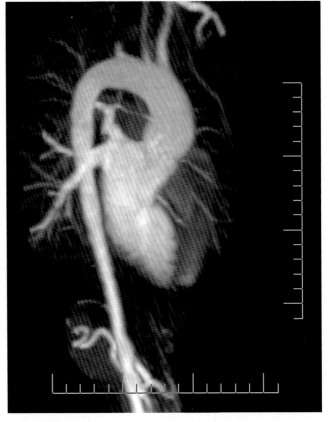

Figure 3-34. MRA. This gadolinium-enhanced image reveals narrowing of the descending aorta and left subclavian ostial occlusion due to Takayasu's disease.

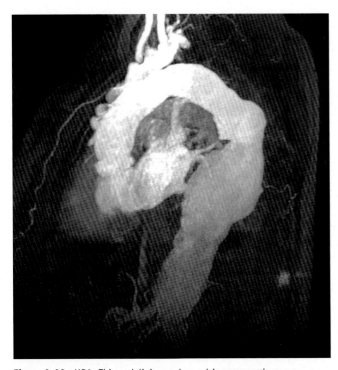

Figure 3-33. MRA. This gadolinium-enhanced image reveals a thoracoabdominal aneurysm and many branch vessels. Some branches are well depicted if they are projected clear of other contrast-enhanced structures (such as an internal thoracic artery), whereas other branch vessels are superimposed and ambiguous (such as the arch vessels).

Most often used are MRA scout images and transverse (8-mm-thick), longitudinal scans. Oblique views are acquired if necessary. Time of image acquisition for spin echo sequences is 25 minutes; for cine MRA, 15 minutes; and for contrast-enhanced MRA, 10 minutes.

Image Reformatting and Post-Processing

MRA-acquired data can be reformatted to yield 2D images along any plane and 3D images. Reformatting and post-processing modalities that are commonly and easily preformed are reformatted 2D images, multiplanar image reformatting to display along nonaxial planes (e.g., sagittal or any other plane or planes that image the aorta and its branches well), and maximum intensity projection, which enhances the maximum signal on any image slice. Reformatted 3D images can be obtained by shaded-surface display and volume rendering. Diagnoses are primarily based on raw data images; post-processing images assist with display but may introduce inaccuracies.

CONTRAST AORTOGRAPHY

As a primary diagnostic test for aortic diseases, aortography has been superseded by TEE, ultrasonography, CTA, and MRA for the detection of dissection, aneurysms, intramural hematomas, pen-

Table 3-3. Comparison of Imaging Modalities for Assessment of the Aorta

	TTE	Vascular Ultrasonography	TEE	CT	MRI and MRA	Contrast Aortography
Utility to image anatomic section						
Aortic root	Good	NA	Excellent	Excellent	Excellent	Excellent
Ascending aorta	Good-fair	NA	Fair-good	Excellent	Excellent	Excellent
Aortic arch	Fair	NA	Fair	Excellent	Excellent	Excellent
Descending aorta	Poor	NA	Excellent	Excellent	Excellent	Excellent
Branch vessel involvement	Nil	Good	Poor	Excellent	Excellent	Excellent
Utility to image pathologic changes						
Dissection flaps	Fair	Excellent (abdominal)	Excellent	Excellent	Excellent	Very good
Dissection tears	Very poor	NA	Very good	Very good	Fair	Good
Cardiac complications	Excellent	NA	Excellent	Fair	Good	Good
Intramural hematomas	Very little	Good (abdominal)	Excellent	Very good	Very good	Very poor
Penetrating ulcers	Nil	NA	Good	Very good	Good	Good
Aneurysms	Fair-good	Excellent	Excellent	Excellent	Excellent	Good
Mural thrombus	Poor	Excellent	Excellent	Excellent	Excellent	Nil
Ruptured aorta	Nil	Fair	Poor	Excellent	Good	Poor
Extra-aortic anatomy	Very poor	Poor	Very poor	Excellent	Excellent	Very poor
Risks						
Contrast	No	No	No	Yes	Minimal	Yes
Radiation	No	No	No	Yes	No	Yes
Access	No	No	No	No	No	Yes
Airway, esophageal	No	No	Yes	No	No	No
Modalities						
Multiplanar imaging	No	No	Yes	Yes	Yes	No
3D rendering	Yes	Poor	Yes	Yes	Yes	Yes
Portable	Yes	Yes	Yes	No	No	No
Suitable for critically ill patients	Yes	Yes	Yes	Yes	No	Yes
Suitable for guiding interventions	No	Somewhat	Yes	Yes	Yes	Yes

CT, computed tomography; MRA, magnetic resonance aortography; MRI, magnetic resonance imaging; NA, not applicable; TEE, transesophageal echocardiography; TTE, transthoracic echocardiography.

etrating ulcers, branch vessel involvement, and associated atherosclerotic disease. In addition to contrast risks and radiation risks, contrast aortography entails access risks and atherothrombosis embolization risks. Aortography retains a small role for diagnosis of aortic diseases, such as traumatic disruption and penetrating ulcers, and for branch vessel assessment. Contrast aortography, although less of a diagnostic test, has gained the central role in guiding aortic endovascular (EVAR) interventional procedures.

Technique and Modalities

For contrast aortography, 20 to 40 mL of contrast material is injected by power injector, and multiple x-ray views (± cine) are recorded. Standard digital subtraction angiography has excellent resolution and is therefore a suitable technique to guide interventions (Fig. 3-35). Spatial resolution is 3 or 4 lines/mm, which is slightly less than plain films, and is obtained on image intensifiers up to 16 inches in diameter. Post-processing and image-

reformatting modalities include diameter analysis, 3D rendering, and rotational 3D rendering. Flat panel technology has substantially increased image resolution.

SURGICAL INSPECTION

Formerly, surgical inspection of the aorta was relatively common, as diagnostic imaging was less reliable. The remarkable advances of diagnostic imaging, though, have not entirely eliminated the role of surgical inspection for aortic diseases.

SUMMARY

- Clinical assessment by way of careful *history and physical examination* is often overlooked, although it may help distin-

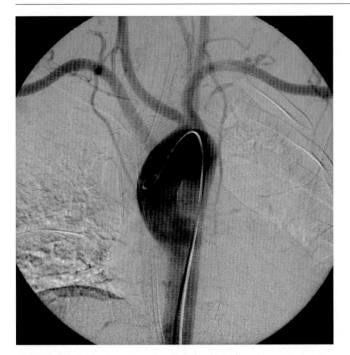

Figure 3-35. Contrast aortography. Digital subtraction contrast aortogram. The aorta and its branches are depicted. Overlap of structures, as seen on one projection, necessitates multiple projections to view complex lesions.

guish aortic disease from other disease. It establishes the clinical urgency of an aortic case better than anything else, and often the background cause. Hypertension remains the greatest risk factor for the development and progression of aortic diseases. Knowing the difference between chest pain of acute aortic syndromes and chest pain of acute ischemic syndromes is invaluable.

- *Plain radiography* offers diagnostic clues. At the very least, chest radiographic evidence of an abnormal aorta is cautionary with regard to interpreting the cause of chest pain.

- *Echocardiography and vascular ultrasonography.* TTE has limited value for the assessment of the aorta but is a strong test to evaluate cardiac complications of dissection, and in some cases it can be diagnostic for proximal dissection. TEE is a practical and powerful tool to assess disease of the thoracic aorta, although with variable availability and user experience.

- *CT aortography (CTA)* is an enormously powerful and widely available test to image all forms of diseases of the aorta. New technology has pushed CT into the vanguard of all testing for aortic diseases. Contrast toxicity is an issue in some patients.

- *MR aortography (MRA)* is perhaps the most sophisticated test for imaging of the aorta. However, it has variable availability and is poorly suited to assessment of critically ill patients because of long test times and difficulty in monitoring patients. Some forms of implanted hardware, such as ICDs and pacemakers, are contraindications to CMR. Lack of significant contrast toxicity is the only advantage of CMR over CT.

- *Contrast aortography* is no longer a first-line diagnostic test for most aortic diseases and has never been a good test to determine maximal luminal diameter in descending thoracic and abdominal aneurysms. The same information now can be obtained from CT scanning. The new role of aortography for aortic disease is not diagnostic but rather to guide aortic interventions.

- Detailed comparison of advanced imaging modalities for assessment of the aorta is presented in Table 3-3.

References

1. Lynch RM: Accuracy of abdominal examination in the diagnosis of non-ruptured abdominal aortic aneurysm. Accid Emerg Nurs 2004;12:99-107.
2. Karkos CD, Mukhopadhyay U, Papakostas I, et al: Abdominal aortic aneurysm: the role of clinical examination and opportunistic detection. Eur J Vasc Endovasc Surg 2000;19:299-303.
3. Fink HA, Lederle FA, Roth CS, et al: The accuracy of physical examination to detect abdominal aortic aneurysm. Arch Intern Med 2000;160:833-836.

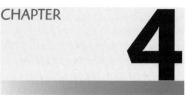
Acute Aortic Dissection

DEFINITIONS AND TERMINOLOGY OF ACUTE AORTIC SYNDROMES

Aortic dissection is a tearing through the intima into the aortic wall (intimal tear), with entry of luminal blood into the wall, resulting in the formation of a false lumen partitioned from the true lumen by the intimal flap. *Acute aortic dissection* is an aortic dissection occurring less than 2 weeks since the attributable pain episode. (The basis of this definition resides in the fact that the preponderant mortality occurs within 2 weeks. However, classification into acute, subacute, and chronic is arbitrary and neither diagnostically nor therapeutically useful.[1])

Laennec's original treatise used the term *anévrisme disséquante* (dissecting aneurysm) to describe aortic dissection. Dissecting aneurysm, however, is not an accurate term and should not be used because of the differences in pathogenesis, course, complications, imaging, and treatment of dissections and aneurysms and the rampant confusion that already exists. The preferred term is *acute aortic dissection*. A *dissection* is the tearing through intima into the wall, with formation of a new lumen, the false lumen, whose wall consists of only partial thickness. An *aneurysm* is pathologically defined as a dilation of the aorta, with the wall consisting of all the normal layers. Clinically (by imaging), it is defined by a transverse diameter more than 1.5 times expected.

A *false aneurysm* (pseudoaneurysm) is pathologically defined as dilation of a cavity or vessel, with the wall consisting of only partial thickness. Clinically (by imaging), it is presumed to be present when the neck connecting the main chamber or vessel to the dilated chamber is less than 50% of the diameter of the dilated segment. These definitions and terminology are suitable for both pathologists and clinicians.

Acute aortic dissections, rupturing aneurysms, rupturing pseudoaneurysms, and the variants of intramural hematomas and penetrating ulcers of the aortic wall are all acute aortic syndromes. There is some potential overlap among them—an intramural hematoma may evolve into an acute aortic dissection, an aneurysm may dissect, a penetrating ulcer may lead to an intramural hematoma or to rupture.

ETIOLOGY AND INCIDENCE

Acute aortic dissection (AAD) is the most common catastrophic aortic disease. The estimated prevalence is 10 to 30 per million per year, greater than for any other catastrophic form of disease of the aorta and twice that of abdominal aortic aneurysm rupture. Most cases involve persons older than 40 years, typically with a background of hypertension. There is a strong male predominance (twofold to threefold), although AAD in women has a higher mortality rate, operated on or unoperated on.[2] Signs of rupture, such as periaortic hematoma and pleural and pericardial effusions, are seen more frequently in women.[2]

Seven percent of AAD cases occur in persons younger than 40 years without gender predominance and are typically related to hereditary conditions (e.g., Marfan syndrome), congenital causes (e.g., bicuspid aortic valve), prior cardiac or aortic surgery, enlarged aorta,[3] or pregnancy. Mortality among AAD patients younger than 40 years is comparable to that among patients older than 40 years.[3] Crack cocaine abuse is more common as a cause of AAD in younger patients[4] and appears more likely to be associated with dissection of the distal aorta.[5] Fortunately, few cases (0.2%) of AAD occur in pregnancy; but within the small subset of AAD occurrences in female patients younger than 40 years, 12% are associated with pregnancy.

Patients with type A AAD with prior cardiac surgery are less likely to have presenting chest pain, to have tamponade on presentation, or to undergo surgical repair. Predictors of death include age older than 70 years, prior aortic valve replacement, hypotension and shock, and renal failure.[6]

Encouragingly, the mortality from AAD has fallen by half during the last 20 years.

NATURAL HISTORY

As with other cardiovascular disorders, there is a striking circadian and seasonal variation to the incidence of AAD, with higher incidence between 6 AM and noon, a peak at 8 to 9 AM, and greater incidence in winter months.[7] The winter peak of AAD occurrence is independent of climate.[8] The mortality of untreated AAD depends on (1) the time since onset; (2) site of involvement of the aorta (proximal versus distal), which is the principal risk determinant, as ascending involvement carries much greater risk than involvement of the descending aorta; (3) development of complications, such as rupture (intrapericardial or elsewhere), aortic valve incompetence, branch vessel or organ compromise, hypotension, and shock; (4) age; and (5) comorbidities.

Unrepaired type A AAD has a mortality of 20% at 24 hours, 30% by 48 hours, 40% by 1 week, and 50% by 1 month,[1] rendering type A AAD a surgical emergency. International Registry of Aortic Dissection data demonstrate that in the current era, unrepaired proximal (type A) AAD still has far greater mortality than unrepaired distal (type B) AAD (58% versus 11%).[9,10]

The in-hospital mortality for type A AAD is 32.5%. For type A AAD, predictors of in-hospital mortality are age older than 70 years, abrupt onset of pain, hypotension-shock-tamponade, pulse deficit, and abnormal electrocardiogram.[10] Elderly patients with type A AAD are subject to less typical chest pain and fewer signs and an increased incidence of hypotension, stroke, and mortality.[11]

COMPLICATIONS

The mortality of AAD is a consequence of complications of AAD (Table 4-1). Complications such as rupture, tamponade, acute aortic insufficiency (AI), and myocardial ischemia confer hemodynamic instability, which remains the dominant predictor of

Table 4-1. Complications of Acute Aortic Dissection and Causes of Mortality

Complications at Presentation	Causes of Death
Tamponade (12%)	Rupture into the pericardial space (fulminant tamponade)
Limb ischemia (8%)	Torrential aortic insufficiency
Mesenteric ischemia (8%)	Myocardial infarction
Myocardial ischemia (8%)	Rupture into the left pleural space (exsanguination)
Acute pulmonary edema (6%)	Rupture into the retroperitoneum or mediastinum
Stroke (2%)	Stroke
	Organ failure
	Multiple concurrent complications

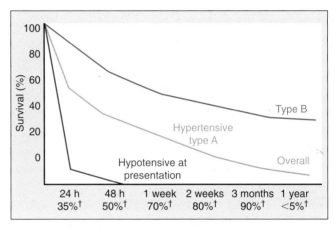

Figure 4-1. Natural history of untreated AAD. AAD patients hypotensive at presentation have already developed major complications and are at extremely high risk. One quarter of patients fall into this group. Most are type A AAD with tamponade, AI, or coronary occlusion. †Death.

untreated and surgical mortality (Fig. 4-1).[12] Early diagnosis of and surgery for type A AAD is critical to avoid hemodynamic instability. Complications confer high risk and must be identified to manage cases appropriately: proximal AAD with complications must be considered for a hastened surgical repair; distal AAD cases with complications should be considered for prompt surgical (and potentially endovascular) repair, rather than ongoing medical management. Rupture is a dreaded occurrence with any form of aortic dissection. As both proximal and distal dissection is likely to extend distally to the aortoiliac bifurcation, the incidence of renal and mesenteric complications is approximately equal between type A and type B AAD. Type A (proximal) AAD is more likely to become complicated and exposes the heart to the development of life-threatening complications.

PATHOGENESIS

The initiating event of AAD is held to be a tear through the intima into the mid or deep media, setting the stage for propagation of

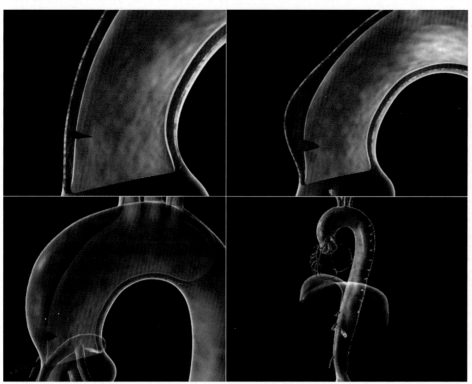

Figure 4-2. Type A AAD pathogenesis. The most common form of AAD originates in the aortic root; typically, a tear develops 2 cm above the right cusp of the aortic valve on the outside curvature of the aorta and allows entry of luminal blood into the wall, with formation and propagation of a false lumen that cleaves between concentric layers of elastin sheets, distally down to the aortic bifurcation, usually into the common iliac artery. The intimal flap is typically very mobile.

the dissection along intramedia planes (Figs. 4-2 to 4-4). An intimal tear may occur spontaneously or with manipulation of the aorta (as with percutaneous coronary intervention, diagnostic catheterization, intra-aortic balloon counterpulsation, aortocoronary bypass, valve surgery, aortic surgery, or coarctation or other peripheral arterial stenting). The underlying causes of mural weakness and susceptibility to dissection are not well understood at present. More than one form of susceptibility (repeated hemodynamic stress from hypertension; intrinsic connective tissue deficiency, such as biglycan deficiency in mice[13]; damage from inflammatory aortitis; trauma) is likely.

The initiating and principally responsible tear is referred to as the primary or the entry (of blood) tear (Fig. 4-5). Pressurized blood in the media dissects the media longitudinally between concentric layers of elastin sheets, forming the false lumen. For poorly understood reasons, the dissection of the aortic wall propagates more anterogradely than retrogradely. Cleavage of the media between concentric sheets of elastin occurs usually one half to two thirds of the way around the circumference of the wall of the aorta. Most commonly, the dissection extends distally to or beyond the iliac bifurcation into the left iliac artery. The false lumen typically runs along the greater curvature of the aorta; hence, in the descending aorta, the false lumen is usually lateral to the true lumen, but it may spiral in a "barber pole" fashion.

For type A AAD, approximately 70% of tears are in the ascending aorta. Most (>80%) are usually within the first 4 cm above the right coronary cusp along the outside curvature of the aorta (the site of the greatest hydrodynamic and torsional forces of the aorta); almost all of the remainder occur within the next 4 cm. Approximately 20% of tears are located in the proximal distal aorta (just distal to the junction of left subclavian artery to descending aorta at ligamentum arteriosum insertion—the typical

tear of a type B dissection) and represent retrograde extension (Fig. 4-6). Similarly, 10% of tears originate at the arch level and with retrograde dissection of the false lumen generate type A AAD. Thus, for type A AAD, surgical intervention on the ascending aorta is likely to eliminate the entry tear in most cases, although the operation may have to be extended into the arch to remedy a primary tear in that location. Tears may also occur in the arch or in the abdominal aorta, and extend variably anteriorly or posteriorly, or occur in branch vessels, and extend retrograde back into the aorta.

Small aortic branch vessels, such as intercostal and spinal arteries, are commonly torn off the intimal flap, leading to smaller secondary (entry) tears that may allow entry or exit flow and often contribute to the persistence of a false lumen.

The false lumen may reconnect distally through a re-entry tear back into the lumen. This will partially depressurize the false lumen (it is therefore less likely to balloon and to occlude branch vessels), will increase flow through it (lessening the chance of thrombosis of the false lumen), and may decrease the pulsatility of the false lumen.

If the false lumen is more pressurized than the true lumen, branch vessels may be occluded, leading to malperfusion syndromes of any arterial bed (coronary, cerebral, renal, mesenteric). Occlusion of limb vessels may be evident by the presence of a pulse deficit, although migratory pulse deficits are more specific for AAD.

Most primary tears are 1 cm or more (several centimeters) in length (Fig. 4-7). This is the size of tear most likely to be responsible for dissection rather than generated by the dissection as a secondary lesion. Identification of the responsible intimal tear is required to ensure that the surgery or intervention successfully eliminates it and flow into and pressurization of the false lumen.

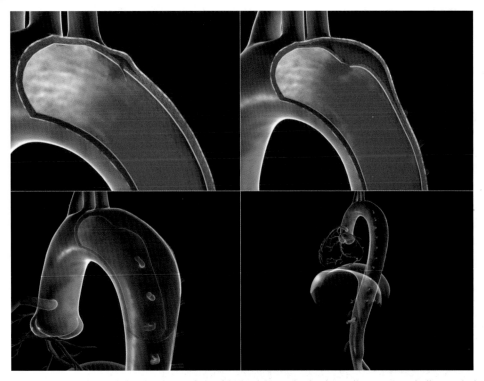

Figure 4-3. Type B AAD pathogenesis. The second most common form of AAD originates in the descending aorta; typically, a tear develops a few centimeters distal to the left subclavian artery origin and allows entry of luminal blood into the wall, with formation and propagation of a false lumen, usually down to the aortic bifurcation. The false lumen typically extends retrograde only a few centimeters to the left subclavian artery ostium. The intimal flap is typically very mobile.

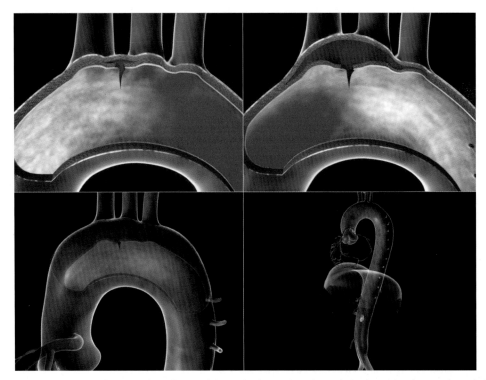

Figure 4-4. Arch AAD pathogenesis. An important variant of AAD originates in the aortic arch. An intimal tear develops at the arch level, forming a false lumen that extends both proximally and distally, resulting in a long false lumen channel that appears similar to that of most "type A" dissections. Importantly, though, at surgery, the repair of the root portion will not address the entry tear unless the repair is extended into the arch—a longer and riskier operation.

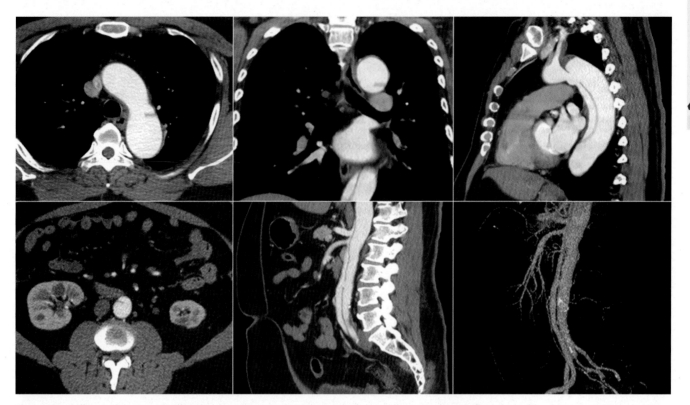

Figure 4-5. Different CT images revealing the primary entry tear in the proximal descending aorta (type B dissection) with a large re-entry tear in the mid abdominal aorta. There was always continuous flow through the false lumen in this case and stability of the false lumen.

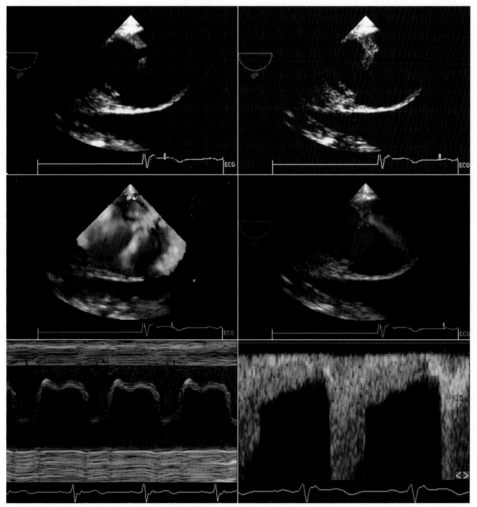

Figure 4-6. TEE short-axis view of the proximal descending aorta (type B AAD). UPPER IMAGES, Two-dimensional view in systole (LEFT) and diastole (RIGHT). The intimal tear, the intimal flaps, and the true and false lumens can be seen. The intimal tear distends in systole as the pressure in the true lumen rises. MIDDLE IMAGES, Color Doppler flow mapping of blood flow through the intimal tear. Flow can be seen streaming across the tear from the true lumen into the false lumen in systole (LEFT) and in diastole (RIGHT). The flow accentuates in systole, with the pressure rise in the true lumen. LEFT LOWER IMAGE, Color M-mode study through a dissected aorta. There is systolic bulging of the intimal flap as the true lumen receives more blood flow and pressure (note more color Doppler signal) in systole, and therefore it rapidly expands, displacing the intimal flap. In systole, the false lumen receives less flow (note less color Doppler signal). At the end of systole, the true lumen decompresses, allowing the flap returns to be displaced more centrally. The mobility of the flap is a prominent feature of dissection pathology. The spectral Doppler mapping of flow at the site of the tear (RIGHT LOWER IMAGE) shows the continuous flow through the tear, accentuated in systole. This patient had a large re-entry tear distally, allowing continuous flow. The false lumen never thrombosed.

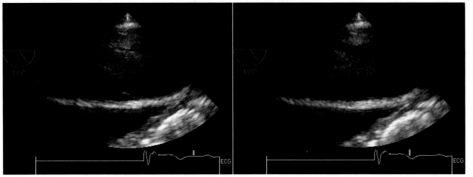

Figure 4-7. Intimal tear motion. In this TEE vertical view of the proximal descending aorta, aligned tangentially through the intimal flap and tear, the intimal tear is seen closed in diastole (LEFT) and open in systole (RIGHT). The intimal tear is 3 cm long.

RISK FACTORS

One of the most important risk factors is a bicuspid aortic valve (Table 4-2). The risk of dissection is increased 9-fold (range, 7- to 10-fold) in the presence of a bicuspid aortic valve. More dissections occur in the setting of bicuspid aortic valves (12%) than in the setting of Marfan syndrome (8%). The likelihood of dilation of the root and ascending aorta is also increased in the presence of a bicuspid valve.

Pathologic studies debate whether there is a predictable substrate that permits dissection. No pathologic evidence has emerged that helps understand the cause of the intimal tear. The concept of a weakened media resulting from congenital, inheritable, or acquired diseases is appealing, but identification of the substrate of the weakening has proved elusive. The term *cystic medial necrosis,* an antiquated light microscopic term describing fragmentation of elastic fibers, loss of vascular smooth muscle nuclei, increased collagen, and infiltration of basophilic ground substance, originally arose in the context of Marfan syndrome. Similar changes are seen, though, with aging (albeit generally less), and such changes may be scant in patients with Marfan syndrome. Furthermore, there is actually neither necrosis nor cysts. The term and concept were most in vogue as an explanation (a substrate) of weakened media that would permit dissection but have not proved synonymous with dissection, which clearly can happen in normal aortas that are manipulated.

Table 4-2. Risk Factors for Acute Aortic Dissection

Congenital	Bicuspid aortic valve (12% of cases)
	Coarctation of the aorta
Hereditary	Marfan syndrome (8% of type A cases)
	Ehlers-Danlos syndrome type IV
	Turner syndrome
	Polycystic kidney disease
	Osteogenesis imperfecta
Acquired	Hypertension (>75% of cases)
	Aneurysms (15% of cases)
	Atherosclerosis
	Inflammatory diseases (giant cell aortitis, Takayasu's aortitis, arthropathies, systemic lupus erythematosus, rheumatoid arthritis)
	Pregnancy
	Crack cocaine abuse (<1% of cases)[5]
Iatrogenic[14]	Cardiac surgery caused (69% of all iatrogenic and 10% of all AAD cases)
	Catheter caused (27%)
	Other (4%)

AAD, acute aortic dissection.

CLASSIFICATION

There are several classifications of AAD based on site of involvement. None is perfect, and all engender some confusion and apply poorly in some cases. The Stanford classification emphasizes whether or not there is involvement by the flap of the ascending aorta. The logic of the classification is its simplicity and the ability of diagnostic testing to identify the presence or absence of a flap in the ascending aorta (which has the highest risk and is surgically treated). The intimal flap is the easiest component of an AAD to image, much easier than the intimal tear (Fig. 4-8). The Stanford classification uses the location of the flap, which can be imaged by all imaging modalities, rather than the tear, which is less successfully imaged. Therefore, the Stanford classification's popularity and success are based on simple and generally quite reliable issues, as flaps are easily imaged, and flaps in the ascending aorta are surgically managed when they are located in the distal aorta.

Stanford type A includes all dissections involving the ascending aorta (Fig. 4-9), regardless of site of origin or the location of the intimal tear. *Stanford type B* includes all dissections not involving the ascending aorta (Fig. 4-10).

Confusion begins to arise with arch dissections because they fall into an unclaimed middle ground. Surgery for ascending dissection is usually successful in achieving resection of the entry tear, as the tear, being just above the sinotubular junction in most cases, is excised with the root excision. Therefore, the anastomosis to the upper ascending aorta excludes the true and false lumens, and the false lumen is likely, without flow, to thrombose, and being excluded from pulsatile flow, it is unlikely to progressively dilate into a false aneurysm. However, if the flap in the ascending aorta represents a retrograde extension from an intimal tear in the aortic arch or descending aorta, surgery to protect the aortic valve and coronary arteries with a tube graft replacement in the ascending aorta position will not exclude the false aneurysm from flow and pressure. Such retrograde dissection cases compose up

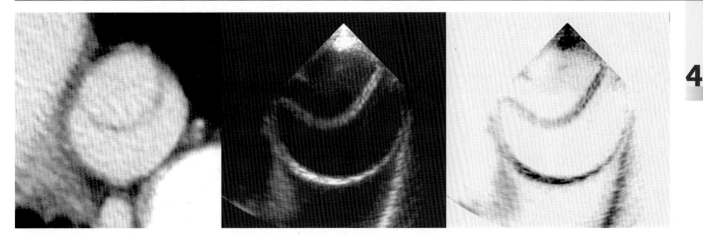

Figure 4-8. The intimal flap: CT and TEE images of the intimal flap, true and false lumens. LEFT IMAGE, Contrast-enhanced CT image. MIDDLE IMAGE, TEE two-dimensional image. RIGHT IMAGE, TEE (color inverted). The flap has a similar appearance by all techniques with good resolution and is the most obvious feature of AAD.

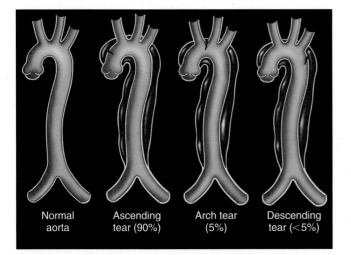

Figure 4-9. Type A dissections with different locations of inciting intimal tears. LEFT IMAGE, Normal aorta. SECOND IMAGE, Usual type A dissection with the flap in the ascending aorta and the responsible tear also in the ascending aorta (90%). THIRD IMAGE, Less common type A dissection with the flap extended retrograde to the ascending aorta from a tear in the arch (5%). Root replacement will exclude the false lumen only if it is extended to include the arch, often requiring circulatory arrest. FOURTH IMAGE, Less common type A dissection with the flap extended all the way retrograde to the ascending aorta from a tear in the proximal descending aorta (<5%). Root replacement will not fully exclude the false lumen in this case.

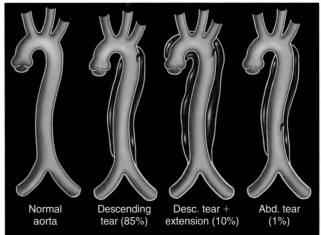

Figure 4-10. LEFT IMAGE, Normal aorta. SECOND IMAGE, Usual type B dissection with the flap in the descending aorta and the responsible tear in the descending aorta (85%). Usually, there is slight retrograde extension of the flap to the left subclavian artery ostium. THIRD IMAGE, Uncommon but important complication of distal dissection—the flap has extended far proximally into the ascending aorta from a tear in the descending aorta (10% of cases with a distal tear); this would be classified a type A dissection. FOURTH IMAGE, Less common type B dissection with the flap extended retrograde to the descending thoracic aorta from a tear in the abdominal aorta (1%).

to 25% of type A AAD cases and may have a better prognosis (in-hospital mortality, 15% versus 38%). The different apparent natural histories and surgical, medical, and interventional factors encourage development of a classification of dissection that describes the proximal extent of the flap and the location of the tear.

The dichotomization of type A and type B cases, in addition to describing untreated risk and usual surgical indication, is revealing of different associations and different patient profiles. Type A patients are more likely to be younger than type B patients (average age, 60 years versus 70 years) and have a predisposing congenital (bicuspid aortic valve), hereditary (Marfan syndrome), or inflammatory (giant cell aortitis or Takayasu's aortitis) condi-tion. Type A patients are less likely to have a history of hyperten-sion than are type B patients (30% versus 71%).[11]

VARIANTS AND DIAGNOSTIC CHALLENGE

Although TEE, CT, and MRI are robust techniques to identify the presence of dissection, and all have been reported to have 100% sensitivity, many series have exhibited intrinsic limitation because they were restricted to classic dissection pathology,

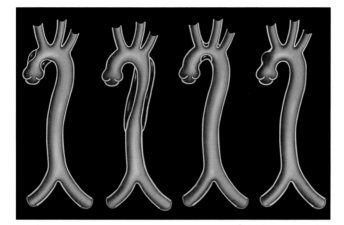

Figure 4-11. Variant lesions of AAD. The three images on the left are depictions of intramural hematoma—hemorrhage into the wall without an intimal tear and without the extensive mobility of the intimal flap. The lesion on the right is an ulcer-like projection or ulcer without hematoma.

single-center experience, or small size. Furthermore, most seminal AAD imaging studies are more than a decade old and are not representative of contemporary advances in CT and MRI technology.

There are significant variant lesions to AAD that have imaging features different from those of AAD (Fig. 4-11). The concern of ruling out AAD fails to address and potentially to identify AAD variant lesions, such as intramural hematoma. Variant dissection lesions without full-fledged findings are more likely to occur in Marfan syndrome and in aortitis.[15]

Variant lesions of dissection are multiple and do include subtle but clinically important pathologic changes, such as the following:

- Intramural hematoma: hematoma without intimal tear
  - 5% to 10% of AAD-like pathologic processes
  - Mural, not luminal, components
- Intimal tear without hematoma, ulcer-like projection
  - 5% to 10% of AAD-like pathologic processes responsible for ascending or arch replacement
  - An intimal tear without hematoma is an acute lesion with risk of mortality but without prominent findings as are sought in pursuing the diagnosis of dissection.
  - Because the findings are far less obvious than the intimal flap of dissection, they are readily missed preoperatively, especially by TEE and MRI, and particularly if the tear site is occluded by clot and the wall is minimally thickened.
  - Aortography with multiple views appears to be the most sensitive means to identify small intimal tears or bulges typical of such lesions that are without prominent flaps, undermined flaps, or intramural hematoma.
  - CT aortography may be able to offer what standard aortography can, if the diagnosis is pursued and multiplanar reconstruction formatting is used.
  - The term *ulcer-like projection* is increasingly used to describe small, generally smooth-walled luminal extensions, without intimal overhangings, believed to represent intimal disruption (intimal tear without hematoma).
- Penetrating ulcers
- Traumatic disruption

Table 4-3. Clinical Presentation of Acute Aortic Dissection

Presenting Symptoms	Description and Cause
Pain	Chest, back, abdominal, flank
	Intense, abrupt onset
Pulmonary edema	Acute aortic insufficiency
	Coronary artery compromise
Cardiogenic shock	Tamponade
	Acute massive aortic insufficiency
	Coronary artery occlusion
Hypovolemic shock	Rupture
Hypertensive crisis	Renal artery occlusion or renal ischemia
	Hyperadrenergic response to pain
Neurologic	Syncope (often due to tamponade)
	Stroke
	Coma
	Paraplegia
	Horner syndrome
Branch occlusion	Left leg pulse deficit (most common)

CLINICAL PRESENTATION

Although most AAD presents with clinically impressive chest pain, it is critical to recall that there are many other presentations that may be distracting from the underlying diagnosis of AAD (Table 4-3). Presentations of aortic dissection may be as subtle as fever of unknown origin[16] or as calamitous as sudden death. Importantly, *not all AAD patients experience pain.*

The pain of AAD is characteristically sudden in onset and severe and maximal at onset (Table 4-4). The relation of pain location to dissection anatomic location is only fair. Although it is said that the location of AAD pain correlates with its location (ascending AAD is associated with pain in the anterior chest, arch AAD is associated with pain in the neck, distal AAD is associated with back pain), there are many exceptions. As dissection of the entire aorta is the most common form, widely extensive pains are common. Flank extension of the pain suggests renal artery involvement. AAD presenting with abdominal pain has higher mortality (28% versus 10%) because of delay in correct diagnosis.[17]

Perturbing, some AADs are painless. Painless AAD is seen more commonly in older patients and in patients with neurologic presentations (syncope, stroke). The prognosis is worse, as would be expected, because the diagnosis is made later.

PHYSICAL EXAMINATION FINDINGS

Hypertension is usual (80%) and reflects the background of hypertension in most, exacerbated by pain (Table 4-5). Renal ischemia may result from renal artery occlusion from the dissec-

Table 4-4. Presenting Symptoms of Acute Aortic Dissection

	All (%)	Type A (%)	Type B (%)	P Value Type A vs. B
Any pain reported	95.5	93.8	98.3	.02
Abrupt onset	84.8	85.4	83.8	.65
Chest pain	72.2	78.9	62.9	<.001
Anterior chest pain	60.9	71.0	44.1	<.001
Posterior chest pain	35.9	32.8	41	.09
Back pain	53.2	46.6	63.8	<.001
Abdominal pain	29.6	21.6	42.7	<.001
Severity of pain: severe or worst ever	90.6	90.1	90	NA
Quality of pain: sharp	64.4	62	68.3	NA
Quality of pain: tearing or ripping	50.6	49.4	52.3	NA
Radiating	28.3	27.2	30.1	.51
Migrating	16.6	14.9	19.3	.22
Syncope	9.4	12.7	4.1	.002

Table 4-5. Physical Examination Findings in Acute Aortic Dissection

	All (%)	Type A (%)	Type B (%)	P Value Type A vs. B
Hemodynamics (n = 451)				
Hypertensive (SBP ≥ 150 mm Hg)	49	35.7	70.1	<.001
Normotensive (SBP 100-149 mm Hg)	156	39.7	26.4	<.001
Hypotensive (SBP < 100 mm Hg)	36	11.6	2.3	<.001
Shock or tamponade (SBP ≤ 80 mm Hg)	38	13	1.5	<.001
Auscultated murmur of aortic insufficiency	31.6	44	12	<.001
Pulse deficit	15.1	18.7	9.2	.006
Cerebrovascular accident	4.7	6.1	2.3	.07
Congestive heart failure	6.6	8.8	3.0	.02

SBP, systolic blood pressure.
From Hagan PG, Nienaber CA, Isselbacher EM, et al: The International Registry of Acute Aortic Dissection (IRAD): new insights into an old disease. JAMA 2000;283:897-903.

tion, producing a hypertensive crisis. Hypertension propagates dissection and increases the risk of rupture. Normal blood pressure at the time of presentation is abnormal for most AAD patients (given their history of hypertension and the context of pain) and is suggestive of the occurrence of complications. Low blood pressure almost inevitably establishes the presence of severe complications and establishes the highest immediate risk. Other physical findings that are significant in AAD patients include the following:

- Jugular venous distention: strongly suggests intrapericardial rupture.
- Pulsus paradoxus: strongly suggests intrapericardial rupture.
- AI murmur, heard in 50% of type A cases: strongly suggests extension into the root, but prior hypertension may independently have resulted in AI.
- Pericardial friction rub: suggests intrapericardial rupture.

- Left pleural effusion may be a sign of rupture but may also be reactive to aortic hematomas.
- Pulse deficit: suggests branch loss. Loss of perfusion to the left leg is the most common deficit. Pulse deficits are associated with significantly higher in-hospital morbidity (renal failure, limb ischemia, coma, and hypotension) and mortality (41% versus 25%).[18] Branch vessel complications are increased in patients with renal insufficiency.[19] In the presence of any findings that suggest the dissection has produced complications, the survival is directly threatened and the access to surgery must be direct.

About one quarter of AAD cases present hypotensive (12% have blood pressure of 80 to 99 mm Hg) or in shock (13% have blood pressure of less than 80 mm Hg), with hugely increased mortality. The presence of pseudohypotension (a result of pulse deficits) must be considered and an effort made to evaluate all limbs and sites of peripheral pulses.

DIAGNOSTIC TESTING

The goal of diagnostic imaging in suspected AAD is to establish or to exclude the diagnosis of AAD and other acute aortic syndromes, to classify the AAD, and to identify or to exclude complications. To ensure confident diagnosis and identification of all of its complications, the average number of tests used in AAD assessment is two (CT and echocardiography are the two most commonly used tests).

Diagnostic testing has evolved enormously during the last decade, and the current utility may not be expressed by the literature. Studies from more than a decade ago reflect the infancy of TEE equipment and performance and a primitive era of CT using a paucity of detectors poorly suited for delineation of cardiovascular disease. There are no contemporary comparative studies of diagnostic testing for AAD, and existing published studies are dated. TEE use is greater in North America than in Europe. CT scanning is the predominant test at community hospitals. The International Registry of Acute Aortic Dissection reports that CT scanning is the most common initial diagnostic test for AAD (61%), followed by echocardiography (33%), aortography (4%), and MRA (2%) (Fig. 4-12).[9,20]

A reasonable strategy is to ensure verification of AAD diagnosis and to ensure verification of the status of the heart. Thus,

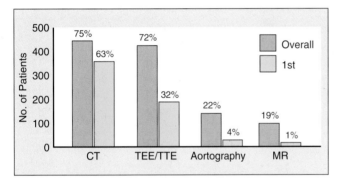

Figure 4-12. Computed tomography (CT) is the most common initial diagnostic test for AAD, followed by echocardiography (TEE, transesophageal echocardiography; TTE, transthoracic echocardiography), aortography, and magnetic resonance (MR). (From Moore AG, Eagle KA, Bruckman D, et al: Choice of computed tomography, transesophageal echocardiography, magnetic resonance imaging, and aortography in acute aortic dissection: International Registry of Acute Aortic Dissection [IRAD]. Am J Cardiol 2002;89:1235-1238, with permission from Elsevier.)

echocardiography is commonly used to supplement the findings of a CT scan performed as the initial diagnostic test. AAD diagnostic strategies should use available tests for their best application, that is, CT for aortic anatomic findings of AAD, signs of aortic hematoma and rupture, and branch vessel involvement. CT is not a suitable test to exclude AI or to establish its relation to an AAD. Conversely, echocardiography, which is excellent to image the heart and potential cardiac complications of AAD, is not a suitable test to delineate branch vessel involvement or distal complications of AAD.

Electrocardiography

Electrocardiography (ECG) has no ability to diagnose AAD, but it may detect ischemic changes suggesting coronary involvement (Table 4-6). Because the ostium of the right coronary artery is involved approximately twice as often as the ostium of the left coronary artery, inferior myocardial ischemic changes are the most common. Unfortunately, the background of hypertension often confers left ventricular hypertrophy (LVH) and renders the baseline ECG recording abnormal, reducing its sensitivity to detection of ischemia and in some cases confusingly associating chest pain with ECG abnormalities and engendering the misdiagnosis of an acute coronary syndrome, which if followed by mistreatment with antiplatelet and anticoagulant medications increases clinical risk for reasons of bleeding and increased time until diagnosis of AAD.[21]

Chest Radiography

The chest radiograph is limited for the diagnosis of AAD and is not an adequate diagnostic test to establish or to refute the diagnosis of AAD. The chest radiograph is usually abnormal in AAD (Table 4-7), but with little likelihood of establishing the specific diagnosis of AAD (Figs. 4-13 and 4-14). There is a disconcerting false-negative rate of the chest radiograph, at least 20% (10% to 35%). A widened superior mediastinum may be due to a dilated aorta, a large false lumen, blood from a ruptured aorta, excess fat, the thymus, or other causes. An enlarged aorta in the clinical context of chest pain should lead to consideration of AAD, intramural hematoma, penetrating ulcer, or ruptured aneurysm and further evaluation with CT, echocardiography, or MRI. The chest radiograph is less sensitive for pathologic

Table 4-6. Electrocardiographic Findings in Acute Aortic Dissection

	All (%)	Type A (%)	Type B (%)	P Value Type A vs. B
Electrocardiographic findings (n = 444)				
No abnormalities noted	31.3	30.8	32.1	.76
Nonspecific ST-segment or T-wave changes	41.1	42.6	42.8	.98
Left ventricular hypertrophy	26.1	25	32.2	.11
Ischemia	15.1	17.3	13.2	.27
Myocardial infarction, old Q waves	7.7	7.1	9.9	.30
Myocardial infarction, new Q waves	3.2	4.8	0.7	.02

From Hagan PG, Nienaber CA, Isselbacher EM, et al: The International Registry of Acute Aortic Dissection (IRAD): new insights into an old disease. JAMA 2000;283:897-903.

Table 4-7. Chest Radiography Findings in Acute Aortic Dissection

	All (%)	Type A (%)	Type B (%)	P Value Type A vs. B
Radiography findings (n = 427)	100	88.6	97.7	
No abnormalities noted	12.4	11.3	15.8	.08
Absence of widened mediastinum or abnormal aortic contour	21.3	17.2	27.5	.01
Widened mediastinum	61.6	62.6	56	.17
Abnormal aortic contour	49.6	46.6	53	.20
Abnormal cardiac contour	25.8	26.9	24.0	.49
Displacement, calcification of aorta	14.1	11.3	18.7	.05
Pleural effusion	19.2	17.3	21.8	.24

From Hagan PG, Nienaber CA, Isselbacher EM, et al: The International Registry of Acute Aortic Dissection (IRAD): new insights into an old disease. JAMA 2000;283:897-903.

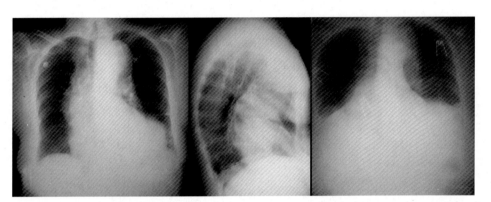

Figure 4-13. A 60-year-old woman presenting to a community hospital with severe chest pain and dyspnea. Pulmonary embolism was considered (no risk factors were present). The V/Q scan was reported as "probable." LEFT AND MIDDLE, At presentation. The lung fields are clear, and there are no pleural effusions. There is remarkable dilation of the ascending aorta and aortic arch, which was not noted initially. Intravenous administration of heparin was started. RIGHT, Same patient on the next day. There has been development of bilateral pleural effusions. Pulmonary infarction was initially considered to be the cause. Eventually, a CT scan was performed; type A AAD was evident. The patient underwent successful surgical repair, albeit with considerable bleeding. The pleural effusions were bloody, bilaterally.

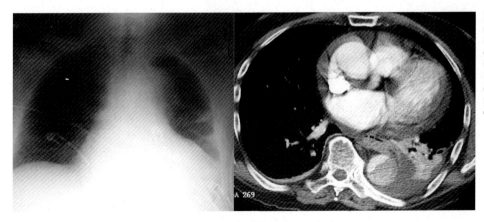

Figure 4-14. LEFT IMAGE, Anteroposterior chest radiograph: widened superior mediastinum, hazy enlarged aortic contour, enlarged cardiopericardial silhouette, and left pleural effusion. RIGHT IMAGE, Differential flow in the descending aorta consistent with true and false lumens, pericardial effusion, and left pleural effusion.

changes in the ascending aorta (47%) versus the descending aorta (77%).[9,22]

Chest radiography findings in AAD include aortic findings (widened superior mediastinum, calcium intimal displacement sign in the arch >1 cm), vascular findings (pulmonary venous congestion suggestive of AI, tamponade, or myocardial infarction), and pleural findings (left effusion bespeaks rupture but is not specific). Cardiac findings are usually normal.

Computed Tomography

Computed tomography (CT) scanning is an excellent test to diagnose AAD and many of its complications (Figs. 4-15 and 4-16). CT has become the de facto first diagnostic test for AAD at most centers because of its availability, its accuracy, its ability to depict rupture, and its ability to identify differential diagnostic concerns (penetrating atherosclerotic ulcer, intramural hematoma, pulmo-

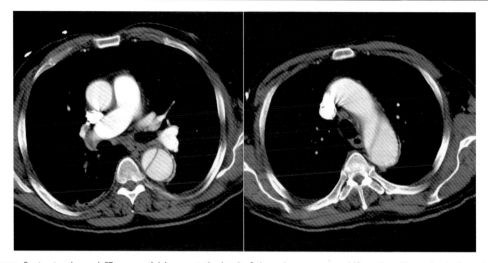

Figure 4-15. LEFT IMAGE, Contrast-enhanced CT scan, axial image at the level of the pulmonary artery bifurcation. There clearly is an intimal flap within the descending aorta but not within the ascending aorta (type B dissection). RIGHT IMAGE, Contrast-enhanced CT scan, axial image at the level of the aortic arch. There is an intimal flap in the mid arch–descending aorta. As well, there are radial streak artifacts arising from the superior vena cava (SVC) because of excess concentration of contrast material in the SVC from upper extremity dye injection. The multiple linear shadows across the ascending aorta are all artifacts, but the thick line in the descending aorta with a different orientation, and not originating from the SVC, is a true intimal flap.

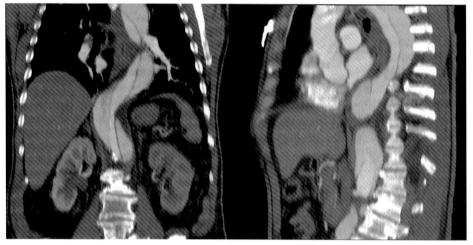

Figure 4-16. Contrast-enhanced CT scan. LEFT, Coronal view. RIGHT, Sagittal view. A dissection flap extends down a very tortuous descending aorta.

nary embolism). Multidetector and multislice CT has shortened scanning time and increased resolution compared with earlier CT technologies.

CT is not well suited for the identification of cardiac complications of AAD. Therefore, commonly, CT as the first test is followed by echocardiography to evaluate the heart better (TTE for evaluation of cardiac complications—AI, tamponade, ischemia; or TEE—AI, tamponade, ischemia, and verification of the aortic findings).

CT dissection findings include intimal flap, intimal tear, false lumen, differential flow lumen : false lumen, pericardial fluid, pleural fluid, extravasated blood indicating rupture, and branch involvement. Intramural hematoma findings include crescentic or annular thickening of the wall of the aorta and higher density (60 to 70 Hounsfield units) on non–contrast-enhanced views.

Validation studies of CT scanning for the detection of AAD are more than 10 years old, with suggested sensitivity of 73% to 93% and specificity of 86% to 100%. Contemporary multidetector spiral CT technology surely increases the sensitivity and specificity, and ECG gating resolves motion artifacts within the aortic root.

Motion artifacts of the ascending aorta have tended to be a significant problem for CT scanning. Older scanners achieved lesser temporal resolution and were susceptible to considerable motion artifact, especially of the ascending aorta, which is subject to 1 cm of translation (as is the nearby pulmonary artery) and 5% pulsatility. Artifacts are seen in more than half of studies before 1999. The mean amplitude and extent of artifacts were both approximately 0.5 cm. The result often was superimposition of diastolic and systolic outlines of the aortic root, slightly askew, yielding a curved line that was plausibly an intimal flap and false lumen. Current 64-slice helical CT scanners are able to perform coronary angiography and hence, with ECG gating and sub-second temporal resolution, enable excellent aortography.

Linear artifacts—as may arise from improper timing of contrast injection–image acquisition, streak artifacts, high-contrast interfaces, and cardiac motion—that project across the aorta may simulate a flap.[23]

The aortic root, ascending aorta, and arch bear the largest burden of artifact. This is due to the motion of these segments of the aorta from cardiac motion and high-attenuation (streak) arti-

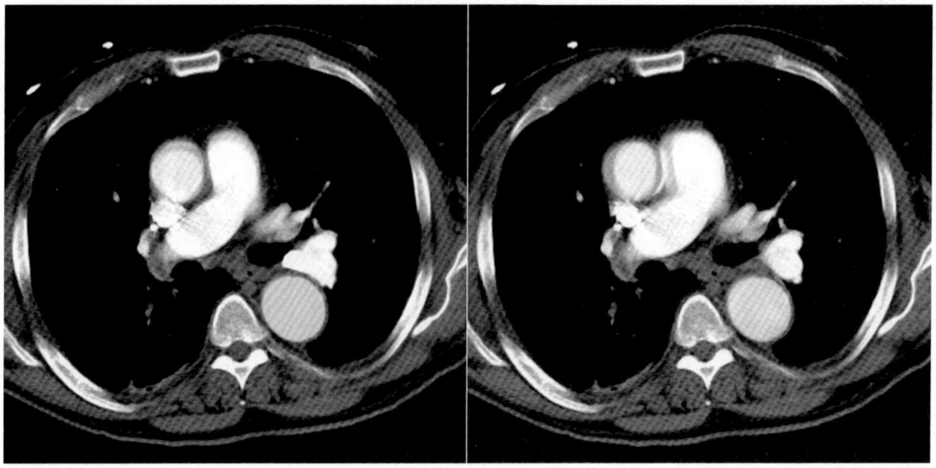

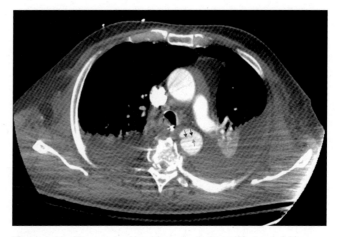

Figure 4-17. Motion artifacts of the ascending aorta and pulmonary artery mimicking intimal flaps. LEFT IMAGE, Anterior motion superimposition artifact simulating a crescentic anterior intimal flap. RIGHT IMAGE, Lateral motion superimposition artifact simulating a crescentic lateral intimal flap.

fact from nondiluted dye in the SVC (Figs. 4-17 to 4-20; Table 4-8).

Computed Tomographic Criteria of Dissection

Identification of a false lumen, to distinguish dissection from intramural hematoma and aneurysm with thrombus[24]:

- *Beak sign.* An acute angle, mimicking an avian beak, is present in the false lumen between its outside wall and the intimal flap. The sign is useful because it is seen in most cases and is reported to have ideal accuracy for the correct identification of a false lumen in both acute and chronic dissections, but it may be limited in the presence of highly mobile intimal flaps and near-circumferential flaps.
- *Cobwebs.* Thin filamentous stranding is seen in the false lumen, usually toward the angle of the outer wall and the intimal flap, in a minority of cases; when seen, it is a useful sign.[24]
- *Wrapping at the level of the aortic arch.* A lumen that wraps around the other is the false lumen; the central lumen, surrounded by the other, is the true lumen.
- *Lumen size.* The false lumen is generally the larger lumen, with the exception of the most proximal part of the dissection. Therefore, the relative size of the lumens is best assessed farther along the dissection: one-quarter along the dissection, 85% of larger lumens are false, whereas halfway along the dissection, that percentage increases to 95%.
- *Outer wall calcification* is a useful sign to identify the true lumen only in acute dissection, as the outer wall of the false lumen may calcify chronically.
- *Thrombosis* is typical of the false lumen in about half of cases, and more chronically. Thrombosis may be present within the true lumen in acute dissection, though, if the dissection arose in an aneurysm that contained mural thrombus.
- *Direction of the flap free edges.* The free edges of the intimal flap on the margins of the primary tear point into the false lumen, passively directed by flow entering the false lumen.

Calcium displacement is a sign of dissection or intramural hematoma, but not all calcium is intimal, and therefore calcium displacement is not invariably intimal displacement. Thrombi may calcify, and the outer wall of a false lumen may calcify in time (Figs. 4-21 and 4-22).

Figure 4-18. CT scan, streak and beam hardening artifacts mimicking intimal flaps. There are numerous linear high-attenuation streak artifacts radiating out of variable contrast regions of the SVC, crossing the ascending aorta. There are numerous linear dark beam hardening artifacts radiating off the spine through structures on both the right and left sides, including the descending aorta. Confusingly, there is an actual intimal disruption *(blue arrow)* contiguous with a beam hardening artifact *(red arrow)* and a nearby second beam hardening artifact *(yellow arrow)*.

Magnetic Resonance Imaging

Magnetic resonance imaging (MRI) and magnetic resonance angiography (MRA) have both been used to image AAD and, more often, chronic aortic dissection (Table 4-9). MRI comprises several different pulse sequences and techniques and has undergone substantial development during the last half-decade, which is not well represented (yet) in the medical literature. Spin echo techniques offer good anatomic detail, although with limited sampling. Steady-state free precession (SSFP) sequences can be cardiac gated. Gadolinium contrast angiography enables rapid acquisition of a large volume of data that can be extensively post-processed. MRA offers superb imaging of AAD and its complications.

Given the availability of other excellent imaging modalities for AAD, in particular of CT scanning, MRI is less commonly performed as a diagnostic test for AAD.

Table 4-8. Computed Tomography Aortic Imaging Artifacts

Artifacts that can produce pseudointimal flaps	Translation artifact, no gating, low temporal resolution
	Adjacent opacified vessel superimposed onto aorta or aorta superimposed onto adjacent opacified vessel. The net effect is that the low-attenuation boundary between the two appears to be an intimal flap.
	Pulmonary artery onto ascending aorta; ascending aorta onto the pulmonary artery
	Pseudoflap on left aspect of ascending aorta
	SVC onto ascending aorta; ascending aorta onto SVC
	Pseudoflap on left aspect of ascending aorta
Beam hardening artifact	Black streak from the spine across the descending aorta
	Black streak from a pacemaker wire in the SVC across the ascending aorta
	Black streak from high contrast in the pulmonary artery across the ascending aorta[23]
Dye streaming artifacts	Dye streaming artifacts in veins must be distinguished from arteries with true and false lumens.
Periaortic structures producing the appearance of an intimal flap or double lumen	Ascending aorta
	Aortic wall motion
	Normal aortic sinuses
	Aortic valve leaflets
	Residual thymus
	Right atrial appendage
	Superior pericardial recess
Arch	Aortic arch branch origins
	Left brachiocephalic vein with injection of contrast material in left arm
Descending aorta	Left superior intercostal vein
	Left inferior pulmonary vein
	Atelectasis
	Left pleural thickening or effusion[23]
Aortic anomalies and lesions that may be confused with dissection	Aortic variations Ductus diverticulum
Aortic lesions	Acquired aortic aneurysm with thrombus
	Penetrating aortic ulcer[23]
	Intramural hematoma

SVC, superior vena cava.

Table 4-9. Magnetic Resonance Imaging for Acute Aortic Dissection

Intimal flap	Sensitivity ~ 100%
	Specificity ~ 100%
Intimal tear	Sensitivity ~ 85%
	Specificity ~ 100%
Detection of aortic insufficiency	Sensitivity ~ 85%
	Specificity ~ 100%
Potential problems	Lack of availability
	Prolonged scanning times
	Difficulty in monitoring critically ill patients during scanning
	Implanted metallic devices are a contraindication
	Claustrophobia

Aortography

Aortography is no longer the key test for AAD, as CT and echocardiography are widely available and are usually the initial, and adequate, diagnostic tests. However, aortography is a useful test to assess for AAD, particularly in cases undergoing angiography or catheterization (Fig. 4-23). In a typical scenario, a case is presumed to be coronary in origin, but on exclusion of coronary artery disease, aortography is performed in the same procedure and identifies the flap and AAD. Another scenario in which aortography is useful is the situation of iatrogenic catheter-related AAD, when the flap can be imaged during the catheterization procedure that had initiated the AAD.

If the intimal flap is not tangential to imaging but is en face, it will likely not be seen, especially if there is equal opacification of the true and false lumens. For the average AAD case, the current diagnostic role of aortography is minimal because it is less sensitive than TEE, CT angiography, and MRI for the

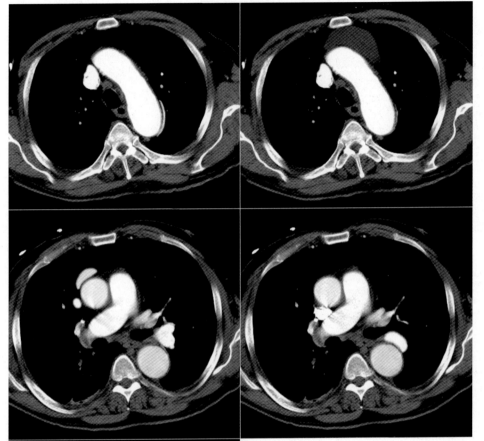

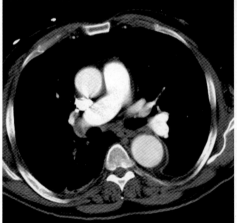

Figure 4-19. Contrast-enhanced CT scans. Periaortic structures producing the appearance of an intimal flap or double lumen. UPPER LEFT IMAGE, Left superior intercostal vein simulating double lumen and intimal flap. UPPER RIGHT IMAGE, Thymus simulating double lumen. MIDDLE LEFT IMAGE, Left brachiocephalic vein simulating double lumen (contrast dye injection of left arm). MIDDLE RIGHT IMAGE, Left inferior pulmonary vein simulating double lumen. LOWER IMAGE, Left pleural effusion and adjacent atelectasis simulating double lumen.

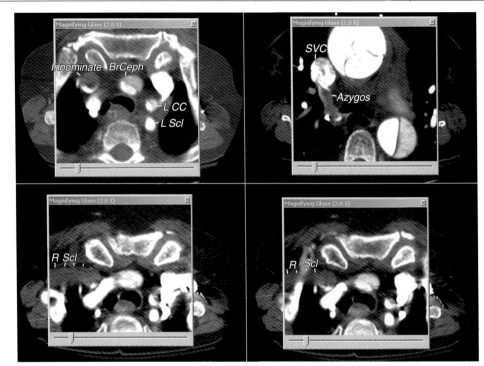

Figure 4-20. Dye streaming artifacts seen on contrast-enhanced CT scanning. This patient had a type A AAD. The left subclavian (L Scl) artery was not involved by the intimal flap, but the left common carotid (L CC) and brachiocephalic (BrCeph) arteries were. The appearance of the superior vena cava (SVC) is actually quite similar to that of the brachiocephalic artery, although it is not due to involvement by the AAD; rather, it is due to dye streaming of contrast material delivered by the innominate vein and of non–contrast-enhanced blood delivered by the right subclavian vein (and right internal jugular vein). RIGHT UPPER IMAGE, The azygos vein delivers non–contrast-enhanced blood that contributes to the complexity of dye streaming in the SVC. The lower images are axial views at slightly different levels that depict the course of the right subclavian artery as it passes under the clavicle and enters the innominate vein. The innominate vein and SVC were dilated and more prominent in this case because there was tamponade due to the AAD. Arch branch vessel variation and dye streaming artifacts require attention.

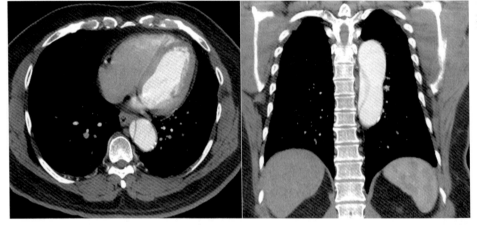

Figure 4-21. Chronic distal dissection (8 years old) with calcification of the outer wall of the false lumen.

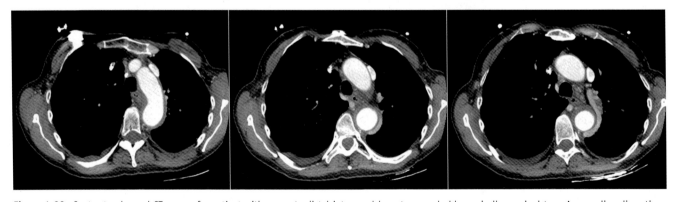

Figure 4-22. Contrast-enhanced CT scans of a patient with an acute distal intramural hematoma and old, surgically repaired type A ascending dissection. LEFT IMAGE, The line across the anterior arch is merely the takeoff of the brachiocephalic artery. There is a contrast-enhancing space anterior to the arch and extending partway to the mid arch (MIDDLE IMAGE), consistent with a chronic false lumen as a sequela of the former type A dissection and surgical repair. The right image reveals the typical crescentic thickening of the wall of the descending aorta due to the intramural hematoma. As well, on the lateral wall, there is a long tubular structure with less enhancement (not the same arterial phase as the aorta), which is actually an enlarged azygos vein due to prior surgery.

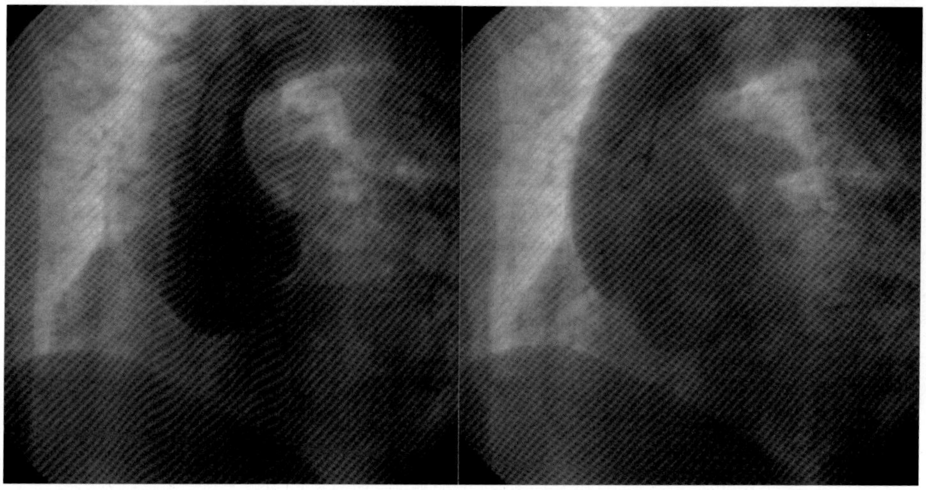

Figure 4-23. Aortography and AAD. Catheter in the aortic root. The intimal flap, which is seen edge-on, partitions the true and false lumens, which have differential contrast because of differential flow. There is AI.

Table 4-10. Aortography for Acute Aortic Dissection

Direct signs of AAD	Double channel, true and false lumens
	Intimal flap
	Entry into false lumen
	Re-entry into true lumen
Indirect signs of AAD	Narrowed true lumen
	Thickened wall (>5 mm)
	Catheter displacement
Other	Aortic insufficiency
	Branch artery involvement
Intramural hematoma signs	Wall thickening
	Indentation of the lumen (crescentic or annular)
20 to 40 mL of contrast material	
Sensitivity	False lumen: 80%-90%
	Intimal flap: 70%
	Intimal tear: 50%
	Overall: 80%-90%
Specificity	90%-100%
Positive predictive value	95%

AAD, acute aortic dissection.

diagnosis of AAD or recognition of the complications of AAD (Table 4-10). Other than branch vessel depiction, it offers nothing beyond TEE, CT angiography, or MRI while incurring time delays and dye risks. What aortography has lost as a diagnostic test for aortic diseases, it has gained as the central imaging modality to guide endovascular interventions for aortic diseases.

Echocardiography

Transthoracic echocardiography (TTE) is less suited for the diagnosis of AAD than it is for the evaluation of the cardiac complications of AAD. Hence, it is extremely well suited to complement CT scanning, which is superb for identification of AAD but less so for identification of the cardiac complications of AAD (pericardial effusion or tamponade, severity and mechanism of aortic valve insufficiency, and wall motion abnormalities indicative of coronary artery occlusion by the intimal flap).

TTE is usually able to depict intimal flaps in the aortic root, especially if the ascending aorta is enlarged (Figs. 4-24 and 4-25). The ascending aorta is usually imperfectly imaged by TTE. The arch and descending aorta may be adequately imaged to visualize intimal flaps, but certainly not in all patients. Artifacts are common from the suprasternal position. The abdominal aorta can often be imaged, revealing the distal extension of a type A or type B dissection.

AAD-like disorders, such as penetrating ulcers and intramural hematoma, are not at all well imaged by TTE.

Transesophageal echocardiography (TEE) is a robust test to identify AAD. Intimal flaps and their mobility can be seen better by TEE than by CT, MRA, or aortography; the intimal tear can be well seen in most type B AAD, but only in about half of type A by TEE (Figs. 4-26 to 4-28). Differential flow between the true and false lumens can be very well imaged by TEE (Fig. 4-29). TEE appears successful in distinguishing patency with flow, even low flow, from thrombosis of the false lumen. Rupture is not well seen by TEE. It is more convincingly seen by CT. TEE is a robust imaging test to identify the mechanism of AI in AAD and also coronary ostial involvement (of the left coronary more easily than the right coronary artery). Inevitably, some portions of the ascending aorta and of the arch are not well seen.

Intramural hematoma findings by TEE differ from those of AAD: regional thickening (>7 mm) in a circular or crescentic shape, with initially low signal (lucency) when the intramural hematoma is acute that resolves in thickness and in brightness during a week. Intramural hematoma that is the result of a penetrating ulcer in an atherosclerotic aorta can be difficult to image through calcified plaque.

The equipment of and experience with TEE have advanced considerably in the last 15 years; in particular, multi(omni)plane probes are standard. False-negative and false-positive results are becoming less common now as there is much greater familiarity with the procedure.

There are significant limitations of echocardiography. Artifacts are still common and engender false-positive and false-

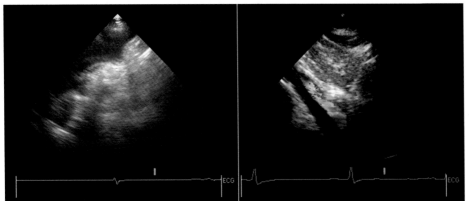

Figure 4-24. TTE. LEFT IMAGE, There is an intimal flap in the ascending aorta and arch from the suprasternal view. RIGHT IMAGE, Subcostal view. The differential flow in the true and false lumens is apparent by color Doppler flow mapping. The abdominal aorta is not dilated. The intimal flap is barely seen. (Type A AAD.)

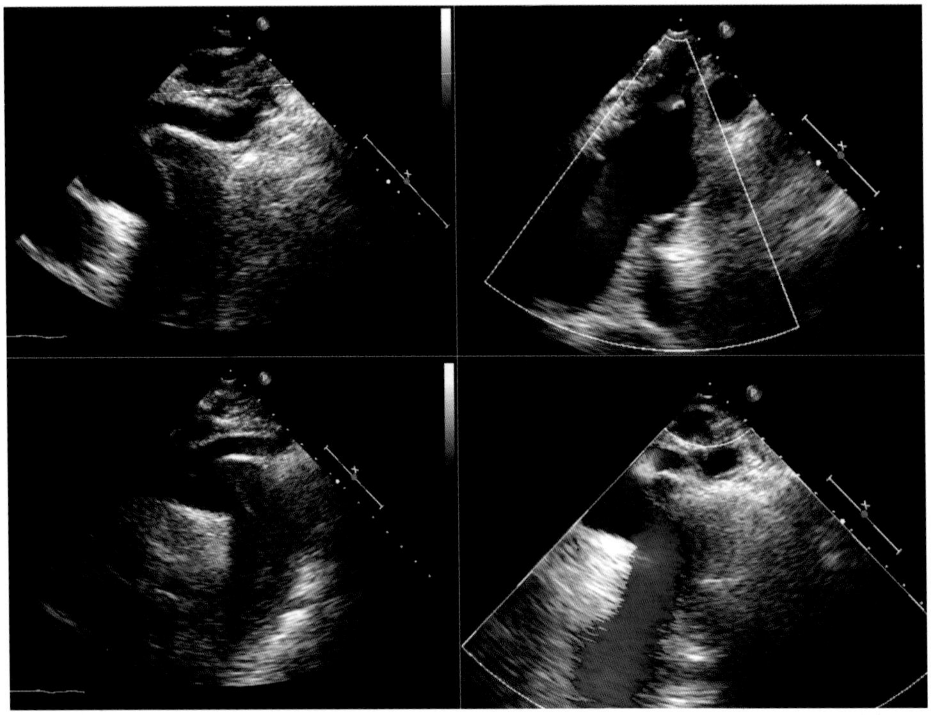

Figure 4-25. TTE (suprasternal views). UPPER LEFT IMAGE, An intimal flap is present, beginning immediately after the left subclavian artery ostium. RIGHT UPPER IMAGE, Color flow mapping reveals the flow into the intimal tear, immediately beside the left subclavian artery ostium. LOWER IMAGES, Intimal flap and partitioning of flow.

negative diagnoses. TTE does not offer adequate visualization of the thoracic aorta in all cases, of the mechanism of AI in all cases, or of any branch vessel complications of almost any cases. Assessment of distal involvement is poor. TEE availability is often limited, and TEE offers almost no visualization of the aortic disease distal to the diaphragm. As imaged by TEE, related pathologic processes, such as aortic valve commissural tears, may emulate AAD.[25]

Pitfalls with TEE include false-positives and false-negatives and potential risks. Reported false-positives include mural thrombus, pseudoaneurysm, ectatic aorta, misreading of near-field arc-artifacts or near-wall calcification reverberating across the lumen, and leiomyosarcoma. Reported false-negatives include localized tear in aortic sinus, short arch dissections occurring in the blind spot hidden by the tracheal air column, artifact obscuring an intimal flap, intramural hematoma in the ascending aorta, and

clotted false lumen in the ascending aorta. Potential risks of serious complications are less than 1%. Death occurs in 1:10,000 procedures. Other risks include esophageal problems (soreness, dysphagia, rupture), pulmonary problems (hypoxemia, bronchospasm, aspiration), cardiovascular risks (hypotension, transient atrioventricular block, nonsustained ventricular tachycardia, transient myocardial ischemia, dissection rupture), blood pressure increase (77%, 16 to 51 mm Hg), heart rate increase (8 bpm), and probe pressure (<17 mm Hg, up to 60 mm Hg). There are no arterial access risks and no contrast risks.

The diagnostic accuracy of TEE as reported by older studies is as follows: sensitivity, 92% to 100%; specificity, 82% to 95%; positive predictive value, 79% to 86%; and negative predictive value, 97% to 100% (Table 4-11).

Table 4-12 gives an overall comparison of various imaging modalities for assessment of AADs.

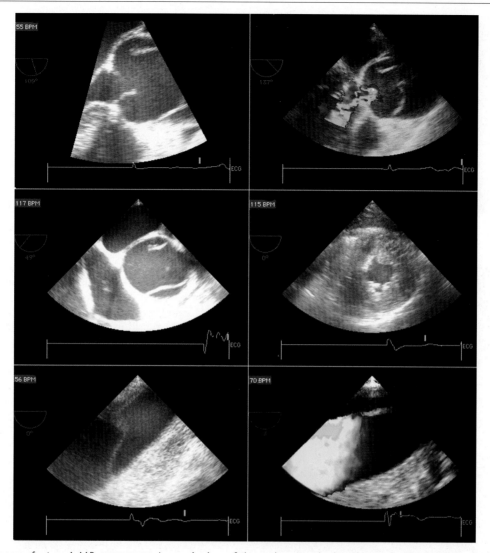

Figure 4-26. TEE images of a type A AAD. UPPER IMAGES, Long-axis views of the aortic root and valve. The root is dilated, and the sinotubular junction is effaced. There is an intimal flap in the aortic root on both the posterior wall and the anterior wall of the aortic root. The intimal tear in this case is on the posterior wall of the aorta. There is moderate AI, from root dilation rather than from direct compromise of the valve by the flap. MIDDLE IMAGE LEFT, Short-axis view of the aortic root. The intimal flap is seen in the aortic root on both the anterior wall and the posterior wall. The intimal tear is again seen to be posterior. MIDDLE IMAGE RIGHT, Transgastric view. LVH with normal wall motion—no compromise of coronary flow. LOWER IMAGES, Horizontal views of the aortic arch. There is an intimal flap within the arch that partitions the flow, resulting in differential flow (more in the true lumen than in the false lumen).

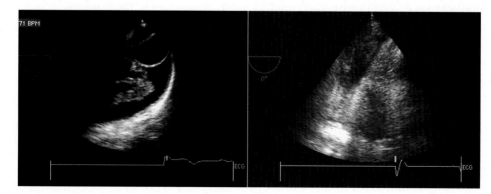

Figure 4-27. LEFT IMAGE, TEE, horizontal view of the mid descending aorta. There is an intimal flap in the descending aorta. There is a significant left pleural effusion as well. RIGHT IMAGE, TEE, view between the descending aorta and the left atrium. Posteriorly there is clot, which appears as gelatinous material with fine specular echoes. The aorta had ruptured into the posterior mediastinum.

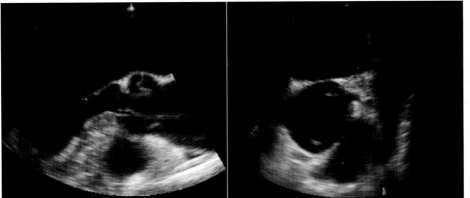

Figure 4-28. LEFT IMAGE, TEE, long-axis view of the aortic valve and root. The intimal flap is prolapsing through the aortic valve, causing severe AI. The root is not dilated. RIGHT IMAGE, TEE, short-axis view of the aortic root. The intimal flap is nearly circumferential within the aortic root and immediately beside the left main coronary artery. In this case, there was myocardial ischemia.

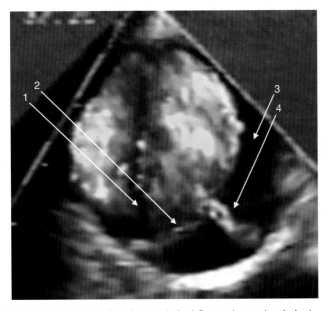

Figure 4-29. True and false lumens, intimal flap, and secondary intimal tears due to avulsed intercostals or spinal branches. The false lumen is located on the outside wall–curvature of the aorta, which is usual. 1, Strong flow signal in the true lumen. 2, Intimal flap. 3, Little flow in the false lumen. 4, Small jet into false lumen through a small secondary tear, probably from a spinal or intercostal artery that tore off the intimal flap.

MANAGEMENT OF ACUTE AORTIC DISSECTION

Prevention of AAD is possible by blood pressure control and elective operation to replace the aneurysmal ascending aorta, particularly in Marfan syndrome.

Once AAD has developed, it is imperative to classify the dissection and to identify whether any complications have occurred. Consideration should be given to taking a patient with AAD and hypotension or shock directly to the operating room for avoidance of any further time delay from diagnostic testing. Intraoperative TEE can be performed within the operating room without adding time. The blood pressure should be stabilized in all cases. A management algorithm for AAD is presented in Figure 4-30. Common exceptions are highlighted in Figure 4-31.

Type A AAD should undergo emergent cardiac surgery; medical management just stabilizes before prompt surgery and does not delay it. A small minority of type A AAD cases, too old or with daunting comorbidities, will be kept on the medical therapy track. For all patients managed medically, serial testing should be performed to determine whether complications are developing.

Medical Management

Medical management is the usual strategy for uncomplicated type B AAD. After rapid control of the blood pressure in the ICU or CCU (target of 110 mm Hg systolic), most patients can be switched to oral medications in 3 days. If they remain well, most can be discharged between 7 and 10 days. Predischarge reimaging is prudent. Comanagement and integrated consultation of cardiology, critical care, anesthesiology, cardiovascular surgery, and radiology specialists is advisable.

The goal of medical management is to control the blood pressure and to prevent rupture. The concept of blood pressure lowering also includes reducing the systolic impulse to the aorta (dP/dt). Hence, intravenous beta-blockers (esmolol, labetalol, metoprolol) should be instituted (in the absence of contraindications such as asthma, hypotension, or heart failure) before other medications, such as sodium nitroprusside (or other pure vasodilators), are started. Analgesics are useful to lower blood pressure, but sedation, as for TEE, may aggravate hypotension.

Severe hypertension, refractory hypertension, or hypertensive crisis occurs in many cases of type B dissection. In most patients, it subsides with time and antihypertensive use, without significant renal distress. The development of oliguria or anuria or a marked rise in creatinine concentration should prompt renal artery imaging and consideration of intervention when it is suitable and feasible.

Surgical Repair of Acute Aortic Dissection

The goal of surgery is to correct or to prevent rupture of the aorta and to correct malperfusion complications and AI when present.

The sites of tube graft replacement are the aortic root for type A AAD and the proximal descending aorta for type B AAD. Tube graft replacement is intended to resect the intimal tear, so

Table 4-11. Review of Published Studies on Acute Aortic Dissection Diagnosis

Year (Study)	Sensitivity (%)	Specificity (%)	PPV (%)	NPV (%)	Classification Error (%)
1989 (Erbel et al[26])					
Type A					
TEE	98	88	97	93	
Angiography	89	87	96	68	
CT	77	100	100	33	
Type B					
TEE	100	100	100	100	
Angiography	85	97	94	92	
CT	93	100	100	98	
Types A and B					
TEE	99	98	99	99	
Angiography	88	94	96	84	
CT	83	100	100	86	
1992 (Nienaber et al[27])					
Type A					
TEE	100	78	74	100	
MRI	100	100	100	100	
TTE	85	78	71	89	
Type B					
TEE	91	98	91	98	
MRI	100	100	100	100	
TTE	55	100	71	89	
All types					
TEE	100	68	82	100	
MRI	100	100	100	100	
TTE	83	63	80	71	
1992 (Nienaber et al[27])					
Type A					
TTE	85	78	71	89	
TEE	100	79	74	100	
MRI	100	100	100	100	
Type B					
TTE	56	100	100	90	
TEE	91	98	100	90	
MRI	100	100	100	100	
1991 (Ballal et al[28])					
TEE	97	100	100	96	0
CT	67	100			33
1996 (Keren et al[29])					
Omniplane TEE					
All patients					
Type A	90	98			
Type B	100	99			
IMH	90	99			
Confirmed by surgery					
Type A	90	94			
Type B	100	98			

1991 (Ballal et al[28])					
TEE	Sensitivity (%)	Specificity (%)	Seen (%)		
LCA	100	100	91		
RCA	75	100	55		
AI	Correct quantization 100%	Detected 100%			

AI, aortic insufficiency; CT, computed tomography; IMH, intramural hematoma; LCA, left coronary artery; MRI, magnetic resonance imaging; NPV, negative predictive value; PPV, positive predictive value; RCA, right coronary artery; TEE, transesophageal echocardiography; TTE, transthoracic echocardiography.

Table 4-12. Comparison of Imaging Modalities for Acute Aortic Dissection

	Chest Radiography	TEE	CT	MRI and MRA	Contrast Aortography
Utility to image anatomic section					
Aortic root	Poor	Good	Excellent	Excellent	Excellent
Ascending aorta	Fair	Good-fair	Excellent	Excellent	Excellent
Aortic arch	Fair	Fair	Excellent	Excellent	Excellent
Descending aorta	Poor	Poor	Excellent	Excellent	Excellent
Branch vessel involvement	Nil	Nil	Excellent	Excellent	Excellent
Utility to image pathologic changes					
Dissection flaps	Nil-poor	Fair	Excellent	Excellent	Very good
Dissection tears	Nil	Very poor	Very good	Fair	Good
Cardiac complications	Poor	Excellent	Poor	Very good	Good
AI	Nil	Excellent	Nil	Very good	Excellent
Tamponade	Nil	Excellent	Poor	Very good	Poor
Myocardial ischemia	Poor	Excellent	Poor	Good	Fair
Intramural hematomas	Poor	Very little	Very good	Very good	Poor
Penetrating ulcers	Poor	Nil	Very good	Good	Good
Aneurysms	Fair	Fair-good	Excellent	Excellent	Good
Mural thrombus	Nil	Poor	Excellent	Excellent	Nil
Ruptured aorta	Fair	Nil	Excellent	Good	Poor
Extra-aortic anatomy		Very poor	Excellent	Excellent	Very poor
Risks					
Contrast	No	No	Yes	No	Yes
Radiation	Scant	No	Yes	No	Yes
Access	No	No	No	No	Yes
Intubation	No	Yes	No	No	No
Modalities					
Multiplanar imaging	No	Yes	Yes	Yes	No
3D rendering	No	Yes	Yes	Yes	Yes
Portable	Yes	Yes	No	No	No
Suitable for critically ill patients	Yes	Yes	Yes	No	Yes
Suitable for guiding interventions	No	Somewhat*	Yes	Yes	Yes

*Can assess intraoperative repair of the aortic valve.
AI, aortic insufficiency; CT, computed tomography; MRA, magnetic resonance angiography; MRI, magnetic resonance imaging; TEE, transesophageal echocardiography.

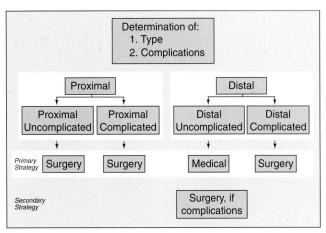

Figure 4-30. Management algorithm for AAD.

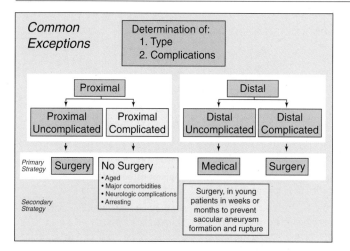

Figure 4-31. Algorithm highlighting the common exceptions in AAD management.

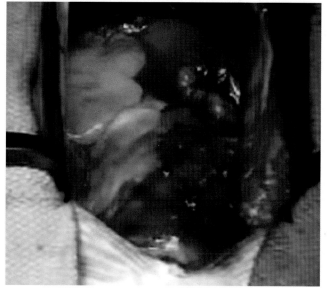

Figure 4-33. AAD surgical specimen. Adventitial hematoma of the ascending aorta, oozing of blood into the pericardial space.

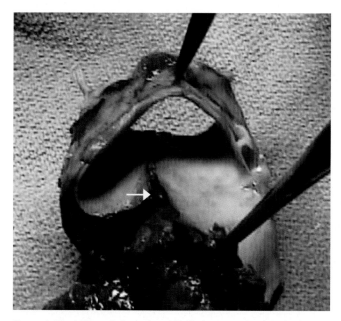

Figure 4-32. AAD surgical specimen. Intimal tear can be seen in the excised segment of aortic root.

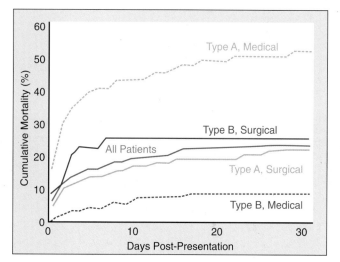

Figure 4-34. Thirty-day mortality of AAD by type of management. (From Hagan PG, Nienaber CA, Isselbacher EM, et al: The International Registry of Acute Aortic Dissection [IRAD]: new insights into an old disease. JAMA 2000;283:897-903.)

that the false lumen does not remain pressurized and vulnerable to late dilation and rupture. The intimal flap is sewn to the outer wall to the distal end of the tube graft, reapproximating the dissected aortic wall. The surgery is not intended to replace the entire length of the aorta that has dissected. Because of secondary tears or failure of the tube graft insertion to eliminate the primary entry tear, a persistence of the false lumen occurs in more than 90% of surgically repaired type A AAD cases.[30] Surgical findings in AAD are shown in Figures 4-32 and 4-33.

Assessed during a 30-year period, the surgical mortality of AAD patients has significantly improved (Fig. 4-34). Earlier detection and operation before development of tamponade, hypotension, shock, and renal failure are likely to underlie the improvement.[31]

Profound hypothermic circulatory arrest during surgical repair of type A AAD to inspect the aortic arch and to repair an intimal tear, if it is located there, is popular. Its use is associated

with comparable early complications, mortality, and long-term reoperation rates, although without evidence of superiority.[32]

Data suggest that patients who present several days after type A AAD can safely undergo semielective surgical repair (rather than emergent repair) and that selected patients with type A AAD who survive the immediate period may be managed with aggressive medical treatment and achieve acceptable short-term outcomes.[33]

Surgical Repair of Type A AAD
Primary goals for surgical repair are replacement of the ascending aorta and replacement or repair of the aortic valve. Secondary goals are elimination of the false lumen and healing and remodeling of the dissected wall. In only 10% of cases of surgically repaired type A AAD is the false lumen eliminated.[30] In the

Table 4-13. Surgical Repair of Acute Aortic Dissection

Ascending Aorta	Arch	Descending Aorta
Procedure	Procedure	Procedure
Midline sternotomy, CPB	Midline sternotomy	Left thoracotomy
Transect ascending aorta.	CPB, cold hypothermic circulatory arrest	CPB, partial CPB
Examine for the presence of an intimal tear. If the tear cannot be seen in the root or ascending portions and is seen in the arch, the best course of management is controversial. In selected patients, type A repair can be extended to replace (usually) part of the arch to resect the responsible intimal tear.	Transect ascending aorta.	Transect descending aorta before tear.
	Examine the arch for site of intimal tear.	Excise segment with tear.
	Approximate inner and outer walls of aorta.	Approximate inner and outer walls of aorta.
Approximate inner and outer walls of aorta.	Interposition graft; if the tear is on the inferior wall of the arch, often the arch branch vessels are left on an "island" that is sewn to the graft, rather than being individually sewn on.	For rupture: interposition graft, direct replacement
± Interposition graft, common		For aortic enlargement: interposition graft, direct replacement
Inspect aortic valve: leave if well functioning and root is not dilated; repair (resuspend) if partially dehisced and not dilated; replace if severely dehisced and root is dilated.		For branch occlusion: fenestration
In three fourths of patients, the valve can be spared.		
Coronaries: leave, resuspend if composite graft is being inserted.		
Risk increases with	Indications	Risk increases with
Tamponade	Rupture at the arch level	Age
Renal failure	Accessible tear in the arch in an ascending repair	Rupture
Renal ischemia		Renal failure or ischemia
Visceral ischemia		Visceral ischemia or infarction
Extension of repair to include arch repair		Risk of paraplegia: 30%-35%[35]
Aortocoronary bypass		
Mortality	Mortality	
7% best cases	15%+	
15% usual	25%+ if arch has ruptured	
Stroke	Stroke	
Ascending repair	5%	
Ascending repair extended to include arch repair		

CPB, cardiopulmonary bypass.

remainder, persistence of tears distal to the repair allows pressurization and flow within the false lumen. Table 4-13 gives an overview of the surgical procedure by aortic segment.

Paraplegia is uncommon with type A repair. Valve-sparing root-remodeling (versus root replacement) surgery may not be associated with better early or late outcome because it may be associated with a higher failure rate.[34] Outcomes of type A AAD in the elderly are shown in Figure 4-35.[11]

Surgical Repair of Type B AAD

Conservative approach is indicated for recurrent or intractable pain despite full medical therapy; rapid, localized expansion; rupture, leakage, or threatened rupture; compromise of a major branch vessel or organ; underlying connective tissue disease (Marfan syndrome); or hypertensive crisis. One problem that arises is that if rupture occurs into the pleural space, few patients will survive to be operated on, let alone to be discharged. Aggressive approach is taken by some centers, which perform surgical repair on all type B AADs, with an overall 10% mortality. Some authors have noted very high mortality (28% to 65%) for direct aortic replacement surgery in all type B cases.[35]

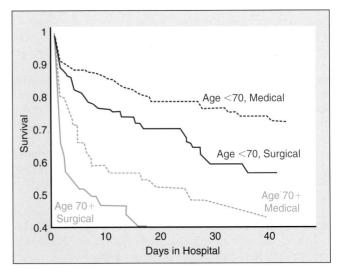

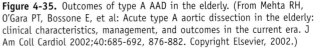

Figure 4-35. Outcomes of type A AAD in the elderly. (From Mehta RH, O'Gara PT, Bossone E, et al: Acute type A aortic dissection in the elderly: clinical characteristics, management, and outcomes in the current era. J Am Coll Cardiol 2002;40:685-692, 876-882. Copyright Elsevier, 2002.)

Surgical repair of type B AAD is associated with in-hospital mortality of approximately 30%.[36] Multivariate predictors of mortality are age older than 70 years (odds ratio, 4.32) and preoperative shock and hypotension (odds ratio, 6.05). Univariate predictors include preoperative coma or altered consciousness, partial thrombosis of the false lumen, evidence of periaortic hematoma on diagnostic imaging, descending aortic diameter of more than 6 cm, and right ventricular dysfunction.[36]

Management of Acute Aortic Dissection Associated with Pericardial Tamponade

The presence of pericardial tamponade, occurring in one fifth of cases of type A AAD, predicts rupture. The optimal management of pericardial tamponade in the context of AAD is unclear. Routine drainage risks aggravating the leak or rupture by restoring arterial pressure that then exacerbates the tear and the driving pressure of the leak, increasing mortality.[37] Deferral of drainage until the time of surgery, though, may forfeit survival of extreme cases of tamponade. A cautious approach adopted by many is to defer drainage until the operating room in cases that appear sustainable; the access to the operating room is accelerated for drainage of cases that appear nonviable otherwise. Autotransfusion has been performed. Pericardial tamponade is a considerable risk when anesthesia is induced, as preload reduction by anesthetic agents may precipitate electromechanical dissociation.

Endovascular Therapy for Acute Aortic Dissection: Stent Grafting and Fenestration

Surgery for AAD corrects more than 90% of pulse deficits. A minority of patients suffer from malperfusion syndrome resulting from persistent pressurization of the false lumen. Renal and bowel ischemia are associated with high in-hospital mortality. Surgical fenestration or reconstruction is associated with significant mortality; hence, interventional strategies have been explored and are under development.

Stenting (covered and bare) and fenestration (intentional laceration of the intimal flap to allow communication of flow between the true and false lumens) depressurize the false lumen so that it is less likely to be occluding branch vessels.

Percutaneous stent grafting has been performed in hundreds of patients with dissection; therefore, it is feasible. Its role is evolving and variable, depending on a center's experience. Covered stent graft deployment over the intimal tear to exclude the false lumen from flow and pressure facilitates thrombosis of the false lumen.[38-40] Anatomically, distal aortic dissections are more amenable to stenting. Chronic dissections are easier to intervene on, as the stent graft can be tailor-made; however, nonimmediate endovascular repair of distal AAD is rendered potentially more difficult because of progression of the false lumen (Fig. 4-36).[41]

Stenting has been performed in both acute type A and type B AAD with high technical success and low complications. Among 16 patients with acute type B AAD and 21 patients with chronic type B AAD, the overall in-hospital mortality was 2.7%: 6.3% in type B AAD with complications, and 0% in type B AAD without complications. The primary success rate was 94%, and there was no mortality during 24 months of follow-up. New intimal tears caused by stents developed in 3 patients.[42]

Percutaneous noncovered stents may be used to maintain flow into branch vessels. There are few long-term outcomes data. Catheter fenestration of occlusive dissection flaps may be used to restore flow in malperfusion syndromes due to AAD.

Patients with acute limb ischemia (malperfusion) due to type B AAD are usually salvaged (>90%) with endovascular repair, with surgical bypass used in only a minority. Stenting and fenestration have a high procedural success rate and sustained limb salvage during 18 months (93%).[43] Ischemic complications of interventional procedures do occur (approximately 10%), but success is above 90%.[1]

In a 1999 study, complete thrombosis of the false lumen occurred in 79%, partial thrombosis in 21%, and revascularization of occluded branches in 76%.[40] Thirty-day mortality was 16%, whereas late mortality (13 months) was 0%.

OUTCOMES AND FOLLOW-UP

In the current era, 90% of type A AAD cases are managed surgically. Of patients surviving initial hospitalization, 1- and 3-year

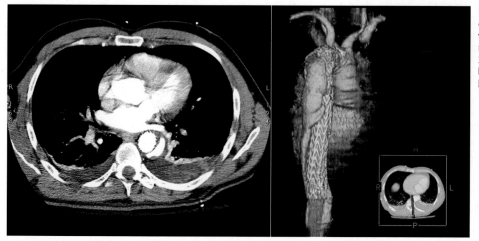

Figure 4-36. Contrast-enhanced CT scans of a stented type B dissection. The axial view (LEFT) and the 3D reconstruction reveal persistence of the false lumen. The 3D reconstruction reveals that the false lumen spirals around the true lumen in barber pole fashion.

survivals of type A AAD are 96.1% ± 2.4% and 90.5 ± 3.9% for patients treated surgically and 88.6% ± 12.2% and 68.7% ± 19.8% for patients treated medically. Predictors of mortality in follow-up are older age, atherosclerosis, and prior cardiac surgery.[44]

In the current era, 3-year survival of type B dissection is 77.6% ± 6.6% treated medically, 82.8% ± 18.9% treated surgically, and 76.2% ± 25.2% after endovascular treatment.[45] Predictors of mortality in follow-up include female gender, prior aortic aneurysm, atherosclerosis, in-hospital renal failure, preoperative pleural effusion, and preoperative hypotension and shock. Given the significant mortality in the years after type B AAD, follow-up is important.[46]

CASE 1

History and Physical Examination

▸ A 44-year-old man with a history of hypertension presented with a sudden onset of severe chest pain between his shoulder blades and was transferred for management.
▸ At transfer: BP 210/110 mm Hg; no pericardial rub; no murmur of AI; no signs of tamponade or of left-sided heart failure
▸ 30 mm Hg BP difference between the arms

Evolution and Management

▸ BP control with IV nitroprusside initially and multiple antihypertensives subsequently led to resolution of pain and stabilization of the dissection.
▸ Part of the left kidney was infarcted because of interrupted blood supply and led to a second wave of severe hypertension while the kidney was ischemic.
▸ Left lower lobe bronchopneumonia developed, requiring mechanical ventilation. After extubation, it was evident that bilateral foot numbness had developed, which persisted. CT scanning of the head excluded cerebral infarction. Spinal ischemia was believed to have been the cause.
▸ A pericardial rub developed. Reimaging determined that the dissection flap was stable and was still confined to the distal aortic arch–descending aorta. The pericarditis was presumed to be reactive to left-sided pneumonia.
▸ Eventually, the complications resolved except for foot numbness, and he was discharged well with good BP control.
▸ During 5 years, he has been stable clinically, as has been the dissection by imaging. The arm BP difference persists.

Comments

▸ Distal (type B) dissection in a previously hypertensive patient
▸ Typical sudden onset with severe chest pain, maximal at onset
▸ No significant abnormality to the aorta on the chest radiograph
▸ Multiple complications developed, some attributable to the dissection, and some to hospitalization.

  ▸ Dissection-related complications were renal ischemia and infarction, with hypertensive crisis for 3 days, spinal cord ischemia (the proximal descending aorta supplies important feeder vessels to the anterior spinal arteries), and left subclavian narrowing seen on CT scanning, the cause of the pulse deficit to that arm.
  ▸ Hospitalization-related complications were bronchopneumonia and unexplained pericarditis.
▸ The false lumen, with its continuous flow, has never thrombosed or dilated.
▸ Long-term survival, medically managed

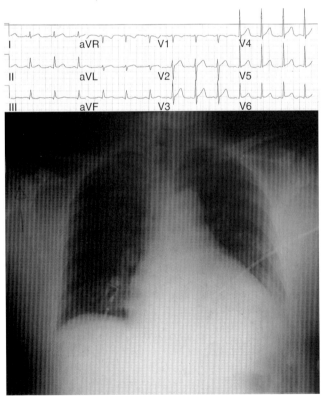

Figure 4-37. ECG: sinus rhythm. No prominent signs of LVH, ischemia, infarction, or pericarditis. Chest radiograph: cardiomegaly. No obvious dilation of the ascending aorta or increased width of the aortic arch. No pleural effusions.

4

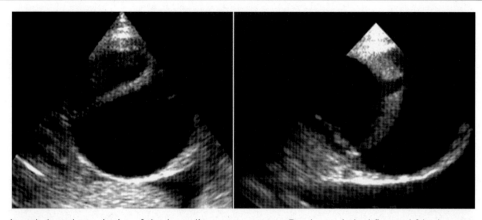

Figure 4-38. TEE, horizontal plane short-axis view of the descending aorta. LEFT PANEL, True lumen, intimal flap, and false lumen. RIGHT PANEL, True lumen, intimal tear and intimal flap, and false lumen.

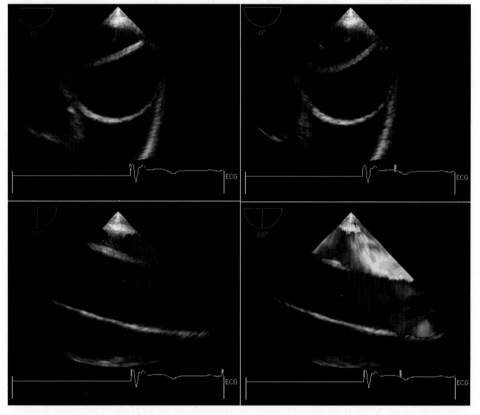

Figure 4-39. TEE. LEFT IMAGES, Diastole. RIGHT IMAGES, Systole. UPPER IMAGES, Short-axis views of the descending aorta. The intimal flap pulses outward to the more lateral false lumen with the pressure rise from systole. LOWER IMAGES, Long-axis views. In systole, the pressure increase and flow in the true lumen exceed those in the false lumen.

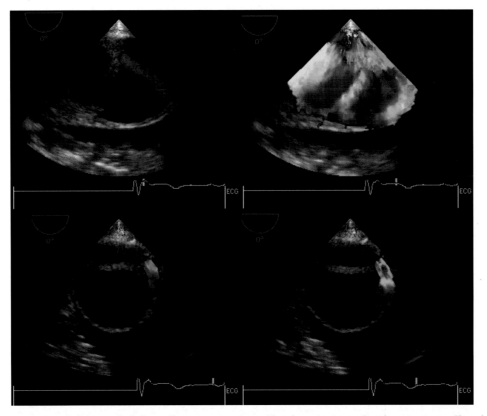

Figure 4-40. TTE, short-axis images of the proximal descending aorta. LEFT IMAGES, Diastole. RIGHT IMAGES, Systole. UPPER IMAGES, The primary intimal tear. In diastole, there is flow through the intimal tear and flap into the false lumen. With the pressure rise in the true lumen in systole, there is a prominent rise in the flow across the intimal tear into the false lumen. LOWER IMAGES, A secondary tear (due to avulsion of a small branch artery). Again, there is slight flow from the true lumen into the false lumen, which increases prominently in systole.

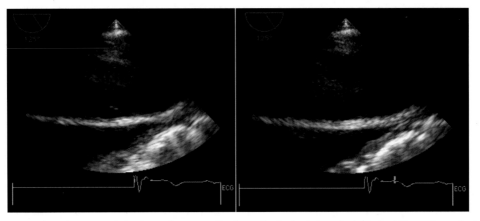

Figure 4-41. Vertical plane, longitudinal view of the descending aorta. The image is obtained through the intimal flap and reveals the opening and closing of the tear through the cardiac cycle as well as the 3-cm length of the tear.

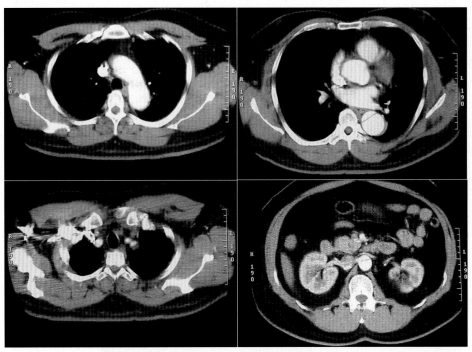

Figure 4-42. Contrast-enhanced CT scan, axial images. LEFT UPPER IMAGE, Arch level. There is no intimal tear. RIGHT UPPER IMAGE, Aortic root level. There is an intimal tear in the descending aorta but not in the ascending aorta: type B AAD. LOWER LEFT IMAGE, The dissection has extended up the left subclavian artery; there are both true (enhanced) and false (less enhanced) lumens. RIGHT LOWER IMAGE, The intimal flap is present at the level of the renal arteries. There is a wedge of nonenhancement of the left kidney, consistent with ischemia.

CASE 2

History and Physical Examination

▸ A 74-year-old man with a history of hypertension presented with abrupt severe pains in the mid back with some radiation to the front.
▸ BP 179/100 mm Hg, HR 100 bpm
▸ No venous distention, no rub
▸ Normal heart sounds; AI murmur
▸ Normal air entry, no pulse deficits

Evolution

▸ Abrupt asystole developed. The patient could not be resuscitated.

Comments

▸ Type B dissection in a previously hypertensive man. The AI pertained to hypertension, rather than to the dissection, as the flap was nowhere near the aortic valve.
▸ Initial appearance, with hypertension at presentation, ready BP control, and pain relief with IV labetalol, was favorable. Initial

management strategy was medical, and the patient was stable clinically and on a follow-up CT scan. Clinically, there were no signs that conservative management of this type B dissection was inappropriate.
▸ Sudden unheralded (by pain) rupture into the left pleural space occurred, followed by asystole. This is the worst-case scenario of medical management strategy. The adventitial hematoma seen on TEE 2 hours earlier probably indicated progression. Rupture in type B AAD may develop without warning, leaving virtually no means to salvage the patient.
▸ By imaging, there were, albeit in retrospect, indications of potential leakage (periaortic hematoma). Adventitial hematoma in the context of AAD is imperfectly understood. It is increasingly believed to be a sign of higher mortality risk. Whether that justifies intervention is unknown.
▸ Fulminant rupture of the aorta in seemingly stable type B AAD is usually fatal because of the combination of abrupt massive hypovolemia and concurrent asystole.
▸ Conservative management for type B AAD is usually successful; but when it fails, it fails definitively. This is the downside of the strategy—it is committing and unforgiving.

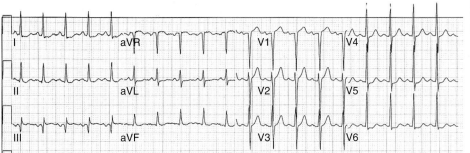

Figure 4-43. ECG: sinus tachycardia. Voltage signs of LVH. Nonspecific repolarization abnormalities.

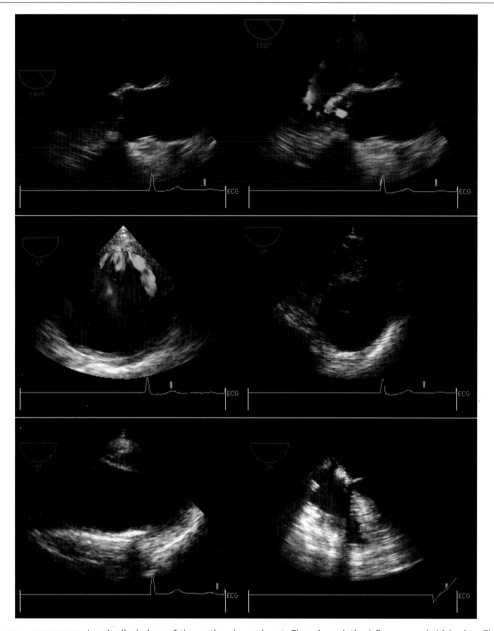

Figure 4-44. TEE images. UPPER IMAGES, Longitudinal views of the aortic valve and root. There is no intimal flap or mural thickening. There is AI, which is not due to dissection but probably relates to the antecedent hypertension. MIDDLE LEFT IMAGE, The mid descending aorta in cross section. There is an intimal flap. Color Doppler flow mapping reveals partitioning of flow and a flow into the false lumen through an entrance tear (at the 12-o'clock position). The intimal flap is faintly seen. MIDDLE RIGHT IMAGE, The proximal descending aorta in cross section. The intimal flap is seen, faintly. LOWER LEFT IMAGE, Horizontal plane image of the aortic arch. The intimal flap extends retrograde onto the posterior wall of the arch. LOWER RIGHT IMAGE, Partial 4-chamber view. The right-sided heart chambers appear collapsed. There is no pericardial effusion. The collapse of the chambers was due to exsanguinations.

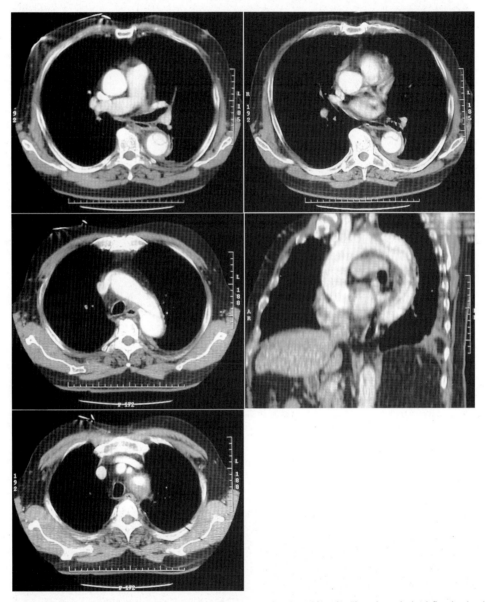

Figure 4-45. Contrast-enhanced CT scan images. LEFT UPPER IMAGE, Systole. RIGHT UPPER IMAGE, Diastole. There is an intimal flap in the descending aorta, not in the ascending aorta. The true lumen distends in systole and collapses in diastole. There is a very small left pleural effusion. The appearance of the periaortic soft tissue is abnormally thick and marbled. MIDDLE LEFT IMAGE, The intimal flap extends back to the mid arch. MIDDLE RIGHT IMAGE, Sagittal view. The intimal flap is present in the descending thoracic aorta and extends to involve the left subclavian artery origin. LOWER LEFT IMAGE, Aortic arch branch vessels. The dissection involves the left subclavian with either thrombosis of the false lumen, mural, or adventitial hematoma.

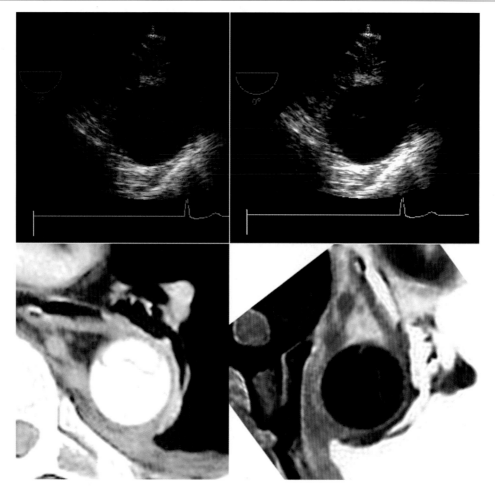

Figure 4-46. UPPER IMAGES, TEE view of the proximal descending aorta. The image on the right simply has the brightness increased. Although it is apparent on the darker image, it is far more obvious on the brightened image that there are several centimeters of soft tissue interposed between the TEE probe and the descending aorta. The nature of the tissue (fine specular echoes) suggests blood clot, which in this context prompts consideration of periaortic or mediastinal hematoma. LOWER IMAGES, Corresponding contrast-enhanced CT scan of the same area. Medial to the descending aorta, there is increased soft tissue with a complex appearance. The right lower image is black-white inverted and rotated to match the TEE images above. The esophagus, from where the TEE image sector originates, is the small black slit at the 12-o'clock position. The marbled appearance of the increased soft tissue closely matches that of the TEE image.

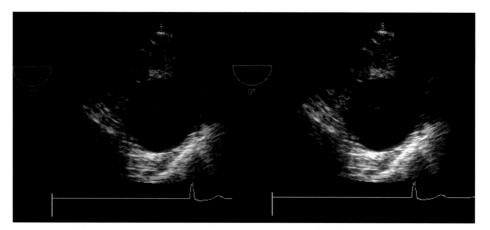

Figure 4-47. TEE, horizontal plane view of the heart. The heart is asystolic. The chambers are collapsed, consistent with volume depletion due to exsanguination. A large amount of left pleural fluid was seen and tapped, yielding blood.

4

CASE 3

History

▸ A 74-year-old male smoker with a history of borderline hypertension developed sudden severe chest pain.
▸ At referring hospital: BP 225/130 mm Hg; no pericardial rub; no signs of tamponade; no AI murmur or signs of left-sided heart failure; no pulse deficits or BP differential. AAD was suspected, and low-dose labetalol was started. The patient was transferred.
▸ On transfer: BP 90/50 mm Hg, HR 100 bpm, dyspneic
▸ No pericardial rub, no signs of tamponade, no pulse deficits or BP differential
▸ AI murmur was present, as were crepitations and increased respiratory rate and effort.

Impression and Management

▸ Type A AAD complicated by severe AI and left-sided heart failure
▸ Patient was referred for an emergent surgery.

Surgical Procedure

▸ Bentall procedure: composite (aortic valve replacement + Dacron tube) graft, with coronary artery implantation

▸ Low output and elevated central venous pressure developed 13 days postoperatively. Echocardiography showed a pericardial effusion and blood clot in the pericardial space. The patient underwent exploration, evacuation of fluid and clots, and drainage (chest tube insertion into the pericardial space). Bleeding from needle holes in the Dacron tube graft was the cause. Ventilator and ICU time was prolonged, but progressive improvement led to eventual recovery.

Comments

▸ Type A AAD in a previously hypertensive man, managed with emergency surgery, with an eventual successful outcome
▸ Hypotension at presentation (transfer) was consistent with a major complication to the AAD—severe AI and heart failure. Hypotension is a major clinical indicator in AAD cases.
▸ The severe AI had developed during a 4-hour window in transfer from the referring hospital.
▸ Postoperative problems are common (in this case, pericardial tamponade with clots) and underrepresented in the literature because despite their mortality risk, most are managed successfully and do not culminate in tabulated mortality.

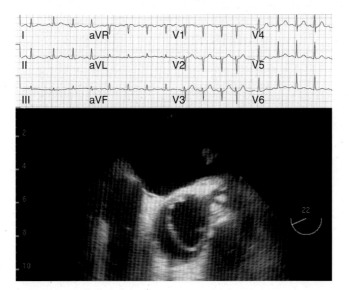

Figure 4-48. ECG: sinus tachycardia, borderline repolarization abnormalities. The lower image reveals that the intimal flap, although close to the left main coronary artery, does not involve it. The right coronary artery is not seen on this plane.

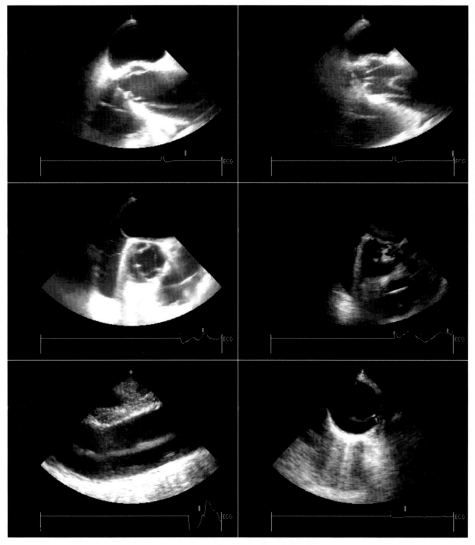

Figure 4-49. TEE images. UPPER IMAGES, Longitudinal view of the ascending aorta. A highly mobile intimal flap is present in the aortic root and ascending aorta; in diastole, the flap prolapses into the aortic valve. MIDDLE IMAGES, Cross-sectional view at the aortic root–valve level. The flap extends down around the right posterior half of the root. Color Doppler flow mapping reveals AI. LEFT LOWER IMAGE, The proximal descending aorta in longitudinal plane. There is an intimal flap and a large amount of soft tissue interposed between the TEE probe and the aorta. RIGHT LOWER IMAGE, Distal thoracic aorta in cross section. There is an intimal flap and a small secondary intimal tear. The flow is partitioned by the intimal flap.

CASE 4

History and Physical Examination

▸ A 60-year-old man with a history of hypertension presented to the emergency department with sudden-onset severe anterior chest, back, and abdominal pain.
▸ BP 230/110 mm Hg; no pericardial rub; no signs of tamponade; no pulse deficits or BP differential
▸ AI murmur was present, but no signs of left-sided heart failure.

Surgical Findings

▸ On arrival in the operating room, the patient developed prominent ST changes and hypotension. Urgent cardiopulmonary bypass was performed. Hematoma was seen on the outside of the ascending aorta, which was very dilated.
▸ An intimal flap extended down the aortic root around both coronary ostia to partially involve the noncoronary cusp of the aortic valve. The intimal tear was two thirds of the circumference of the aorta 2 cm above the aortic valve.

Surgical Procedure

▸ Dacron tube graft was inserted down to the aortic sinuses to resuspend the aortic valve (especially the noncoronary sinus and leaflet). The coronary arteries were resuspended on buttons to the tube graft.

▸ Anterior wall hypokinesis was apparent coming off bypass but resolved during 15 minutes. It was presumed that the anterior wall had been ischemic on arrival to the operating room because of intimal flap compromise of the left coronary ostium and responsible for the hemodynamic instability at that time. There was very little AI after repair.

Comments

▸ Type A AAD in a previously hypertensive man, complicated by mild to moderate AI due to malsuspension of a commissure, left coronary ostial occlusion from the intimal flap, with resulting myocardial ischemia and progressive development of complications
▸ Complications occurred despite BP control (normal wall motion on the initial diagnostic TEE and no significant ST shifts; but 90 minutes later, ST shifts and hypotension, with persisting hypokinesis), underscoring the need for urgent surgery, especially once complications have been identified in type A AAD, which are usually progressive.
▸ The hypertension at presentation militated against hemodynamically severe complications at that time, but there was already some AI, and the flap was in the proximity of the coronary arteries.
▸ Development of hypotension resulted from worsening complications.
▸ No neurologic complications developed despite evidence of carotid obstruction from the flap, presumably because of adequate collateralization from the circle of Willis.

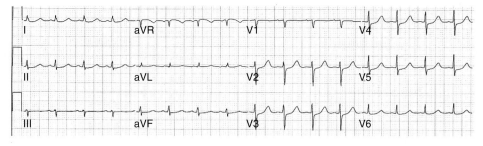

Figure 4-50. ECG showing sinus rhythm, nonspecific repolarization abnormalities, and no definite signs of ischemia or pericarditis.

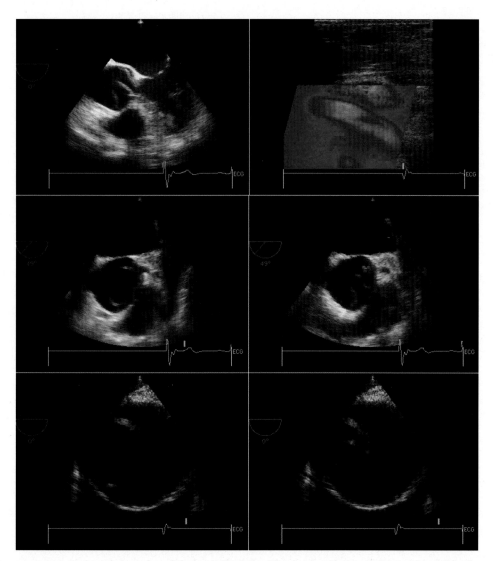

Figure 4-51. TEE images. TOP LEFT, Horizontal plane view of the heart. The intimal flap involves the low root and prolapses into the aortic valve. There is no pericardial effusion. The left ventricle was dynamic. Despite the flap's being low in the root, there is no apparent wall motion abnormality. TOP RIGHT, Carotid ultrasonography. There is an intimal flap in the common carotid artery. This extended down to the ostium of the carotid. The flow in the artery was of a high-resistance pattern, distinctly abnormal and indicative of obstruction. MIDDLE, Cross-sectional views of the aortic root showing the intimal flap's mobility and proximity to the ostium of the left main coronary artery. BOTTOM, Descending thoracic aorta in cross section during systole (LEFT) and diastole (RIGHT). The true lumen is the smaller lumen, and the false lumen is the larger crescentic lumen that runs on the outside. There is pressurization of the false lumen such that it compresses the true lumen in diastole.

CASE 5

History

▸ A 53-year-old man with hypertension presented to an emergency department with severe chest pain.
▸ Borderline ST elevation was noted, and a fibrinolytic was administered.
▸ Some increase and sharpening of the pain occurred and left-sided heart failure developed, prompting consideration of other innumerable diagnoses.

Physical Examination

▸ BP 130/80 mm Hg
▸ No pericardial rub, but the jugular veins were distended
▸ AI murmur
▸ Initially, there were no complaints or signs of left-sided heart failure, but dyspnea, crepitations, and hypoxemia did develop.
▸ No pulse deficits or BP differential

Surgical Findings

▸ Bloody pericardial effusion under pressure, consistent with tamponade
▸ Sanguineous left pleural effusion
▸ Near-circumferential intimal tear just above the aortic valve; extensive involvement of the right coronary ostium
▸ Extensive dehiscence of all commissures of the aortic valve. With detailed inspection, a second intimal tear was found in the mid arch just before the left subclavian artery ostium.

Surgical Procedure

▸ Bentall procedure (composite graft) extending to the mid distal arch to exclude both intimal tears. Aortic valve replacement because of the extensive involvement of the aortic valve. Reimplantation of the left coronary artery. Saphenous grafting to the right coronary artery was needed because of compromise of the ostium of the right coronary artery.
▸ Cardiopulmonary bypass time, 209 minutes; cross-clamp time, 162 minutes; hypothermic circulatory arrest time, 36 minutes

Comments

▸ Type A dissection in a previously hypertensive patient complicated by AI and pericardial tamponade (the left pleural effusion was sanguineous, suggestive of rupture)
▸ Although the coronary artery ostia were involved (especially the right, as is typical of dissection), the AAD was probably the perpetrator of the myocardial ischemic event.
▸ The presentation of chest pain and an abnormal ECG (which was probably LVH) led to algorithmic administration of a fibrinolytic. An echocardiogram at presentation to verify the presence of a wall motion abnormality would likely have looked beyond the ECG. The ECG pattern never changed.
▸ Uneventful course, and remarkably little bleeding despite recent administration of fibrinolytics

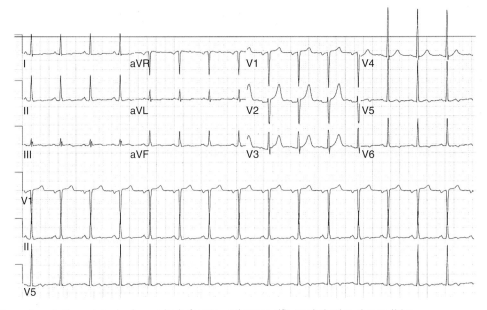

Figure 4-52. ECG shows sinus rhythm, minimal voltage criteria for LVH, and nonspecific repolarization abnormalities.

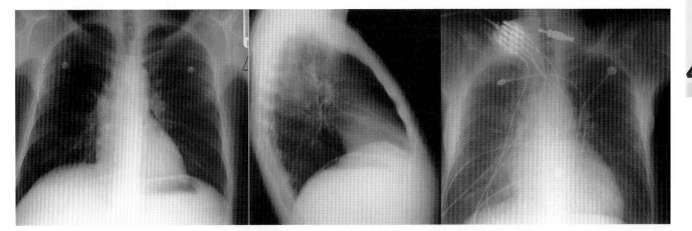

Figure 4-53. LEFT AND MIDDLE, Chest radiographs on arrival in the emergency department show enlargement of the ascending aorta. RIGHT, Chest radiograph taken 2 hours later, showing the development of interstitial pulmonary edema.

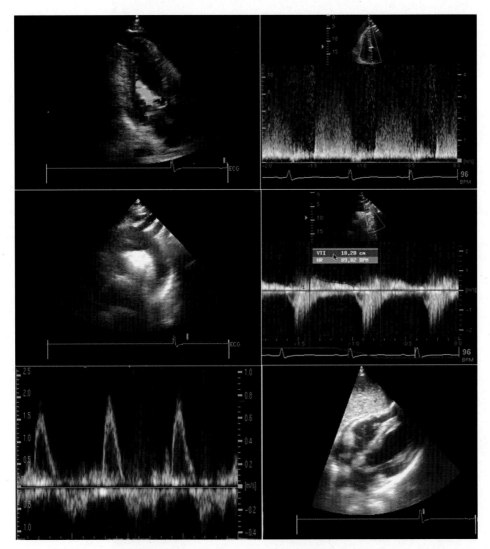

Figure 4-54. TTE. TOP LEFT, Apical 3-chamber view with color Doppler mapping. Prominent AI flow is seen. TOP RIGHT, Continuous wave Doppler spectral display of AI flow. The AI jet has a steep deceleration time, lower early and particularly late diastolic velocities, consistent with low blood pressure and near-equilibration of the aortic and left ventricular pressure by end-diastole, consistent with severe AI. MIDDLE LEFT, Suprasternal view. An intimal flap is seen at the aortic arch level. MIDDLE RIGHT, Suprasternal view. Spectral display of flow in the proximal descending aorta. A large (VTI > 13 cm) amount of flow reversal is seen at the distal arch level, consistent with severe AI. BOTTOM LEFT, Subcostal spectral display of flow in the abdominal aorta. There is diastolic reversal of flow in the abdominal aorta (seen beneath the baseline) indicative of severe AI. BOTTOM RIGHT, Subcostal view. A circumferential pericardial effusion is present, with right atrial collapse. On this view, the right ventricle is small but is not collapsing.

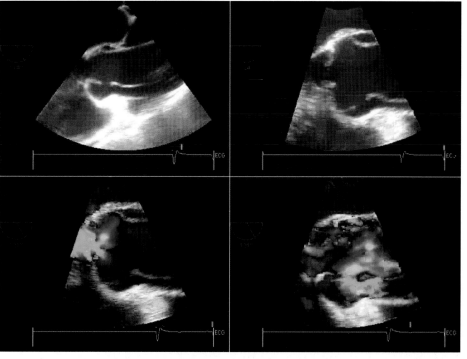

Figure 4-55. TEE. Longitudinal views of the aortic valve and root. TOP IMAGES, The intimal flap extends down into the root, and the intimal tear is located at the level of the sinotubular junction on the anterior aspect of the aorta. BOTTOM LEFT, Diastolic image shows severe aortic valve insufficiency. BOTTOM RIGHT, Entry of blood through the intimal tear into the false lumen is demonstrated.

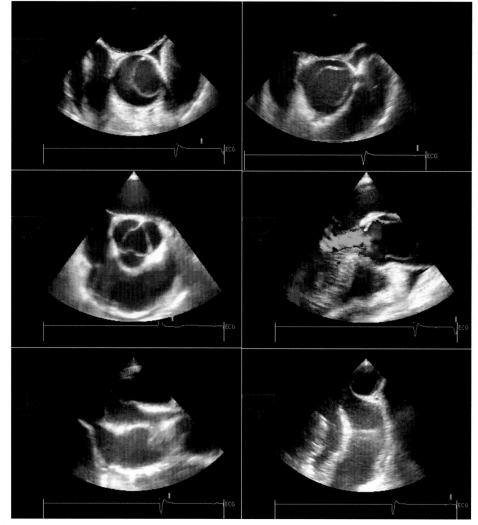

Figure 4-56. TEE. TOP LEFT, Cross-sectional view of the aortic root. The intimal flap involves two thirds of the circumference of the aortic root. TOP RIGHT, Cross-sectional view of the aortic root. A near-circumferential dissection flap at the root level is present. The flap is very close to the left main coronary artery seen at the 3-o'clock position from the root. MIDDLE LEFT, Short-axis view of the aortic valve. The aortic valve is clearly trileaflet. The false lumen does not extend down to this level, nor is the flap seen to prolapse into the valve orifice. The pericardial effusion is seen, with a very small amount of diastolic collapse. MIDDLE RIGHT, Longitudinal view of the aortic valve and root. The intimal flap extends down into the root, and there is severe AI. BOTTOM LEFT, Bicaval view showing right atrium and cavae. A pericardial effusion causing right atrial collapse is present. BOTTOM RIGHT, Cross-sectional view of the descending aorta. No intimal flap is seen in the mid descending aorta. A large left pleural effusion is present.

CASE 6

History

▸ A 76-year-old woman with hypertension presented to a community hospital emergency department with chest pain.
▸ Pulmonary embolism was suspected, and heparin and clopidogrel were started.
▸ An echocardiogram detected an intimal flap, confirmed by CT scanning, and she was transferred for further evaluation and management.

Physical Examination

▸ BP 180/90 mm Hg
▸ No pericardial rub or signs of tamponade
▸ No AI murmur or signs of left-sided heart failure
▸ No pulse deficits or BP differential

Comments

▸ Type A AAD in a previously hypertensive patient
▸ Ambiguous presentation, mistaken initial diagnosis and treatment
▸ Entry tear seen in the arch
▸ Surgery involved tube graft replacement down to the aortic sinuses (valve sparing) and replacement of half of the arch (hemiarch) to exclude the intimal tear from the aorta. As the tear was on the inferior aspect of the arch, the arch vessels were left on an island that was sewn as a single piece into the tube graft.
▸ Surprisingly, despite the clopidogrel, hemostasis was not a problem. Steady recovery—discharged eventually, with better BP control.

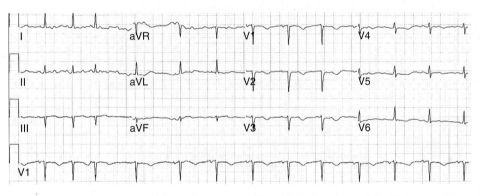

Figure 4-57. ECG shows sinus rhythm with premature atrial complexes, nonspecific repolarization abnormalities that are consistent with ischemia. There is a possible septal infarct and a prolonged QT.

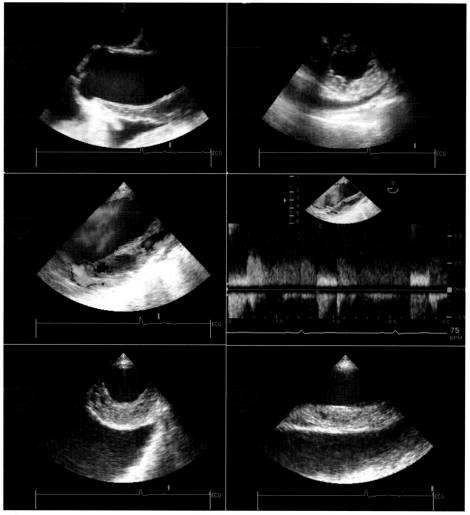

Figure 4-58. TEE images. TOP LEFT, Longitudinal view of the aortic valve and root. The aorta is dilated in its root and ascending portions. The anterior wall is thickened and appears thrombosed: intramural hematoma versus thrombosed false lumen. There is a pericardial effusion. TOP RIGHT, Transgastric short-axis view of the heart. There is LVH and a small pericardial effusion. MIDDLE LEFT, Horizontal plane view of the arch. There is a flap in the anterior arch with a partially thrombosed false lumen. The entry tear into the false lumen is depicted. There is a small amount of flow in the nonthrombosed false lumen. MIDDLE RIGHT, Spectral display of flow at the entry tear. In systole, there is flow into the false lumen. In diastole, the flow reciprocates and exits through the intimal tear. To-and-fro flow. BOTTOM LEFT, Cross-sectional view of the descending aorta. The false lumen is predominantly thrombosed. Left pleural effusion. BOTTOM RIGHT, Longitudinal view of the descending aorta. There is a predominantly thrombosed false lumen (or adventitial hematoma) in the descending aorta. Left pleural effusion.

CASE 7

History and Physical Examination

▸ A 75-year-old man with a history of hypertension treated with monotherapy presented with sudden onset of severe chest and back pain associated with dyspnea.
▸ BP 110/70 mm Hg, HR 90 bpm, RR 20/min
▸ No pericardial rub, no signs of tamponade
▸ AI murmur present
▸ Crepitations bilaterally and increased respiratory effort
▸ No pulse deficits or BP differential

Management and Outcome

▸ Given the cardiogenic shock and ongoing deterioration, the patient was taken directly to the operating room within 75 minutes of arrival.
▸ Surgical findings were a type A dissection, flail aortic valve leaflets, and dissection flap extending into the left main coronary artery.

▸ Bentall procedure (composite tube graft, aortic valve replacement) with reimplantation of the coronaries was performed.
▸ Perioperative stroke prolonged ventilator time, but the patient survived.

Comments

▸ Type A AAD in a previously hypertensive man complicated by severe left main coronary artery disruption, myocardial ischemia, and cardiogenic shock
▸ The myocardial ischemia was not present initially but developed within an hour of arrival, underscoring the progressive nature of complications of type A AAD.
▸ The low-normal initial BP and the pulmonary edema attest to the severity of the AI and the elevation of clinical risk in this previously hypertensive patient.
▸ The hemodynamic deterioration underscores the need for rapid evaluation and treatment of AAD cases, especially those with complications.

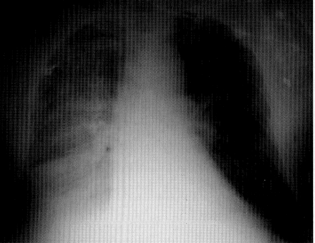

Figure 4-59. Chest radiograph shows a normal cardiopericardial silhouette, no definite aortic abnormalities, and interstitial infiltrates.

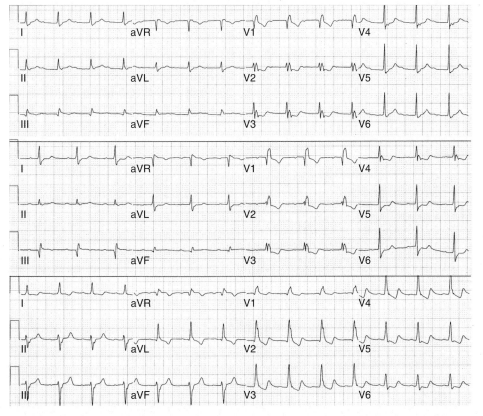

Figure 4-60. ECG evolution. TOP, At arrival in the emergency department, the ECG shows sinus rhythm with first-degree atrioventricular block and right bundle branch block (RBBB) with secondary repolarization disturbances. MIDDLE, Thirty minutes later, the tracing shows sinus rhythm with first-degree atrioventricular block, RBBB with secondary repolarization disturbances, and evolving lateral repolarization abnormalities not secondary to the RBBB, indicative of possible myocardial ischemia. BOTTOM, Sixty minutes later, there is sinus rhythm with first-degree atrioventricular block, RBBB with secondary repolarization disturbances, and worsened lateral repolarization abnormalities not secondary to the RBBB, consistent with myocardial ischemia.

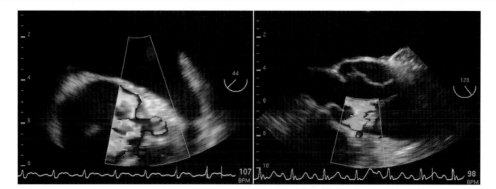

Figure 4-61. TEE views of the aortic root. LEFT, Oblique plane to image the flow into the left main coronary artery. The intimal flap extends to the ostium of the left main coronary artery. RIGHT, Vertical view of the anterior wall of the aorta to image the right coronary ostium. The intimal flap also extends to the right coronary artery.

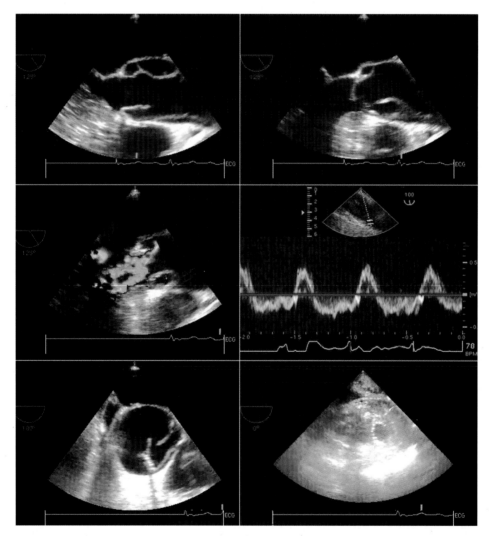

Figure 4-62. TEE images. TOP, Longitudinal views of the aortic valve and root. The intimal flap extends down through the root into the aortic valve annulus. In systole (LEFT), the true lumen is pressurized and the intimal flap is away from the aortic valve. In diastole (RIGHT), the true lumen depressurizes (partly due to AI), and the flap moves into the aortic valve. One cusp of the aortic valve is severely prolapsing and flail from dehiscence because of the intimal flap extension into its sinus of Valsalva. MIDDLE LEFT, Severe AI arising from aortic leaflet cusp prolapse and flail. MIDDLE RIGHT, Spectral display of flow in the abdominal aorta. There is holodiastolic flow reversal consistent with severe AI. BOTTOM LEFT, The aortic root in cross section. The intimal tear and the intimal flap are imaged. BOTTOM RIGHT, Transgastric short-axis view of the left ventricle shows concentric LVH and no significant pericardial effusion.

4

CASE 8

History and Physical Examination

▸ A 73-year-old man with a history of hypertension presented with severe sudden-onset chest and back pain, with dyspnea and presyncope.
▸ On physical examination, the patient was distressed, with cool extremities.
▸ BP 100/60 mm Hg, HR 110 bpm
▸ Short murmur of AI
▸ No pericardial rub or signs of tamponade
▸ No crepitations, pulse deficits, or BP differential

Evolution and Outcome

▸ Severe and refractory cardiogenic shock
▸ The patient died within 3 hours of presentation and within 4 hours of pain onset.

Comments

▸ Type A AAD in a previously hypertensive patient complicated by acute severe AI, left coronary artery disruption with myocardial ischemia, and cardiogenic shock
▸ The patient died within 4 hours of pain onset despite resuscitation efforts, underscoring the instability of a subset of AAD cases.
▸ The systolic BP of 100 mm Hg on presentation was misleading in regard to the actual tissue perfusion and severity of pulmonary edema, particularly in a previously hypertensive patient with pain.
▸ Presentation of AAD *without hypertension* predicts high early mortality.

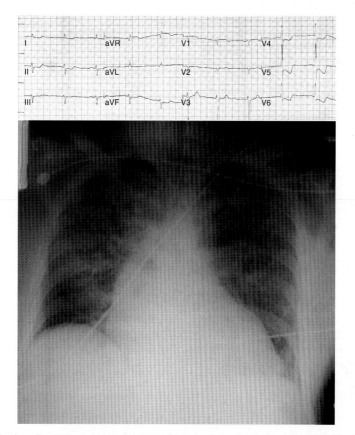

Figure 4-63. TOP, ECG shows sinus bradycardia, ST depression consistent with ischemia and subendocardial infarction. The ST depression is not characteristic of strain from LVH. BOTTOM, Chest radiograph shows an increased cardiopericardial silhouette and severe interstitial and alveolar pulmonary edema.

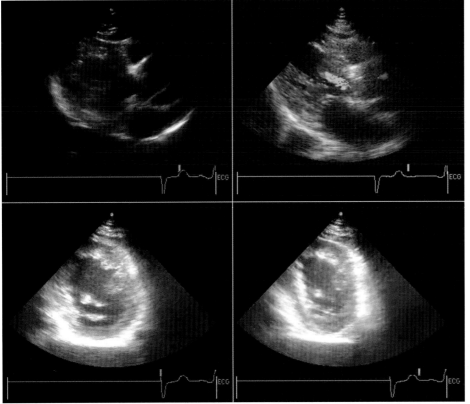

Figure 4-64. TOP LEFT, TTE parasternal long-axis views. The aorta is dilated in its root and ascending portions, and there is effacement of the sinotubular junction. A flap is present in the root. There is anteroseptal akinesis. TOP RIGHT, TTE with color Doppler mapping shows AI. BOTTOM, Parasternal short-axis views in diastole (LEFT) and systole (RIGHT). The entire anterior and lateral territories are akinetic. The inferior wall is hypokinetic.

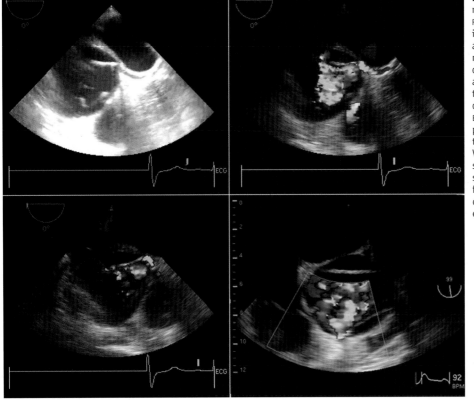

Figure 4-65. TEE images of the aortic root. TOP LEFT, Two-dimensional image. TOP RIGHT, With color Doppler mapping. The intimal flap extends down into the root and is directly at the ostium to the left main coronary artery. Systolic flow is detected within the left main coronary artery. The intimal flap partitions flow in the root. Flow across the entry tear is just depicted (at the 12-o'clock position). BOTTOM LEFT, Diastolic frame shows a less prominent flow in the true lumen and in the left main coronary. BOTTOM RIGHT, Vertical plane view of the aortic root to show the anterior wall. The intimal flap is seen both posteriorly and anteriorly. The flap extends to the ostium of the right coronary artery on the anterior wall, whose entrant flow is depicted.

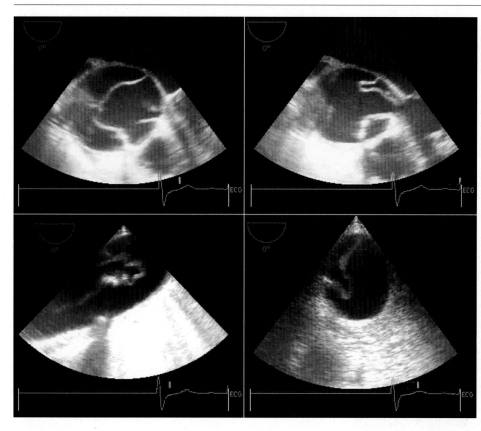

Figure 4-66. TEE images. TOP LEFT, Systole. The intimal flap extends around most of the circumference of the aortic root. TOP RIGHT, Diastole. The intimal flap prolapses into the aortic valve in diastole. BOTTOM LEFT, Horizontal plane view of the aortic arch. The intimal flap is extensive. There is intimal (luminal) displacement of a large calcified plaque in the distal arch. BOTTOM RIGHT, Cross-sectional view of the mid descending thoracic aorta. The intimal flap is present. No pleural effusion.

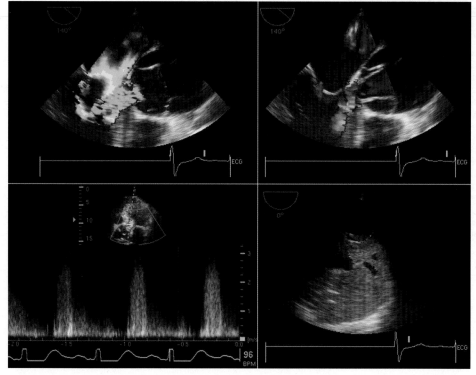

Figure 4-67. TEE images. TOP, Longitudinal views of the aortic valve and root in early diastole (LEFT) and late diastole (RIGHT). In early diastole, the intimal flap is away from the aortic valve and there is severe AI. In late diastole, the flap has prolapsed into the aortic valve and there is little AI. BOTTOM LEFT, Spectral display of AI. The velocities are very low, caused by shock, and the deceleration time is extremely steep because of diastolic equilibration of aortic and left ventricular diastolic pressures. Furthermore, the signal intensity diminishes abruptly, interestingly when the flap prolapsed into and plugged the aortic valve. BOTTOM RIGHT, Horizontal view of the left hemithorax and the left pleural cavity. The left lung is so edematous that it has the same appearance that liver usually does (hepatization). The flow within the pulmonary artery and veins is seen as the extreme pulmonary edema is transmitting ultrasound signal and Doppler shift.

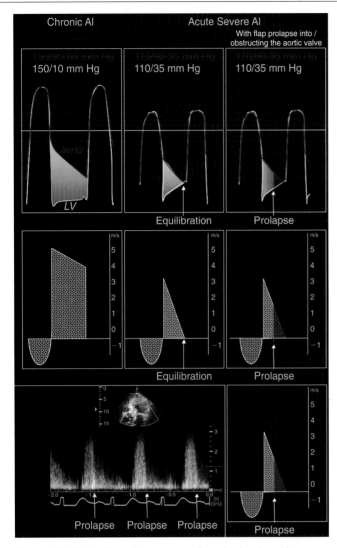

Figure 4-68. Illustrations of pressure waveforms in chronic aortic insufficiency (AI) and in severe (torrential) acute AI. The illustrations on the left side depict the unusual AI spectral flow pattern seen in this case (BOTTOM LEFT). In usual chronic AI, there is a sustained aorta to left ventricle (LV) gradient through diastole, and the aortic and LV pressures do not approximate as the compliance of the LV is adequate to receive the volume, which is not excessive. As the aortic pressure remains above the LV pressure, the sustained gradient results in a Doppler spectral profile (MIDDLE) that is sustained through diastole, that has a relatively shallow slope, and that has high velocity due to the magnitude of the driving gradient. In acute severe torrential AI, the magnitude of the regurgitant volume of AI and the limited LV compliance result in rapidly falling aortic pressure and rapidly rising LV pressure that equilibrate and eliminate the driving gradient. The spectral profile reflects the rapid decay in aortic to LV gradient and has a steep slope. In this case, the torrential AI drew the aortic intimal flap into the aortic valve, obstructing it in mid-diastole. The spectral profile weakens at the time of prolapse, resulting in a distinctly short murmur of AI.

CASE 9

History and Physical Examination

▸ An 87-year-old man with a history of hypertension presented with fatigue and dyspnea 5 days after a chest pain episode.
▸ BP 120/70 mm Hg, HR 60 bpm
▸ AI murmur present
▸ No venous distention, pulsus, or rub; no pulse deficits
▸ No signs of left-sided heart failure

Evolution and Outcome

▸ Given the advanced age of the patient and the "self-selection" of a survivor of 5 days, medical therapy was adopted.
▸ The patient survived to hospital discharge, lived for 3 additional years, and died of other causes.

Comments

▸ Late presentation type A dissection in a previously hypertensive patient
▸ The entry tear may have been in the arch as seen on the CT image.
▸ The intimal displacement was particularly obvious as the age-related intimal calcification was more advanced than in most (younger) patients.
▸ Despite many side branches being involved, there was no organ or tissue underperfusion.
▸ There was no in-hospital progression of the AI or the pericardial effusion.
▸ The previous hypertension appeared to be gone as a result of the AI.

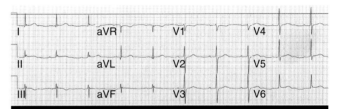

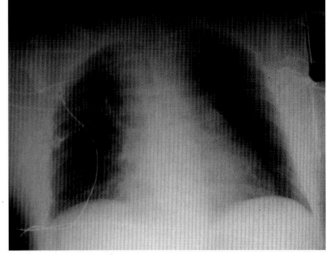

Figure 4-69. TOP, The 12-lead ECG shows sinus bradycardia with nonspecific repolarization abnormalities and no definite criteria of LVH. BOTTOM, Anteroposterior chest radiograph. The cardiopericardial silhouette is mildly enlarged, as the mediastinum is mildly widened. No left pleural effusion, and no radiographic signs of left-sided heart failure.

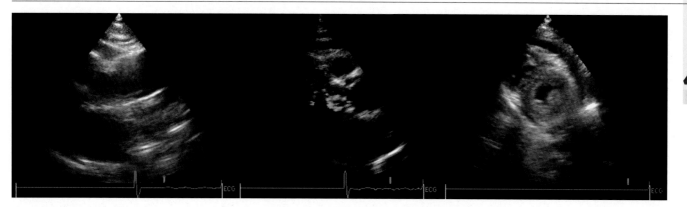

Figure 4-70. TTE. LEFT, Parasternal long-axis view. There is a flap in the aortic root along the posterior wall. There is concentric LVH. MIDDLE, Parasternal long-axis view with color Doppler mapping. There is AI. The mechanism is unclear. RIGHT, Parasternal short-axis view. The LV is clearly dynamic. There is a small pericardial effusion.

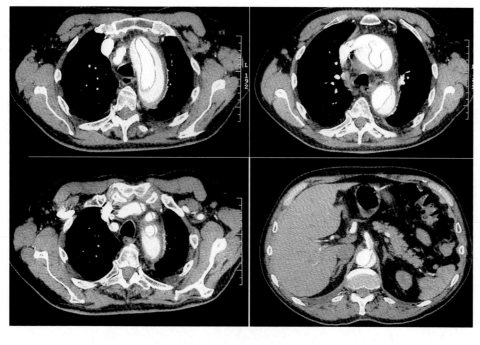

Figure 4-71. Contrast-enhanced axial CT scans. TOP, An intimal flap is present in the arch, the ascending and descending thoracic and abdominal aorta. There is a tear at the arch level. The flap has extended up the arch branch vessels (BOTTOM RIGHT) and up the superior mesenteric artery (BOTTOM LEFT). No pleural effusion.

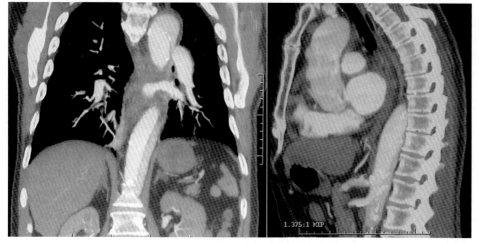

Figure 4-72. Contrast-enhanced CT scans. LEFT, Coronal image. RIGHT, Sagittal image. The intimal flap and the true and false lumens can be well seen. There is obvious displacement of intimal calcification, especially in the proximal descending aorta and abdominal aorta.

CASE 10

History and Physical Examination

▸ A 45-year-old man with a long history of IV drug and alcohol abuse presented with an aphasia after using crack cocaine.
▸ He was known to have hepatitis A, B, C, and D and cirrhosis and chronic hypertension.
▸ A non–contrast-enhanced head CT scan ordered in the emergency department identified an intimal flap in both carotid arteries that was confirmed with contrast-enhanced images.
▸ There was a 40 mm Hg BP differential between the arms (R > L).

Evolution and Outcome

▸ Surgical repair was not offered because of the advanced cirrhosis.
▸ The neurologic deficits resolved entirely within a week, and repeated imaging did not demonstrate evolution or complication.

Comments

▸ Type A AAD with neurologic sequelae
▸ Chest radiograph findings normal
▸ Intimal tear in the ascending aorta, with false lumen extension into the arch and arch vessels
▸ AAD associated with crack cocaine abuse
▸ Survival, unoperated on

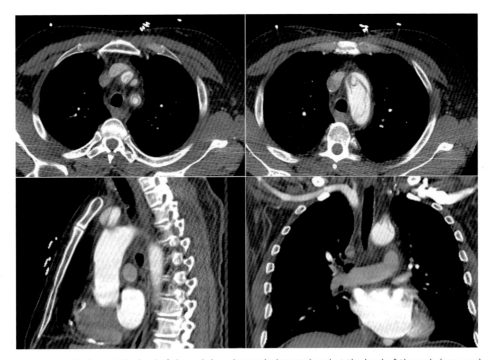

Figure 4-73. Contrast-enhanced axial views at the level of the arch branch vessels (TOP LEFT) and at the level of the arch (TOP RIGHT). Circumferential intimal flaps are present in the innominate artery and the left subclavian artery. BOTTOM LEFT, Sagittal view of the arch and the innominate artery revealing the intimal flap extending into the innominate artery. BOTTOM RIGHT, Coronal view again revealing the aortic intimal tear intussuscepting into the innominate artery.

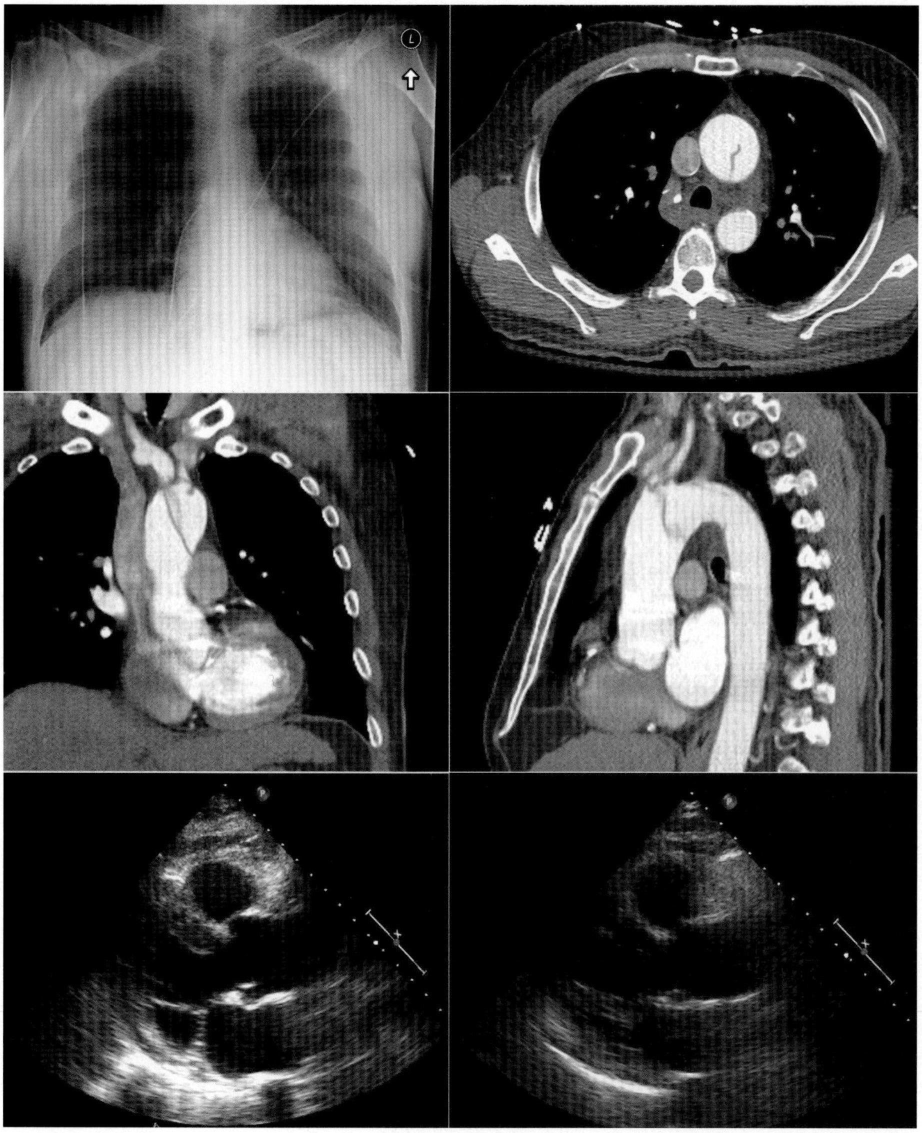

Figure 4-74. TOP LEFT, Chest radiograph. The aortic size and contour are normal. There are no signs of dissection. TOP RIGHT, Contrast-enhanced axial CT scan revealing the intimal tear and flap in the upper ascending aorta. MIDDLE, Coronal view (LEFT) and sagittal view (RIGHT) again show the intimal flap in the upper ascending aorta and arch but not in the descending aorta. BOTTOM, TTE, which did not image an intimal flap in the root or ascending aorta because of the flap's being located in the upper ascending aorta away from the field of view.

CASE 11

History and Physical Examination

▶ A 55-year-old man with chronic hypertension presented with aphasia and may have had chest pain at the onset.
▶ There was a right radial pulse deficit.
▶ He rapidly obtunded, requiring airway support.

Evolution

▶ Progressive brain death due to cerebral infarction and uncal herniation, by hour 40

Comments

▶ Type A AAD with cerebral infarction
▶ Painless dissection associated with cerebral ischemia

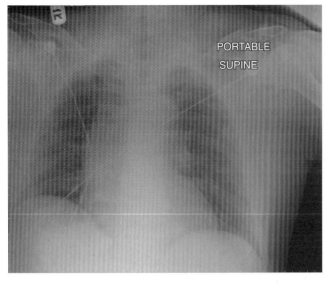

Figure 4-75. Chest radiograph shows a widened mediastinum. There are no pleural effusions or pleural cap.

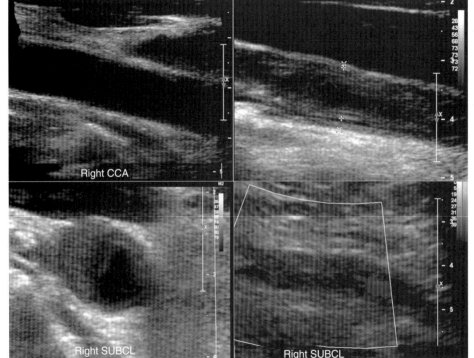

Figure 4-76. Carotid artery ultrasound images. TOP LEFT, The upper right common carotid artery (CCA) is normal. TOP RIGHT, The lower right common artery is obstructed by a thrombosed false lumen, leaving a minimal slit of a lumen. BOTTOM LEFT, Cross-sectional view of the right subclavian artery revealing a thrombosed false lumen occupying more than half of the lumen. BOTTOM RIGHT, There is an absence of flow in the right subclavian artery.

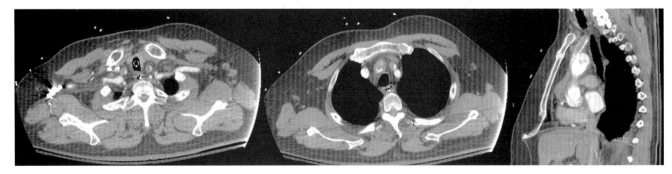

Figure 4-77. Contrast-enhanced CT scans. LEFT, Axial cut at the level of the arch branch vessels. The carotid arteries are partially occluded bilaterally. MIDDLE, The innominate artery and the left carotid artery are both partially obstructed. RIGHT, Sagittal view revealing an intimal flap in the aortic root and ascending aorta, extending into the innominate artery, with thrombosis of the false lumen.

4

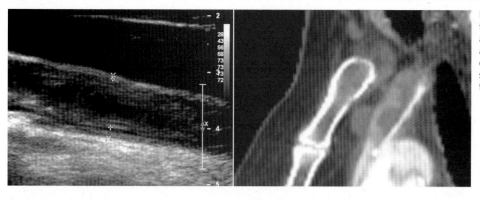

Figure 4-78. Views of the dissected and thrombosed innominate and right carotid arteries. LEFT, Ultrasound image. RIGHT, CT angiogram. In both images, the thrombosis of the false lumen is apparent, and there is some similarity of the texture of the thrombosed false lumen.

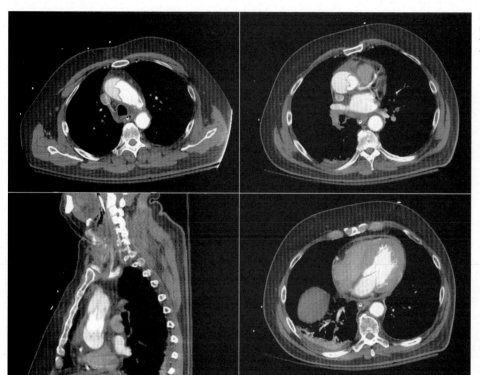

Figure 4-79. Contrast-enhanced CT scans revealing the intimal flap and false lumen in the ascending aorta and arch, but not in the descending aorta.

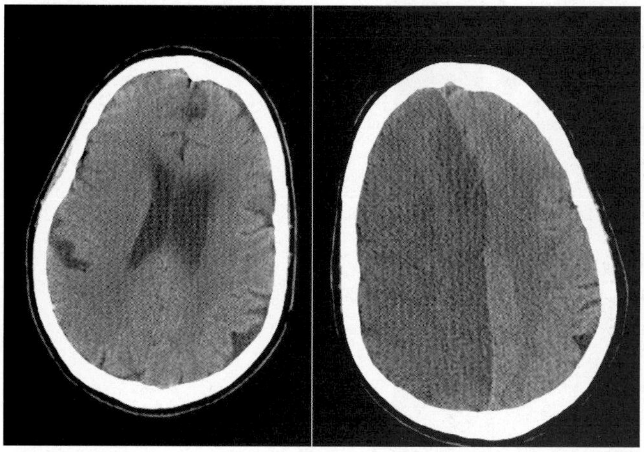

Figure 4-80. Non–contrast-enhanced axial CT scans of the head at presentation with aphasia (LEFT) and 36 hours later (RIGHT). Within this period, there has been hemispheric infarction with gross edema; effacement of the sulci, gyri, and ventricles; and midline shift.

CASE 12

History and Physical Examination

▸ A 63-year-old woman with polycystic kidneys, hypertension, and renal failure was evaluated for ischemic heart disease, which identified CCS class II angina and a low-risk perfusion abnormality on nuclear testing.

▸ The ascending aorta was also noted to be dilated, and the aortic valve was trileaflet and moderately insufficient.

▸ As the aortic valve was not severely insufficient and the ascending aorta was dilated less than 55 mm, no surgery was offered.

Evolution and Outcome

▸ Six months later, she was received in transfer with severe chest pain and hypotension (75/50 mm Hg).

▸ She underwent emergency surgery that identified a poorly contracting right ventricle, the intimal tear above the right coronary artery, and tamponade due to blood.

▸ Surgical repair was performed, but the right ventricle was entirely akinetic postoperatively, leading to insufficient output and early death.

Comments

▸ The asymptomatic dilation of the aortic root, confirmed by both echocardiography and CT to be below the standard surgical threshold of 55 mm, proceeded to dissect, demonstrating that the 55-mm threshold does not apply perfectly to all cases.

▸ Further considerations of the 55-mm threshold should include indexing it to body size (the patient was petite in stature) and allowing a degree of intertest and intratest variability in determining the diameter of the aorta as well as systolic:diastolic variations of the diameter. The validity of the 55-mm threshold was recently questioned.[47]

▸ The patient's blood pressure was also known to be variable, imperfectly controlled. Hypotension is predictive of high mortality, which in this case was due to both tamponade and right ventricular systolic dysfunction. The right ventricular dysfunction was due to right coronary ischemia, which was compounded by poor pump protection.

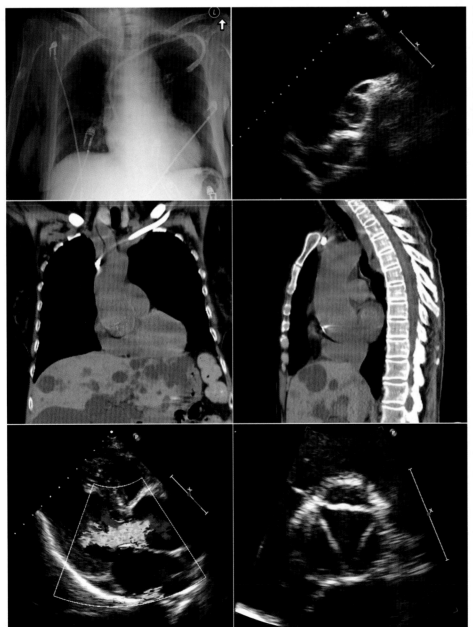

Figure 4-81. TOP LEFT, Chest radiograph revealing dilation of the ascending aorta and a dialysis catheter. TOP RIGHT, Transthoracic (right) parasternal image revealing the dilated ascending aorta and absence of an intimal flap or wall hematoma. MIDDLE, Non–contrast-enhanced CT scans revealing the dilated ascending aorta. BOTTOM, TTE images confirming that the aortic valve is trileaflet and insufficient.

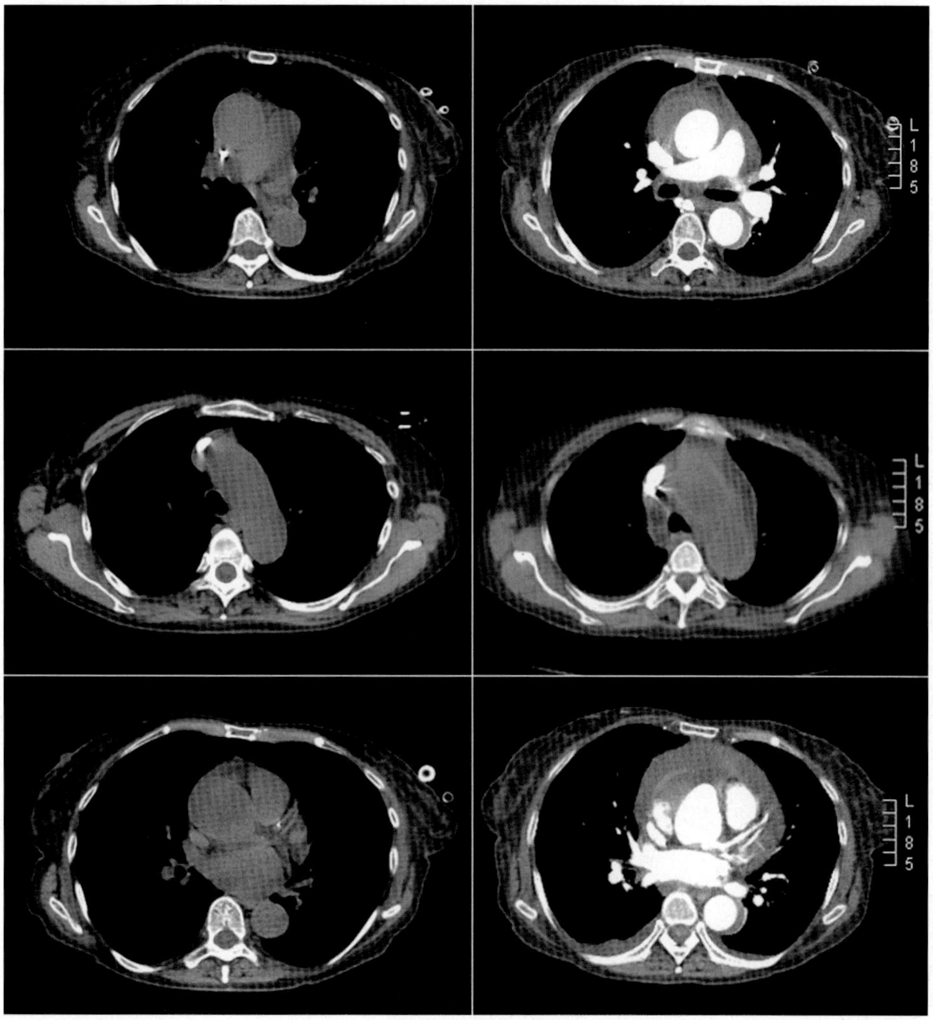

Figure 4-82. CT scans before (LEFT IMAGES) and after (RIGHT IMAGES) AAD. Because of renal insufficiency, the pre-AAD scan was performed without the administration of contrast material. The pre-AAD images demonstrate dilation (50 to 52 mm) of the ascending aorta. There is only mild dilation of the aortic arch. The contrast-enhanced images obtained at the presentation with AAD reveal a crescentic thrombosed false lumen in the aortic root, in the arch, and also in the proximal descending aorta. There is adventitial hematoma along the aortic arch anterior wall. The proximal left coronary artery is unremarkable. The proximal right coronary artery has been partially avulsed off the intimal flap, resulting in the small area of opacification of the false lumen adjacent to its origin.

CASE 13

History and Physical Examination

▸ A 46-year-old man collapsed after taking a large amount of crack cocaine.
▸ He had a long history of drinking, smoking, and drug abuse as well as hepatitis, cirrhosis, and COPD.
▸ After regaining consciousness, he had an expressive aphasia.
▸ On physical examination, he was hypertensive (220/120 mm Hg) and tachycardic (140 bpm).
▸ No murmurs or pulse deficits were noted.
▸ His chest radiograph and TTE were unremarkable.
▸ On the second hospital day, he was able to communicate that he had chest pain, which prompted a CT scan.

Management and Evolution

▸ Clinical impression was that of a type A AAD, with associated stroke.
▸ The neurologic deficits improved steadily and resolved by day 10.
▸ The patient was declined for surgery because of the advanced cirrhosis.

Comments

▸ Crack cocaine–associated AAD
▸ Syncope presentation
▸ Initially painless dissection due to the syncope, and subsequent aphasia
▸ Delay in diagnosis due to painless presentation
▸ Survival to discharge on medical treatment alone

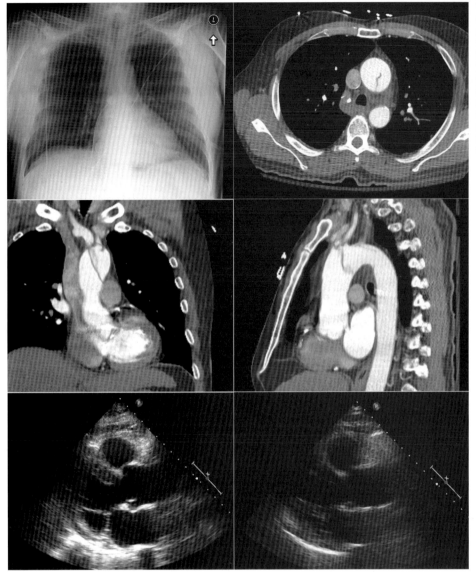

Figure 4-83. TOP LEFT, Normal anteroposterior chest radiograph, without an enlarged aorta, abnormal contour, or pleural effusions. TOP RIGHT AND MIDDLE, Contrast-enhanced CT scans reveal an intimal flap and tear in the upper ascending aorta extending into the arch but not into the descending aorta. A standard parasternal echocardiographic view (BOTTOM LEFT) and a high parasternal view (BOTTOM RIGHT) do not reveal the intimal flap located more distally. Arch views were not useful in this case.

CASE 14

History and Physical Examination

▸ A 67-year-old woman with a history of smoking and hypertension collapsed on getting up from bed.
▸ She regained consciousness 30 minutes later and complained of chest pain.
▸ No murmurs, pulse deficits, or venous distention initially
▸ BP was low at 80/50 mm Hg.

Management and Evolution

▸ Pulmonary embolism was considered, as the chest radiograph was clear.
▸ A CT scan of the chest detected an intimal flap beginning in the ascending aorta, a pericardial effusion, and underperfusion of one kidney.
▸ She was transferred for surgery.
▸ AI murmur, asymmetric arm pulses, and jugular venous distention were now present.
▸ Arterial line was inserted into the arm with lower blood pressure (35 mm Hg less).

Comments

▸ Type A AAD with multiple complications: AI, tamponade, myocardial ischemia, and malperfusion (renal, limb, and probably cerebral)
▸ No physical diagnosis findings (murmur of AI, venous distention, and pulse deficits) were noted initially.
▸ Syncope presentation caused a delay in diagnosis.
▸ Although it is attractive, valve-sparing surgery does have early and late failures.

4

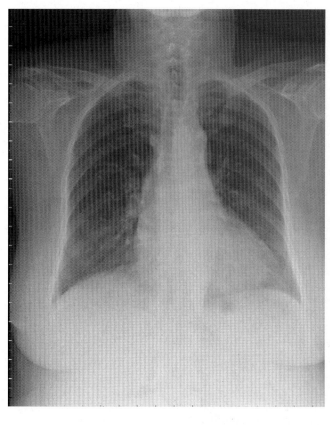

Figure 4-84. Chest radiograph shows that the ascending aorta is mildly dilated, but the arch is not, nor is the descending portion. There is no apparent intimal displacement and no pleural effusion.

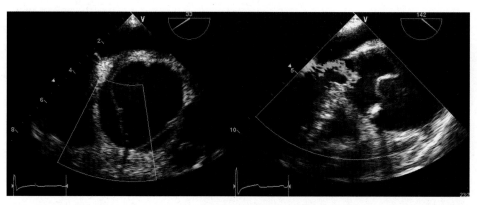

Figure 4-85. TEE images. Short-axis view at the aortic root level (LEFT IMAGE) and long-axis view also at the aortic root level (RIGHT IMAGE). The intimal flap has extended down into half of the circumference of the aortic root. There is severe AI. The intimal flap has displaced calcium into the root.

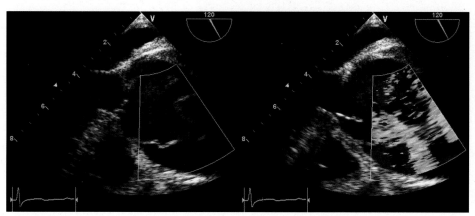

Figure 4-86. TEE images reveal that the intimal tear is located in the ascending aorta over the anterior wall. With systole, there is a jet of flow into the false lumen through the intimal tear.

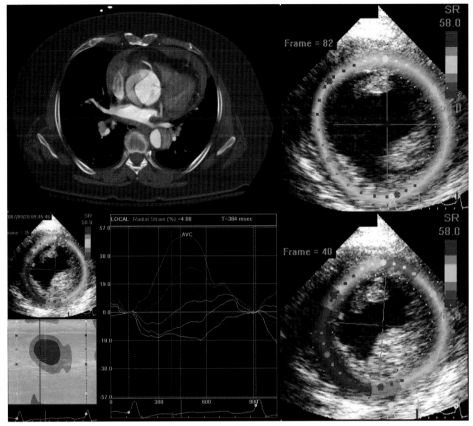

Figure 4-87. TOP LEFT, Contrast-enhanced CT scan at the aortic root level demonstrating the intimal flap extending to the origin of the right coronary artery. TOP RIGHT, Color-coded short-axis radial strain in diastole is normal. BOTTOM RIGHT, image in systole. There is dyskinesis of the inferior and inferolateral walls. BOTTOM LEFT, Radial strain tracing demonstrating negative radial strain in the inferoposterior walls.

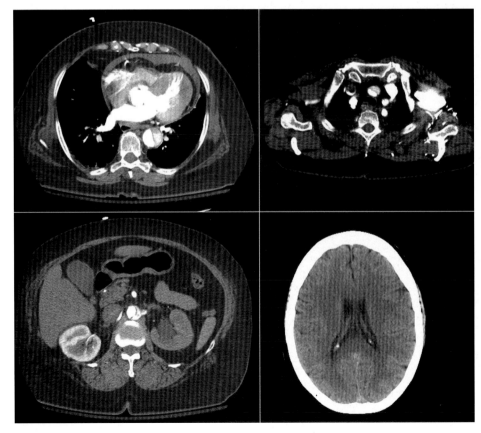

Figure 4-88. Contrast-enhanced axial CT scans. TOP LEFT, At the level of the outflow tracts. There is a prominent pericardial effusion and collapse of the right ventricular free wall. The intimal flap and the true and false lumens are obvious in the descending aorta. TOP RIGHT, At the level of the arch vessels. Intimal flaps are present in the brachiocephalic and left common carotid arteries but not in the left subclavian artery. There is prominent dye streaming in the SVC. BOTTOM LEFT, The left renal artery arises from the false lumen. The left kidney opacifies far less than does the right kidney. BOTTOM RIGHT, No bleed or early signs of infarction.

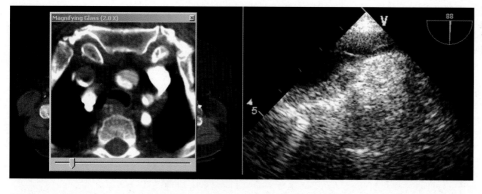

Figure 4-89. The contrast-enhanced CT scan (LEFT) does not demonstrate a flap into the left subclavian artery, but the TEE performed 6 hours later (RIGHT) does.

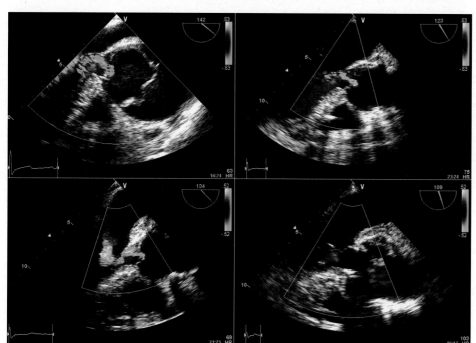

Figure 4-90. TEE images taken at four different times. TOP LEFT, Before the first surgery. The aortic root but even more the ascending aorta are dilated, and there is effacement of the sinotubular junction. There is severe AI. TOP RIGHT, After the first surgery (tube graft replacement of the ascending aorta and resuspension of the aortic valve), there is mild AI. The bottom images were taken on the following day. BOTTOM LEFT, Before the second surgery. The AI is severe again. BOTTOM RIGHT, After aortic valve replacement. There is no more AI.

References

1. Nienaber CA, Eagle KA: Aortic dissection: new frontiers in diagnosis and management: Part I: from etiology to diagnostic strategies. Circulation 2003;108:628-635.

2. Nienaber CA, Fattori R, Mehta RH, et al: Gender-related differences in acute aortic dissection. Circulation 2004;109:3014-3021.

3. Januzzi JL, Isselbacher EM, Fattori R, et al: Characterizing the young patient with aortic dissection: results from the International Registry of Aortic Dissection (IRAD). J Am Coll Cardiol 2004;43:665-669.

4. Hsue PY, Salinas CL, Bolger AF, et al: Acute aortic dissection related to crack cocaine. Circulation 2002;105:1592-1595.

5. Eagle KA, Isselbacher EM, DeSanctis RW: Cocaine-related aortic dissection in perspective. Circulation 2002;105:1529-1530.

6. Collins JS, Evangelista A, Nienaber CA, et al: Differences in clinical presentation, management, and outcomes of acute type a aortic dissection in patients with and without previous cardiac surgery. Circulation 2004; 110(Suppl 1):II237-II242.

7. Mehta RH, Manfredini R, Hassan F, et al: Chronobiological patterns of acute aortic dissection. Circulation 2002;106:1110-1115.

8. Mehta RH, Manfredini R, Bossone E, et al: The winter peak in the occurrence of acute aortic dissection is independent of climate. Chronobiol Int 2005;22:723-729.

9. Hagan PG, Nienaber CA, Isselbacher EM, et al: The International Registry of Acute Aortic Dissection (IRAD): new insights into an old disease. JAMA 2000;283:897-903.

10. Mehta RH, Suzuki T, Hagan PG, et al: Predicting death in patients with acute type a aortic dissection. Circulation 2002;105:200-206.

11. Mehta RH, O'Gara PT, Bossone E, et al: Acute type A aortic dissection in the elderly: clinical characteristics, management, and outcomes in the current era. J Am Coll Cardiol 2002;40:685-692.

12. Ehrlich MP, Schillinger M, Grabenwoger M, et al: Predictors of adverse outcome and transient neurological dysfunction following surgical treatment of acute type A dissections. Circulation 2003;108(Suppl 1):II318-II323.

13. Heegaard AM, Corsi A, Danielsen CC, et al: Biglycan deficiency causes spontaneous aortic dissection and rupture in mice. Circulation 2007;115:2731-2738.

14. Januzzi JL, Sabatine MS, Eagle KA, et al: Iatrogenic aortic dissection. Am J Cardiol 2002;89:623-626.

15. Svensson LG, Labib SB, Eisenhauer AC, Butterly JR: Intimal tear without hematoma: an important variant of aortic dissection that can elude current imaging techniques. Circulation 1999;99:1331-1336.

16. Gorospe L, Sendino A, Pacheco R, et al: Chronic aortic dissection as a cause of fever of unknown origin. South Med J 2002;95:1067-1070.

17. Upchurch GR Jr, Nienaber C, Fattori R, et al: Acute aortic dissection presenting with primarily abdominal pain: a rare manifestation of a deadly disease. Ann Vasc Surg 2005;19:367-373.

18. Bossone E, Rampoldi V, Nienaber CA, et al: Usefulness of pulse deficit to predict in-hospital complications and mortality in patients with acute type A aortic dissection. Am J Cardiol 2002;89:851-855.

19. Beckman JA, Mehta RH, Isselbacher EM, et al: Branch vessel complications are increased in aortic dissection patients with renal insufficiency. Vasc Med 2004 November;9(4):267-270.

20. Moore AG, Eagle KA, Bruckman D, et al: Choice of computed tomography, transesophageal echocardiography, magnetic resonance imaging, and aortography in acute aortic dissection: International Registry of Acute Aortic Dissection (IRAD). Am J Cardiol 2002;89:1235-1238.

21. Hansen MS, Nogareda GJ, Hutchison SJ: Frequency of and inappropriate treatment of misdiagnosis of acute aortic dissection. Am J Cardiol 2007;99: 852-856.

22. von Kodolitsch Y, Nienaber CA, Dieckmann C, et al: Chest radiography for the diagnosis of acute aortic syndrome. Am J Med 2004;116:73-77.

23. Batra P, Bigoni B, Manning J, et al: Pitfalls in the diagnosis of thoracic aortic dissection at CT angiography. Radiographics 2000;20:309-320.

24. LePage MA, Quint LE, Sonnad SS, et al: Aortic dissection: CT features that distinguish true lumen from false lumen. AJR Am J Roentgenol 2001;177: 207-211.

25. Kupersmith AC, Belkin RN, McClung JA, Moggio RA: Aortic valve commissural tear mimicking type A aortic dissection. J Am Soc Echocardiogr 2002;15:658-660.

26. Erbel R, Engberding R, Daniel W, et al: Echocardiography in diagnosis of aortic dissection. Lancet 1989;1:457-461.

27. Nienaber CA, Spielmann RP, von Kodolitsch Y, et al: Diagnosis of thoracic aortic dissection. Magnetic resonance imaging versus transesophageal echocardiography. Circulation 1992;85:434-447.

28. Ballal RS, Nanda NC, Gatewood R, et al: Usefulness of transesophageal echocardiography in assessment of aortic dissection. Circulation 1991;84: 1903-1914.

29. Keren A, Kim CB, Hu BS, et al: Accuracy of biplane and multiplane transesophageal echocardiography in diagnosis of typical acute aortic dissection and intramural hematoma. J Am Coll Cardiol 1996;28:627-636.

30. Bogaert J, Meyns B, Rademakers FE, et al: Follow-up of aortic dissection: contribution of MR angiography for evaluation of the abdominal aorta and its branches. Eur Radiol 1997;7:695-702.

31. Fann JI, Smith JA, Miller DC, et al: Surgical management of aortic dissection during a 30-year period. Circulation 1995;92(Suppl):II113-II121.

32. Lai DT, Robbins RC, Mitchell RS, et al: Does profound hypothermic circulatory arrest improve survival in patients with acute type a aortic dissection? Circulation 2002;106(Suppl 1):I218-I228.

33. Scholl FG, Coady MA, Davies R, et al: Interval or permanent nonoperative management of acute type A aortic dissection. Arch Surg 1999;134: 402-405.

34. Leyh RG, Fischer S, Kallenbach K, et al: High failure rate after valve-sparing aortic root replacement using the remodeling technique in acute type A aortic dissection. Circulation 2002;106(Suppl 1):I229-I233.

35. Elefteriades JA, Lovoulos CJ, Coady MA, et al: Management of descending aortic dissection. Ann Thorac Surg 1999;67:2002-2005.

36. Trimarchi S, Nienaber CA, Rampoldi V, et al: Role and results of surgery in acute type B aortic dissection: insights from the International Registry of Acute Aortic Dissection (IRAD). Circulation 2006;114(Suppl):I357-I364.

37. Isselbacher EM, Cigarroa JE, Eagle KA: Cardiac tamponade complicating proximal aortic dissection. Is pericardiocentesis harmful? Circulation 1994;90:2375-2378.

38. Ince H, Nienaber CA: The concept of interventional therapy in acute aortic syndrome. J Card Surg 2002;17:135-142.

39. Nienaber CA, Fattori R, Lund G, et al: Nonsurgical reconstruction of thoracic aortic dissection by stent-graft placement. N Engl J Med 1999;340: 1539-1545.

40. Dake MD, Kato N, Mitchell RS, et al: Endovascular stent-graft placement for the treatment of acute aortic dissection. N Engl J Med 1999;340:1546-1552.

41. Bortone AS, Schena S, D'Agostino D, et al: Immediate versus delayed endovascular treatment of post-traumatic aortic pseudoaneurysms and type B dissections: retrospective analysis and premises to the upcoming European trial. Circulation 2002;106(Suppl 1):I234-I240.

42. Shimono T, Kato N, Yasuda F, et al: Transluminal stent-graft placements for the treatments of acute onset and chronic aortic dissections. Circulation 2002;106(Suppl 1):I241-I247.

43. Henke PK, Williams DM, Upchurch GR Jr, et al: Acute limb ischemia associated with type B aortic dissection: clinical relevance and therapy. Surgery 2006;140:532-539.

44. Tsai TT, Evangelista A, Nienaber CA, et al: Long-term survival in patients presenting with type A acute aortic dissection: insights from the International Registry of Acute Aortic Dissection (IRAD). Circulation 2006; 114(Suppl):I350-I356.

45. Tsai TT, Fattori R, Trimarchi S, et al: Long-term survival in patients presenting with type B acute aortic dissection: insights from the International Registry of Acute Aortic Dissection. Circulation 2006;114:2226-2231.

46. Movsowitz HD, Levine RA, Hilgenberg AD, Isselbacher EM: Transesophageal echocardiographic description of the mechanisms of aortic regurgitation in acute type A aortic dissection: implications for aortic valve repair. J Am Coll Cardiol 2000;36:884-890.

47. Pape LA, Tsai TT, Isselbacher EM, et al: Aortic diameter ≥5.5 cm is not a good predictor of type A aortic dissection: observations from the International Registry of Acute Aortic Dissection (IRAD). Circulation 2007;116: 1120-1127.

Aortic Intramural Hematoma

DEFINITION OF AORTIC INTRAMURAL HEMATOMA

Aortic intramural hematoma (IMH) is defined as a hematoma within the aortic wall without an intimal flap, demonstrable intimal tear, or direct communication of flow with the lumen. Hence, it constitutes a dissection without luminal components.

PATHOGENESIS OF AORTIC INTRAMURAL HEMATOMA

Aortic IMH was first described by Krukenberg in 1920.[1] The pathogenesis is unknown and controversial. Conventional wisdom invokes that in the usual pathogenesis, hemorrhage into the media by the vasa vasorum initiates the IMH. The cause of the hemorrhage is unclear, except in trauma cases. Importantly, and by definition, an intimal tear allowing luminal blood into the wall is not present. A less common pathogenesis is erosion into the media by a penetrating atherosclerotic ulcer, initiating a hemorrhage into the media (Fig. 5-1).

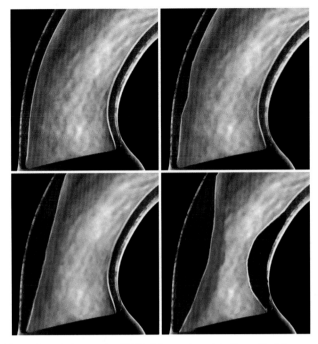

Figure 5-1. Pathogenesis of IMH. A hemorrhage into the wall of the aorta leads to accumulation of a hematoma and displacement of the intima into the lumen, forming an annular or crescentic thickening of the wall of the aorta, with a smooth inner surface, no intimal tear, and no false lumen.

Ascending (48%)   Arch (8%)   Descending (44%)

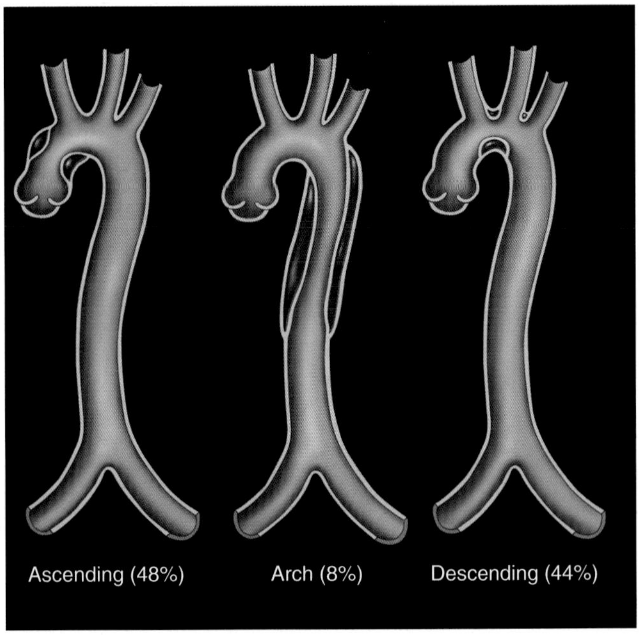

Figure 5-2. Anatomic locations of IMH: ascending (type A), descending (type B), and arch. The length of an IMH lesion is shorter than that of most aortic dissections.

Table 5-1. Anatomic Findings of Aortic Intramural Hematoma

Maximal wall thickness	0.7-3.0 cm
Maximal aortic diameter	3.0-8.4 cm
Maximal length	3.0-20.0 cm
Echo-free space by transesophageal echocardiography	66%
Smooth inner wall to the aorta	26%
Atherosclerotic inner surface	73%

Normal descending aorta (maximal, outside) diameter: 1.45 ± 0.16 cm/m².

Table 5-2. Distal Extent of Intramural Hematoma Versus Acute Aortic Dissection

Distal Extent	IMH	AAD
Distal descending aorta	28%	12%
Supraceliac abdominal aorta	57%	12% (*P* < .0001)
Suprarenal abdominal aorta	4%	7%
Infrarenal abdominal aorta	2%	23% (*P* < .0001)
Common iliac artery	0%	39%

AAD, acute aortic dissection; IMH, intramural hematoma.

INCIDENCE AND PREDISPOSING FACTORS

Predisposing factors for aortic IMH are hypertension (70% to 95%),[2-4] Marfan syndrome (12%), trauma (28%),[2] and penetrating ulcers.[3,5]

IMH accounts for approximately 5% to 10% (range, 3% to 30%) of suspected dissection cases.[2,6,7] Of 1010 patients enrolled in the International Registry of Aortic Dissection (IRAD) presenting with suspected aortic dissection, 5.7% had IMH.[8] The actual incidence is unknown as the diagnosis is potentially overlooked.

ANATOMIC FINDINGS OF AORTIC INTRAMURAL HEMATOMA

Unlike acute aortic dissection (AAD), which consistently demonstrates a 60% ascending and 40% descending incidence, the anatomic locations of IMH are distributed relatively evenly between the ascending and descending aorta: 48% ascending, 8% arch, and 44% descending (Fig. 5-2).

Most IMHs (85%) are circular; a minority (15%) are crescentic.[3] Another difference from AAD is the length of lesions; the lesion of IMH is typically much shorter (average length is 85 ± 5 mm). The average thickness is 20 ± 12 mm (Table 5-1).[2] The distal extent of IMH is less than that of AAD (Table 5-2).[9]

NATURAL HISTORY AND COMPLICATIONS OF INTRAMURAL HEMATOMA

There are no comprehensive studies of the natural history of IMH. Most studies are retrospective analyses. It is clear, though, that a relation of mortality and complications to anatomic location exits that is similar to AAD.[8] IMH involving the ascending aorta has greater mortality risk than does IMH confined to the descending aorta alone. Several series have documented a high incidence of pericardial effusion among patients with ascending IMH, and some have demonstrated pericardial effusion in all ascending cases.[6] It may be that the less conspicuous imaging findings result in later diagnoses, influencing observed complications and survivals.

IMH may undergo progression to either limited or frank AAD, progression to rupture, or regression. Of proximal IMH, about half progress and half regress. Two small series demonstrated similar findings. Of 13 patients with proximal IMH who survived initial hospitalization, regression occurred in 7 of 13, progression to typical aortic dissection occurred in 3 of 13, and progression to focal AAD occurred in 3 of 13.[4] Of 14 patients with IMH (7 ascending and 7 arch or descending), among the ascending cases, there were 1 sudden death and 3 surgeries (due to progressive aortic enlargement in 1 and development of secondary tears in 2). Three ascending IMH cases demonstrated regression. Among 7 arch or descending IMH cases, there was 1 death.[3]

As with proximal AAD, a high proportion of proximal IMH develop complications (pericardial fluid, tamponade, aortic insufficiency, coronary compromise, rupture, progressive enlargement, and intimal tears), and medically managed proximal IMH is associated with high mortality. The development of effusions (pericardial, pleural, and mediastinal) is common.[6] The effusion tends to be anatomically adjacent to the IMH lesion, although not all effusions are bloody.[10] In the initial admission, approximately 20% to 25% of all IMH cases will progress to frank AAD or rupture.[6,11]

Aortic insufficiency and pericardial or mediastinal fluid are associated with 42% of type A and 18% of type B IMH cases.[8] Progression to overt dissection, rupture, or tamponade occurs in up to 33% of cases within 24 to 72 hours.[2,6,12] IRAD reported a progression of 16% of cases.[8]

The presence of a penetrating atherosclerotic ulcer is associated with a significantly greater complication rate. In a retrospective series of 65 cases of IMH, 34 cases were associated with a penetrating ulcer and 31 were not. IMH without penetrating ulcer was more commonly located in the ascending aorta (26% versus 9%). Most cases of IMH with penetrating ulcer were located in the descending aorta (91%), as penetrating ulcers occur most commonly in the descending thoracic aorta or arch. Clinical (recurrent or uncontrollable pain) and radiologic (increasing pleural effusion) instability was significantly more common in IMH with penetrating ulcers. The maximum diameter and maximum depth of the penetrating ulcer were significant predictors of progression. Cases with progressive course had larger average maximum diameters (21 ± 8 mm versus 11.6 ± 4 mm) and larger average depth (13.7 ± 4 versus 7.4 ± 3.5 mm) of penetrating ulcers. Lesions in the proximal descending aorta and arch were more likely to be progressive.[13]

Complications associated with IMH do differ in several regards from those of AAD (Table 5-3). Because few IMH extend beyond the celiac artery, malperfusion of renal, splanchnic, and iliac vessels is less common than in AAD.[9] Arch IMH (by the IRAD study) appears to have a lower complication rate.

MORTALITY OF AORTIC INTRAMURAL HEMATOMA

The mortality of IMH is influenced by the location of the IMH lesions, regardless of whether the course is progressive or not, the development of complications, an associated underlying penetrating ulcer, and the age of the patient (Table 5-4). The IRAD Registry included 1010 patients, of whom 5.7% were found to have IMH (Table 5-5).[8]

Imaging features within 48 hours of symptom onset offer some prediction of development of complications and outcomes. Adverse outcomes (death, surgery, development of frank dissection) among medically treated cases were associated with increased hematoma thickness and area as well as aortic diameter and cross-sectional area (Fig. 5-3; Table 5-6).[14]

One-year survival of aortic IMH was analyzed by Nienaber and colleagues.[2] IMH of an ascending aorta has 20% survival with

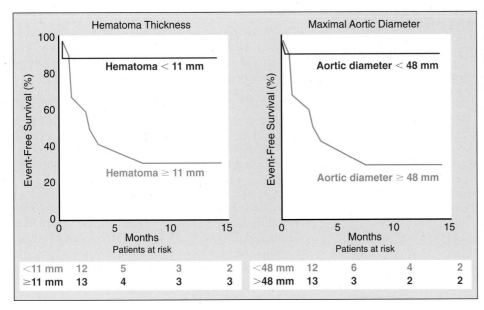

Figure 5-3. Prediction of development of acute type A IMH complications, if medically treated. (From Song JM, Kim HS, Song JK, et al: Usefulness of the initial noninvasive imaging study to predict the adverse outcomes in the medical treatment of acute type A aortic intramural hematoma. Circulation 2003;108[Suppl II]: II324-II328.)

Table 5-3. Complication Rates of Intramural Hematoma and Acute Aortic Dissection

	IMH	AAD	P Value
In-hospital complications			
Death	0%	14%	.006
Mesenteric ischemia	0%	7%	
Renal failure	2%	23%	.001
Leg ischemia	2%	14%	.033
Late complications			
Rupture	0%	2%	
Reoperation	0%	2%	
Others	6%	5%	

AAD, acute aortic dissection; IMH, intramural hematoma.

Table 5-4. Mortality of Intramural Hematoma by Location Involved

Aortic root	60% (3/5)
Sinotubular junction	50% (1/2)
Ascending aorta	33% (4/12)
Aortic arch	0% (0/7)
Left subclavian artery	7% (1/15)
Descending aorta	13% (2/15)
Abdominal aorta	0% (0/1)

Data from Evangelista A, Mukherjee D, Mehta RH, et al: Acute intramural hematoma of the aorta: a mystery in evolution. Circulation 2005;111:1063-1070.

Table 5-5. IRAD Comparison of Intramural Hematoma Versus Acute Aortic Dissection

	IMH	AAD	P Value
Average age of patients	68.7 years	61.7 years	<.001
More distal aortic involvement	60.3%	35.3%	<.001
More severe initial pain			Significant
Ischemic leg pain, AI, pulse deficits			Significant
Longer time to initial diagnosis			Significant
Mortality			
Overall	21%	24%	NS
Type A	39%	30%	NS
Type B	8%	13%	NS
Progression to AAD	16%		

AAD, acute aortic dissection; AI, aortic insufficiency; IMH, intramural hematoma; IRAD, International Registry of Aortic Dissection; NS, not significant.
Data from Evangelista A, Mukherjee D, Mehta RH, et al: Acute intramural hematoma of the aorta: a mystery in evolution. Circulation 2005;111:1063-1070.

Table 5-6. Predictors of Intramural Hematoma Outcome

	Adverse	Uneventful	P Value
Hematoma thickness	14 ± 4 mm	8 ± 4 mm	<.005
Hematoma area	988 ± 316 mm^2	555 ± 352 mm^2	<.01
Aortic diameter	53 ± 6 mm	48 ± 8 mm	.10
Aortic cross-sectional area			.09

Data from Song JM, Kim HS, Song JK, et al: Usefulness of the initial noninvasive imaging study to predict the adverse outcomes in the medical treatment of acute type A aortic intramural hematoma. Circulation 2003;108(Suppl II):II324-II328.

medical therapy and 71% survival with surgery ($P < .05$). Arch IMH survival was half of cases with medical therapy. The 1-year survival of the descending aortic IMH was 80% with medical therapy and 83% with surgical management.[2]

DIAGNOSIS OF INTRAMURAL HEMATOMA

Because the findings are less obvious than with dissection flaps, time to IMH diagnosis is significantly longer than for AAD, and the number of diagnostic tests used is significantly greater.[8] There are no perfect tests for the detection of IMH. The lesion should be imaged by more than one modality to comprehensively assess it.

Basic imaging criteria include circular or crescentic thickening of the wall (>0.7 cm), evidence of hematoma as the cause of the thickening, absence of a flap, absence of communication with the lumen, absence of flow within the area of thickening, and intimal calcium displacement.

Principal differential diagnoses include the following:

- Aortic dissection with thrombosed false lumen. A false lumen, without large exit tears, will tend to thrombose in its more distant and stagnant margins. Characteristically, even if the false lumen is largely thrombosed, there will still be persistence of part of the false lumen near the intimal tear where flow washed in and out, preventing local thrombosis. An intimal flap also is seen in the nonthrombosed parts.
- Aortic aneurysm with extensive mural thrombus. The case of aneurysm with mural thrombus lacks the appearance of an intimal layer, although this can be difficult to resolve. Intimal calcification, if it is present, is very useful to establish the identification of the intima. Central displacement of intimal calcification excludes aneurysm with mural thrombus.
- Aortic false aneurysm with extensive thrombus
- Atherosclerotic wall thickening. Unfortunately, atherosclerotic disease of the aorta can be complicated with ulcer that, if it is penetrating into the wall, can lead to IMH. Because the wall of atherosclerotic aorta is heterogeneous in composition and imaging characteristics, false-positive and false-negative IMH diagnoses are possible.
- Aortic tumor (potentially)

IMAGING OF INTRAMURAL HEMATOMA

Transesophageal Echocardiography

Typical transesophageal echocardiography (TEE) findings in IMH include regional thickening (>7 mm) of the wall with a crescentic or circular shape and an absence of luminal components (Figs. 5-4 to 5-6). Recent "fresh" IMH characteristically has low-intensity signal (echolucency). Some movement (shearing) of the layers of the wall may be observed. Subacute IMH characteristically has crescentic thickening of the wall with signal indistinguishable from the rest of the wall.

TEE utility in IMH may be limited by technical factors, such as limited visualization of the ascending aorta and arch and limited visualization through calcified atherosclerotic plaque, and by operator experience in the context of IMH and penetrating ulcers, as well as availability.

Computed Tomography

Suspected IMH is typically first imaged by non–contrast-enhanced computed tomography (CT), followed by contrast-enhanced CT (Fig. 5-7). Recent fresh IMH characteristically has crescentic thickening of the wall with high-density signal (60-70 Hounsfield units) and absence of luminal components. Subacute (thrombosed) IMH characteristically has crescentic thickening of the wall with variable (increasing, layered) signal density and absence of luminal components. Central displacement of intimal calcification and absence of contrast enhancement within the wall are useful signs on CT.

Magnetic Resonance Imaging

Recent (acute) IMH characteristically appears isodense with vessel wall on T1-weighted imaging; on T2-weighted imaging,

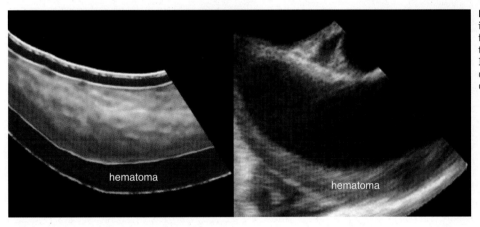

Figure 5-4. IMH of the ascending aorta: illustration and TEE. Typical imaging findings include homogeneous or lucent thickening of the aortic wall due to the IMH, a smooth contour, intimal calcium displacement, and no intimal flap or tear or flow within the hematoma.

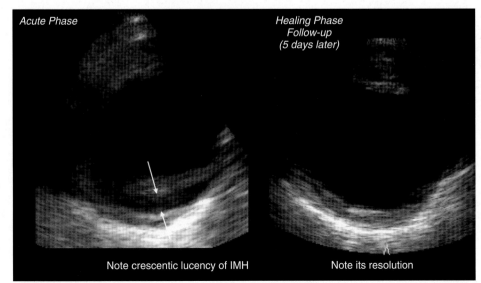

Figure 5-5. TEE short-axis views of the descending aorta. LEFT, Acute IMH. Note the lucency of the wall thickening consistent with fresh hemorrhage. RIGHT, Note the resolution of the wall thickening and the lucency seen within 5 days.

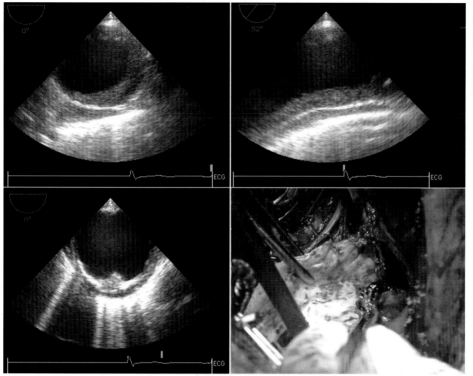

Figure 5-6. TEE of IMH of the proximal descending thoracic aorta. TOP LEFT, Short-axis view. TOP RIGHT, Long-axis view. BOTTOM LEFT, TEE demonstration of a thrombus protruding from an atherosclerotic ulcer associated with the IMH. BOTTOM RIGHT, Surgical view of the same thrombus-ulcer-IMH complex.

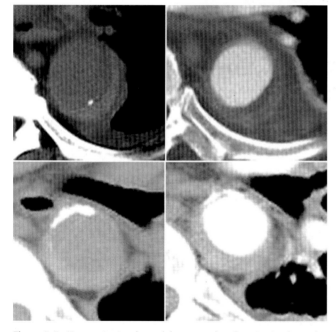

Figure 5-7. Non–contrast-enhanced (LEFT IMAGES) and contrast-enhanced (RIGHT IMAGES) CT. TOP, The phantom-like crescentic thickening of the wall of the aorta is best seen on the left posterior aspect. The intimal calcification is displaced into the lumen (intimal displacement), indicative of mural thickening and dissection. With contrast, the lumen is better seen, and therefore also the wall thickening, but the intimal calcification is obscured by the high signal in the lumen. BOTTOM, In a different patient, the intimal calcification is away from the wall thickening and therefore does not demonstrate intimal displacement indicative of mural thickening and dissection. With contrast, the lumen is better seen, and therefore also the wall thickening opposite to the intimal calcification.

fresh blood has high signal (bright). Day 1 to day 5 IMH characteristically has low signal intensity. Subacute IMH characteristically has high signal on both T1- and T2-weighted imaging because of methemoglobin formation. Crescentic thickening of the wall with an absence of luminal components and absence of blood flow within the wall by cine magnetic resonance (MR) are typical signs of aortic IMH.

Angiographic Imaging

Because CT, TEE, and MRI have more than 96% sensitivity, and angiography is considerably less sensitive (78%), the role of angiography is secondary to that of the other modalities, other than potentially to visualize associated penetrating ulcers.

Angiographic signs of IMH include diameter reduction of the aortic lumen and rectification of the aortic contour. Wall thickening of crescentic nature cannot be reliably depicted by angiography. Angiographic false-negatives are well known: in the study by Bansal and colleagues,[15] there were 15 of 65 false-negatives (13 IMH); and in the study by Vilacosta and associates,[3] there were 17 of 21 false-negatives.

MANAGEMENT OF INTRAMURAL HEMATOMA AND DISSECTION

- Establish type (location) of IMH and dissection; complications, if present; presence or absence of a penetrating ulcer associated with the IMH.
- Stabilize blood pressure in all cases; institute beta-blockers if tolerable.

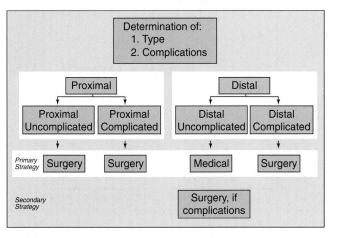

Figure 5-8. Algorithm for initial management of aortic IMH.

Table 5-7. Predictors of Risk in Aortic Intramural Hematoma

In-hospital predictors of risk (death, progression, surgery)	Ascending location
	Greater thickness
	Echolucency
Long-term predictors of risk (death, progression, surgery)	Initial echolucency
	Longitudinal extent
	Larger aortic size (>45 mm)
	Atherosclerotic plaque
	Penetrating ulcer
	Age >70 years
Predictors of regression	Normal-size aorta
	Younger patients
	Absence of penetrating ulcer

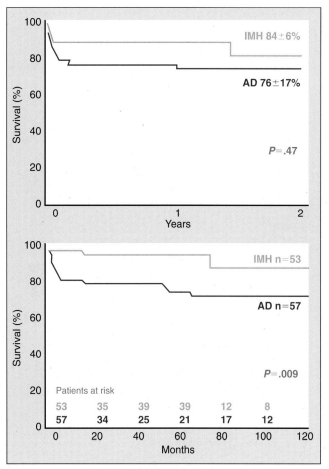

Figure 5-9. Survival of type A (TOP) and type B (BOTTOM) aortic IMH. AD, aortic dissection. (Top panel from Song JK, Kim HS, Kang DH, et al: Different clinical features of aortic intramural hematoma versus dissection involving the ascending aorta. J Am Coll Cardiol 2001;37:1604-1610. Bottom panel from Kaji S, Akasaka T, Katayama M, et al: Long-term prognosis of patients with type B aortic intramural hematoma. Circulation 2003;108[Suppl 1]:II307-II311.)

- Consider initial management strategy similar to that of AAD: type A IMH, if operable, should be managed surgically; type B IMH, if uncomplicated, can be managed medically (Fig. 5-8).
- Consultative and collaborative management (ICU and CCU, cardiology, radiology, anesthesiology, cardiovascular surgery).

LONG-TERM SURVIVAL AND COMPLICATIONS OF INTRAMURAL HEMATOMA

The 2-year survival of ascending IMH may not be different from that of AAD,[4] although the survival of descending IMH may be better than that of AAD[2,4,9] (Figs. 5-9 and 5-10). There is a sub-stantial progression rate to complicated aortic lesions for several years after discharge. Evangelista and coworkers[16] reported a series of 50 IMH cases followed up at 3, 6, and 12 months and then for a mean of 45 months. At 6 months, complete regression occurred in 34% of cases. Another 24% of cases progressed to a pseudoaneurysm, 22% to fusiform aneurysm, 12% to classic dissection, and 8% to saccular aneurysm.

Likelihood of progression to classic dissection relates to initial echolucency and longitudinal extent. Development of aortic diameter of aneurysmal size was more likely if there was atherosclerotic plaque or absence of echolucency.[16] Age older than 70 years and ulcer-like features predict a worse prognosis.[9,13,17]

Several studies have indicated that smaller (<45 mm) aortic diameters are predictors of good prognosis and that the best predictor of regression is a normal aortic diameter (Table 5-7).[16,17] Disappearance of IMH is associated with better survival rates (Fig. 5-11).

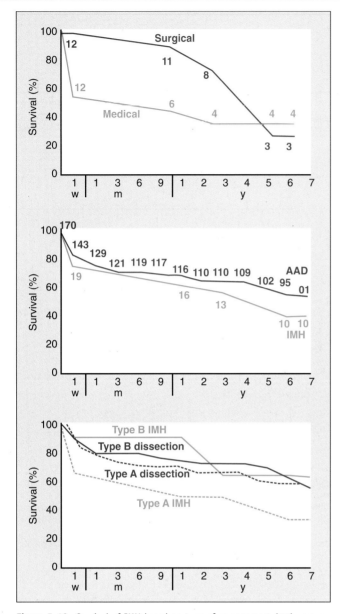

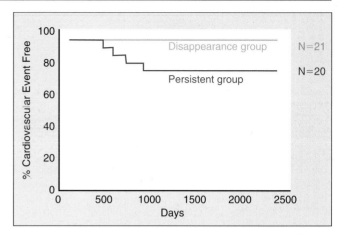

Figure 5-11. Disappearance of IMH is associated with better survival.

Figure 5-10. Survival of IMH based on type of management (TOP) versus AAD (MIDDLE) and by type (BOTTOM). (From Nienaber CA, von Kodolitsch Y, Petersen B, et al: Intramural hemorrhage of the thoracic aorta. Diagnostic and therapeutic implications. Circulation 1995;92:1465-1472.)

CASE 1

History

▸ An 80-year-old man presented with sudden onset of severe chest pain radiating to the back and abdomen.
▸ No prior such pains
▸ Past medical history is significant for aortocoronary bypass 8 years before, abdominal aortic aneurysm resection 8 years before, hypertension, dyslipidemia, and atrial fibrillation with warfarin (therapeutic INR).

Physical Examination

▸ BP 220/100 mm Hg
▸ No pericardial rub, no pulse deficits or bruits
▸ No murmur of aortic insufficiency; no signs of tamponade or left-sided heart failure
▸ 40 mm Hg BP difference between the arms (L < R)

Comments

▸ Distal (descending) aortic IMH occurring in a patient with hypertension and a history of coronary artery disease, aortocoronary bypass grafting, and aneurysms
▸ Blood pressure control (nitroprusside), then multiple antihypertensives (beta-blocker, ACE inhibitor, calcium antagonist, diuretic) and cessation of anticoagulation, led to resolution of symptoms and IMH findings by objective testing.
▸ It is interesting, but unlikely, that the anticoagulation was causal, as IMH is well enough described without the presence of underlying bleeding disorders.
▸ The IMH may have explained the pulse differential as MRI demonstrated involvement of the origin of the left subclavian artery (the arm with the lower blood pressure). Once the IMH clinically and radiographically resolved, the differential blood pressure did as well.

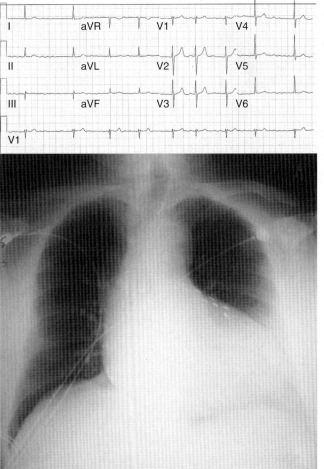

Figure 5-12. TOP, ECG demonstrates atrial fibrillation with a slow average ventricular response of 60 bpm. BOTTOM, Chest radiograph shows cardiomegaly, prior sternotomy, surgical clips along a left internal mammary graft, and a prominent aorta. It is unclear if there is a left pleural effusion.

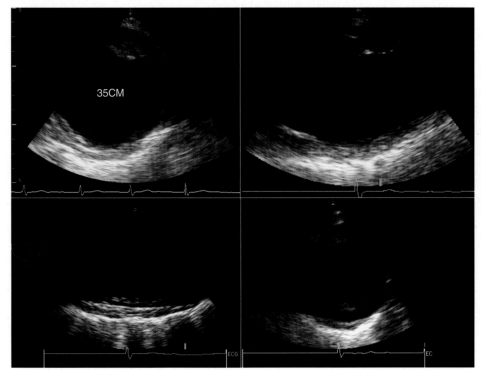

Figure 5-13. TEE. TOP LEFT, Intimal artifact—not intimal flap. From the near wall of the aorta on both the short-axis image (TOP LEFT) and the long-axis image (TOP RIGHT), there is a reverberation artifact that projects across the lumen, potentially generating confusion about an intimal flap being present. TOP RIGHT, Longitudinal plane view of the descending aorta. There is an abnormal thickening of the near wall of the aorta. BOTTOM LEFT, Longitudinal plane view of the descending aorta. Longitudinal lucency within the far wall of the aorta is consistent with an IMH. BOTTOM RIGHT, Cross-sectional view of the descending aorta. There is crescentic thickening and lucency of the far wall of the descending aorta.

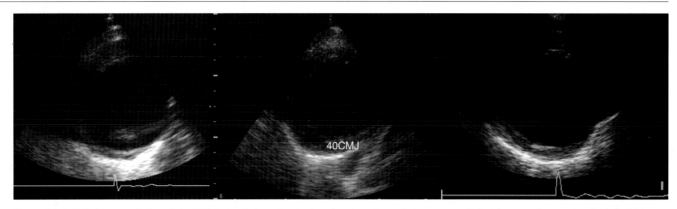

Figure 5-14. TEE shows resolution of the IMH during 3 days. On the first day, there is an obvious crescentic hypolucency that resolves both in thickness and in lucency during 3 days, with blood pressure control.

CASE 2

History

▸ 57-year-old man with sudden onset of severe chest pain and hypertension
▸ Past medical history was significant for untreated borderline hypertension.

Physical Examination

▸ BP 190/110 mm Hg
▸ No pericardial rub; no murmur of aortic insufficiency; no signs of tamponade or of left-sided heart failure
▸ No pulse deficits or BP differential

Comments

▸ Distal (descending) aortic IMH in a hypertensive patient
▸ The description of borderline hypertension was surely an underestimate, given the well-developed left ventricular hypertrophy, the degree of blood pressure elevation that occurred during pain, and the aortic complication.
▸ Resolution of IMH findings with blood pressure control, initially with IV labetalol monotherapy but subsequently with multiple antihypertensives (beta-blocker, ACE inhibitor, calcium antagonist)

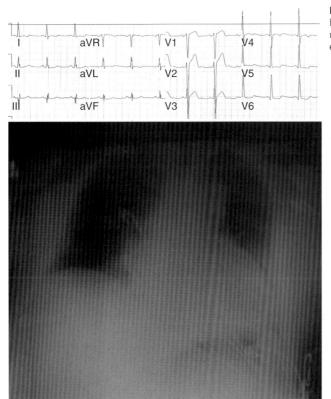

Figure 5-15. TOP, ECG demonstrates sinus rhythm, left ventricular hypertrophy with nonspecific repolarization abnormalities. BOTTOM, Chest radiograph shows cardiomegaly, widened mediastinum, and no pulmonary edema.

5

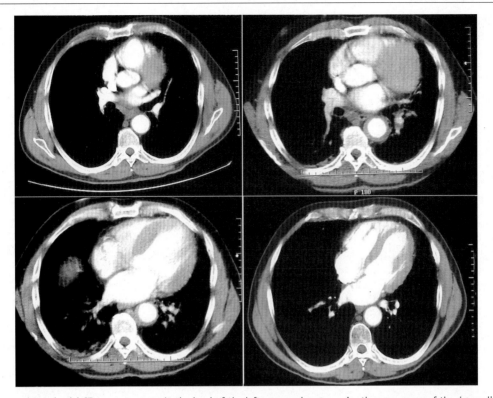

Figure 5-16. Contrast-enhanced axial CT scans. TOP LEFT, At the level of the left upper pulmonary vein, the appearance of the descending aorta is normal. TOP RIGHT, Shortly below, there is annular thickening of the wall of the descending aorta. BOTTOM LEFT, Crescentic thickening of the wall of the descending aorta. BOTTOM RIGHT, Shortly below, the wall of the aorta is normal. There is no left pleural effusion.

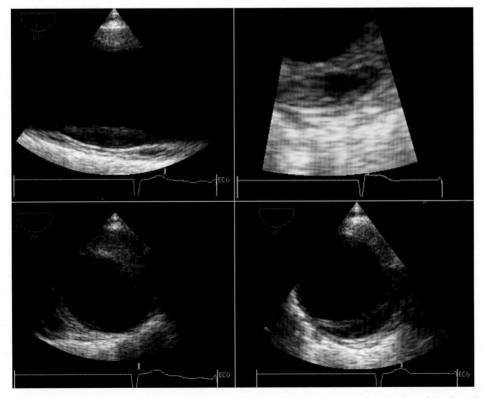

Figure 5-17. TOP LEFT, The proximal descending aorta in longitudinal lane. There are several centimeters of thickening of the far wall of the aorta, with a heterogeneous appearance. TOP RIGHT, Zoom view of the far wall of the aorta. There is echolucency, consistent with blood in the wall of the aorta. BOTTOM LEFT, Descending aorta in cross section. There is crescentic thickening of the near wall of the aorta, with homogeneous appearance, and some narrowing of the lumen. BOTTOM RIGHT, There is crescentic thickening of the left wall of the aorta, with a more lucent layer on the far wall. Note the lesser appreciation of the near wall (near-field) due to the narrowness of the sector, compared with the appreciation of the far wall.

CASE 3

History

▸ A 71-year-old man presented with abrupt onset of sharp chest pain.
▸ Initial CT scan at presenting hospital was negative for pulmonary embolism but established that there was some form of abnormality to the ascending aorta.
▸ He was transferred for evaluation and management.
▸ Past medical history was significant for hypertension.

Physical Examination

▸ BP 200/100 mm Hg; no pericardial rub; no murmur of aortic insufficiency
▸ No signs of tamponade or of left-sided heart failure
▸ No pulse deficits or BP differential

Surgical Findings

▸ Blood within the pericardial space, with obvious pericardial reaction
▸ Bluish discoloration and enlargement of the outside of the root and ascending aorta
▸ Blood clot within the wall of the aorta
▸ Penetrating ulcer of the ascending aorta and very little atherosclerosis
▸ Serosanguineous pleural effusion

Surgical Procedure

▸ Cross-clamping of the aorta, cardiopulmonary bypass, progressive cooling

▸ Opening of the aorta between the cross-clamp and the aortic valve; inspection of the aortic valve and verification of its integrity (mild involvement of the noncoronary cusp); sewing in of the proximal end of a Dacron graft
▸ Once core temperature was below 20° C, circulatory arrest started, and the aorta was opened. The involved aorta (IMH and ulcer) was resected from the sinotubular junction to the mid arch in its entirety and replaced by sewing in the Dacron graft distally.
▸ Cardiopulmonary bypass time, 112 minutes; cross-clamp time, 70 minutes; deep circulatory arrest, 36 minutes

Outcome

▸ Discharged well, without complications, now taking several antihypertensives

Comments

▸ Ascending IMH associated with a penetrating ulcer
▸ Chest pain of dissection-like nature (abrupt and severe)
▸ Prior hypertension may have facilitated the IMH, but the ulcer was the likely inciting factor. In the absence of atherosclerosis, the etiology of the ulcer was difficult to explain.
▸ Complications included pericarditis and pericardial effusion, presumably oozing from the aorta.
▸ Physical examination did not recognize the pericardial effusion, and physical diagnosis and ECG did not recognize pericarditis.
▸ No specific abnormalities were determined on histology that elucidated the cause of the ulcer.

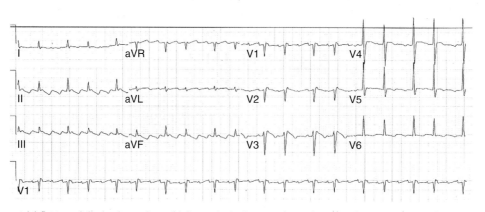

Figure 5-18. ECG shows atrial flutter, minimal voltage signs of left ventricular hypertrophy, and nonspecific repolarization abnormalities.

5

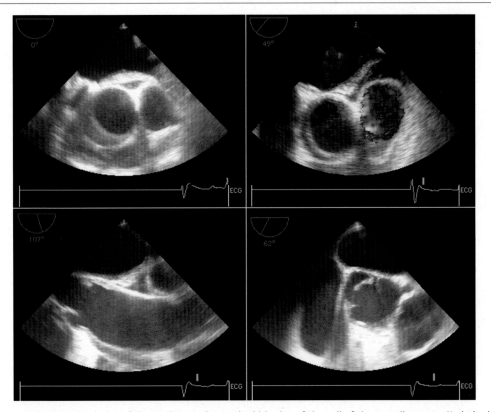

Figure 5-19. TEE. TOP LEFT, Cross-sectional view of the aortic root. Crescentic thickening of the wall of the ascending aorta. No intimal flap. TOP RIGHT, No flow within the crescentic thickening of the aortic root wall. BOTTOM LEFT, Longitudinal view of the ascending aorta. There is homogeneous thickening of the anterior wall of the aorta. BOTTOM RIGHT, Normal-appearing bioprosthetic aortic valve replacement. No obvious involvement of root wall thickening at the left main coronary artery.

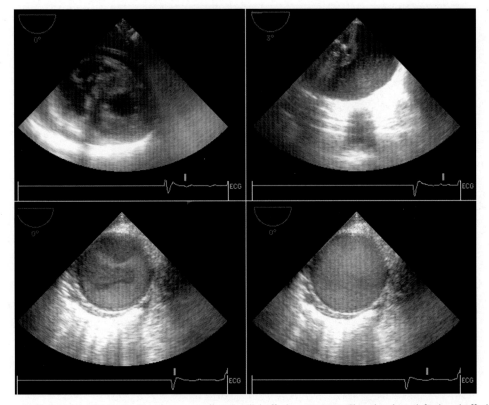

Figure 5-20. TEE. TOP LEFT, Transgastric short-axis view shows a small pericardial effusion. TOP RIGHT, There is a large left pleural effusion with specular echoes suggestive of blood. BOTTOM LEFT, Cross-sectional view of the descending aorta. There is dilation of the aorta, but no flap or mural thickening. BOTTOM RIGHT, There is spontaneous contrast forming in the descending aorta.

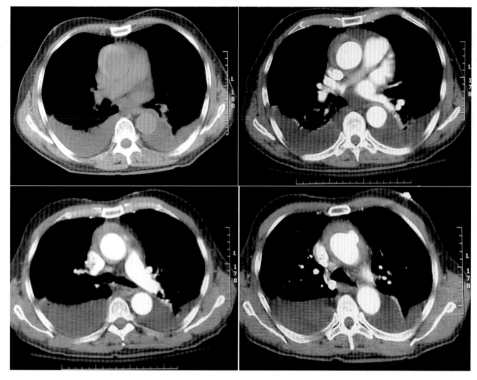

Figure 5-21. TOP LEFT, Non–contrast-enhanced axial CT scan shows a faint crescentic thickening of the lateral wall of the ascending aorta. There are bilateral pleural effusions. TOP RIGHT, Contrast-enhanced axial CT scan at the same level again shows the crescentic thickening of the wall of the ascending aorta. BOTTOM LEFT, There is a cavity with contrast dye located within the wall of the ascending aorta. BOTTOM RIGHT, There is a penetrating ulcer of the wall of the ascending aorta, surrounded with thrombus of IMH.

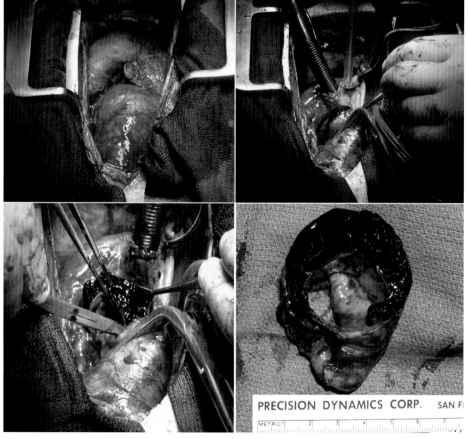

Figure 5-22. Surgical findings. TOP LEFT, Enlarged ascending aorta with hemorrhagic outer surface. TOP RIGHT, The aorta is cross-clamped. There is IMH. BOTTOM LEFT, The aorta has been opened, and there is an IMH in the ascending aorta. BOTTOM RIGHT, There is crescentic thickening of the wall of the aorta due to IMH.

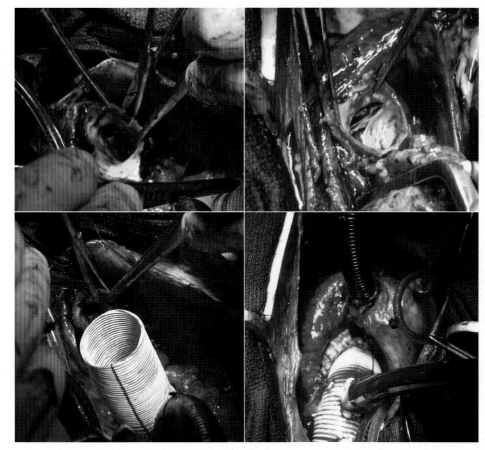

Figure 5-23. TOP LEFT, The ascending aorta has been resected down to where the wall is normal—above the sinotubular junction. The aortic valve is visible. TOP RIGHT, The ascending aorta has been surgically opened. BOTTOM LEFT, A Dacron tube graft has been anastomosed proximally. BOTTOM RIGHT, The Dacron tube graft is in situ, replacing the ascending aorta.

CASE 4

History

▸ A 74-year-old woman presented with severe sharp chest pains in the front and back of the chest.
▸ Past medical history was significant for hypertension managed with two medications.
▸ No known coronary disease

Physical Examination

▸ Elderly and frail appearing for age
▸ BP 195/95 mm Hg, HR 90 bpm, mildly dyspneic
▸ Normal venous pressure
▸ S_1, S_2 normal; S_4 present; no murmur of aortic insufficiency, sustained apex
▸ Chest clear
▸ Prominent peripheral pulses, no bruits

Clinical Impression

▸ Clinical impression was that of an IMH of the proximal aorta developing in a hypertensive patient with atherosclerosis.
▸ Suspicious lesion for penetrating (atheromatous ulcer) and ulcer-like luminal extension into disrupted wall
▸ Radiographic signs suggestive of leakage included complex soft tissue adjacent to the query ulcer, pleural effusions, and specular appearance to the effusion by ultrasound examination.
▸ Poor operative candidate given age and general health

Evolution and Outcome

▸ During 24 hours, the patient was stable and the BP controlled with IV antihypertensives, but there were nagging episodes of chest pain.
▸ Discussions with patient's family and surgeons ongoing, reservations concerning risks
▸ Sudden fall in BP, presumably because of a rupture of the aorta due to the IMH or the penetrating ulcer
▸ The patient lost BP very rapidly and arrested with asystole and could not be resuscitated.

Comments

▸ IMH in association, possibly caused by a penetrating atherosclerotic ulcer or complicated by an ulcer-like extension
▸ Leakage of the aorta suggested by odd complex soft tissue beside the aorta and pleural effusions
▸ Rupture of the aorta into the left pleural cavity was the terminal event, be it from the IMH, the progression of the IMH into dissection, or the progression of the penetration of the ulcer.
▸ Mortality underscores the risk of IMH of the proximal aorta, association with (suspected penetrating) ulcer, and acute aortic syndrome with suspected rupture.

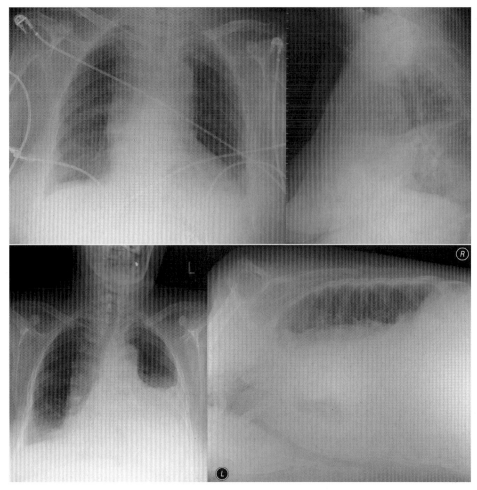

Figure 5-24. TOP, Initial chest radiographs show enlarged ascending aorta, arch, and descending aorta. The heart size is normal. No left-sided heart failure. Probable left pleural effusion. BOTTOM, Chest radiographs during admission. There has been development of a large left pleural effusion.

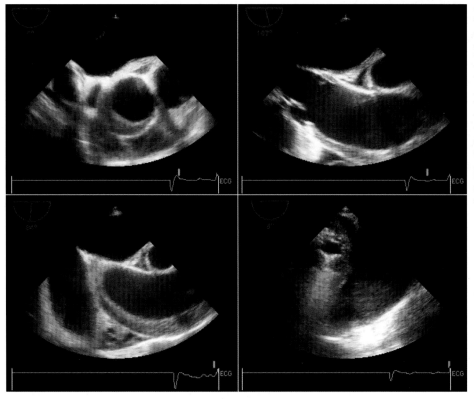

Figure 5-25. TEE. TOP LEFT, Short-axis view of the aortic root. There is obvious crescentic thickening of the wall of the aorta from the 4-o'clock to the 11-o'clock position. TOP RIGHT, Longitudinal view of the aortic root and ascending aorta. Thickening of the anterior wall of the aortic root and ascending aorta. The thickening has a uniform appearance. There is no intimal flap. BOTTOM LEFT, Longitudinal view of the aortic root and ascending aorta. The thickening of the anterior wall of the aortic root and ascending aorta is better seen. BOTTOM RIGHT, There is a large left pleural effusion with specular re-echoes within, which prompted consideration of hemothorax.

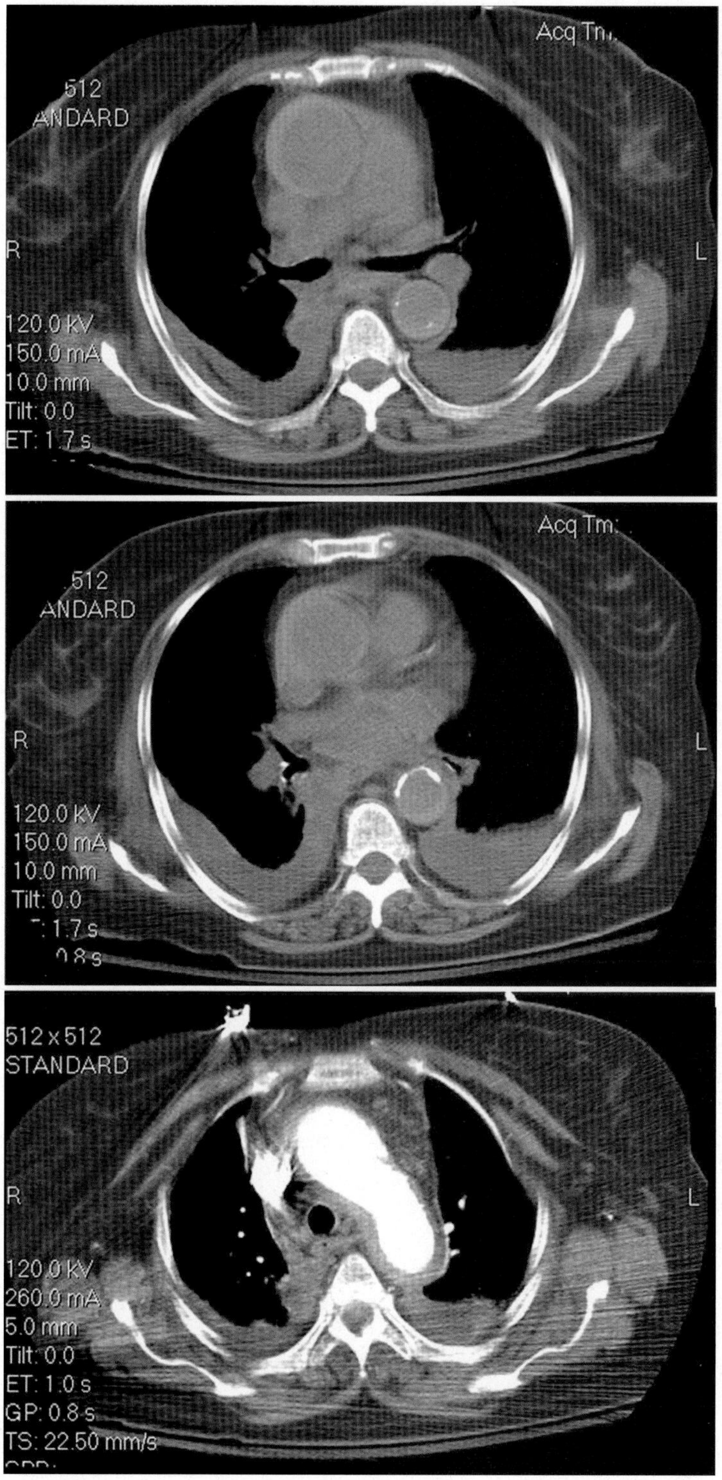

Figure 5-26. TOP AND MIDDLE, Non–contrast-enhanced axial CT scans show faint crescentic thickening of the wall of the ascending aorta, but not the descending aorta. There is intimal calcification of the descending aorta. BOTTOM, Contrast-enhanced axial CT scan at the arch level. The appearance of the wall of the aorta is normal.

5

References

1. Krukenberg E: Beitrage zur Frage des Aneurysma dissecans. Beitr Pathol Anat Allg Pathol 1920;67:329-351.
2. Nienaber CA, von Kodolitsch Y, Petersen B, et al: Intramural hemorrhage of the thoracic aorta. Diagnostic and therapeutic implications. Circulation 1995;92:1465-1472.
3. Vilacosta I, San Román JA, Ferreirós J, et al: Natural history and serial morphology of aortic intramural hematoma: a novel variant of aortic dissection. Am Heart J 1997;134:495-507.
4. Song JK, Kim HS, Kang DH, et al: Different clinical features of aortic intramural hematoma versus dissection involving the ascending aorta. J Am Coll Cardiol 2001;37:1604-1610.
5. Stanson AW, Kazmier FJ, Hollier LH, et al: Penetrating atherosclerotic ulcers of the thoracic aorta: natural history and clinicopathologic correlations. Ann Vasc Surg 1986;1:15-23.
6. Mohr-Kahaly S, Erbel R, Kearney P, et al: Aortic intramural hemorrhage visualized by transesophageal echocardiography: findings and prognostic implications. J Am Coll Cardiol 1994;23:658-664.

7. Hirst AE Jr, Johns VJ Jr, Kime SW Jr: Dissecting aneurysm of the aorta: a review of 505 cases. Medicine (Baltimore) 1958;37:217-279.

8. Evangelista A, Mukherjee D, Mehta RH, et al: Acute intramural hematoma of the aorta: a mystery in evolution. Circulation 2005;111:1063-1070.

9. Kaji S, Akasaka T, Katayama M, et al: Long-term prognosis of patients with type B aortic intramural hematoma. Circulation 2003;108(Suppl 1): II307-II311.

10. Mohr-Kahaly S: Aortic intramural hematoma: from observation to therapeutic strategies. J Am Coll Cardiol 2001;37:1611-1613.

11. Tittle SL, Lynch RJ, Cole PE, et al: Midterm follow-up of penetrating ulcer and intramural hematoma of the aorta. J Thorac Cardiovasc Surg 2002;123:1051-1059.

12. Coady MA, Rizzo JA, Elefteriades JA: Pathologic variants of thoracic aortic dissections. Penetrating atherosclerotic ulcers and intramural hematomas. Cardiol Clin 1999;17:637-657.

13. Ganaha F, Miller DC, Sugimoto K, et al: Prognosis of aortic intramural hematoma with and without penetrating atherosclerotic ulcer: a clinical and radiological analysis. Circulation 2002;106:342-348.

14. Song JM, Kim HS, Song JK, et al: Usefulness of the initial noninvasive imaging study to predict the adverse outcomes in the medical treatment of acute type A aortic intramural hematoma. Circulation 2003;108(Suppl II):II324-II328.

15. Bansal RC, Chandrasekaran K, Ayala K, Smith DC: Frequency and explanation of false negative diagnosis of aortic dissection by aortography and transesophageal echocardiography. J Am Coll Cardiol. 1995;25:1393-1401.

16. Evangelista A, Dominguez R, Sebastia C, et al: Long term follow up of aortic intramural hematoma: predictors of outcome. Circulation 2003;108: 583-589.

17. Nishigami K, Tsuchiya T, Shono H, et al: Disappearance of aortic intramural hematoma and its significance to the prognosis. Circulation 2000;102(Suppl 3):III243-III247.

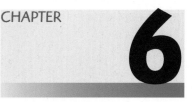

Late Complications of Aortic Dissection

The natural history of untreated acute aortic dissection (AAD) has most of the mortality in the acute phase: 15% die within 15 minutes—sudden death presentations; 35% more die within 48 hours, and 40% more die within 3 months, leaving 10% alive at 3 months. Untreated survivors after 3 months are far more likely to have had type B than type A AAD; 3-month survival of unrepaired AAD is 10% for type A and 75% for type B. Among medically treated patients who survive to 3 months, there is no difference in survival of type A and type B patients during the next 5 years.

Survivors both operated on and unoperated on are susceptible to recurrent dissection, false lumen expansion and rupture (Fig. 6-1), malperfusion syndromes, false aneurysm formation, aortic insufficiency and congestive heart failure, and nonaortic complications of chronic hypertension.

Late deaths (after 3 months) occur from (1) aortic deaths (30%) due to rupture of saccular false aneurysms that formed from a persistently patent (pressurized) aortic false lumen, rupture of dilated aortic false lumen, or dissection or aneurysm rupture of another segment of aorta; (2) other deaths (40%), such as stroke from chronic hypertension, congestive heart failure from severe aortic insufficiency, or coronary deaths, particularly in the iatrogenic AAD subgroup; and (3) undefined sudden deaths (30%) that include some aortic ruptures.

The management of chronic dissection places emphasis on control of blood pressure and surveillance with regular clinical and imaging follow-up. There have been no randomized controlled trials of different antihypertensive regimens after AAD, but retrospective data support that beta-blocker use is associated with improved outcomes (Figs. 6-2 and 6-3).[1,2]

FOLLOW-UP RECOMMENDATIONS FOR SURVIVORS OF ACUTE AORTIC DISSECTION

Imaging surveillance may be performed with several different tests. In general, the combination of computed tomography (CT) and echocardiography allows assessment of the aorta and the aortic valve and heart. In patients with renal insufficiency, magnetic resonance (MR) angiography may be used.

Many complications will occur within 3 months (Figs. 6-4 and 6-5). Therefore, clinical follow-up, blood pressure control, and follow-up imaging should ideally be scheduled for 1, 3, 6, and 12 months. The choice of modality to reimage the aorta includes CT and MR, with the selection determined by patient factors and availability.

At 1 year, if the patient and aorta are stable, follow-up (clinical follow-up, blood pressure check, chest radiograph, reimaging of the aorta) can become yearly. Patients with marked dilation of the aorta should be observed more closely. Implicit in follow-up is comparison of imaging with prior studies, hence the need for longitudinal follow-up.

Determination of the size of the aorta is important, as size represents a threshold to intervention. Axial views may depict the aorta off its shorts axis, overrepresenting diameter. It has been observed that the aorta dilates after type B AAD at the rate of approximately 2 mm/year in the thoracic segment and 1 mm/year in the abdominal segment.[3] Timely recognition of aortic expansion allows timely and more successful reoperation. Reoperation

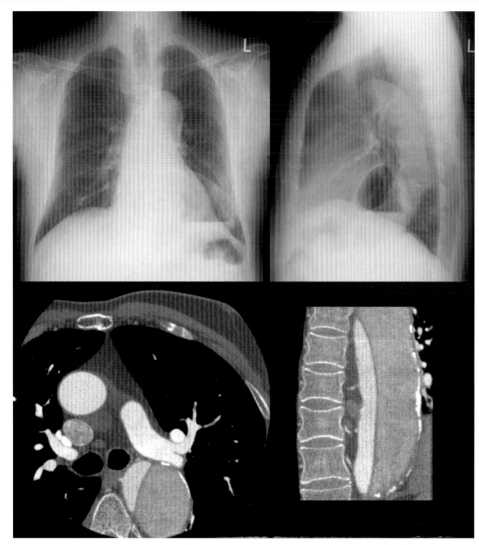

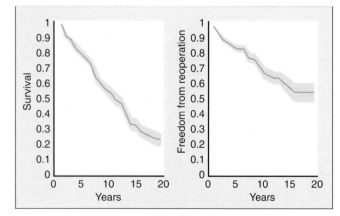

Figure 6-1. This patient had undergone elective aortic root replacement 8 years previously and had experienced a type B aortic dissection 3 years previously. The chest radiographs (TOP LEFT AND TOP RIGHT) show the enlargement of the distal arch and descending aorta and depict some calcification. They also show a large paraesophageal hernia. The axial (BOTTOM LEFT) and coronal (BOTTOM RIGHT) contrast-enhanced CT images reveal patency of the larger false lumen on the outside of the aorta and its extensive wall calcification. Serial CT scanning had not demonstrated progressive enlargement of the false lumen.

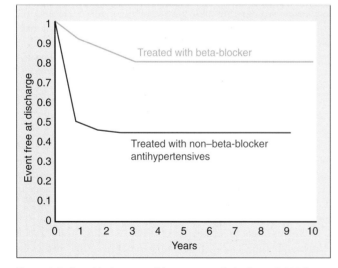

Figure 6-2. Beta-blocker use and long-term survival of type B AAD in a nonrandomized observation study. (From Genoni M, Paul M, Jenni R, et al: Chronic beta-blocker therapy improves outcome and reduces treatment costs in chronic type B aortic dissection. Eur J Cardiothorac Surg 2001;19:606-610, with permission from Elsevier.)

Figure 6-3. Beta-blocker use and long-term survival of type B AAD. (From Fann JI, Smith JA, Miller DC, et al: Surgical management of aortic dissection during a 30-year period. Circulation 1995;92[Suppl]: II113-II121.)

6

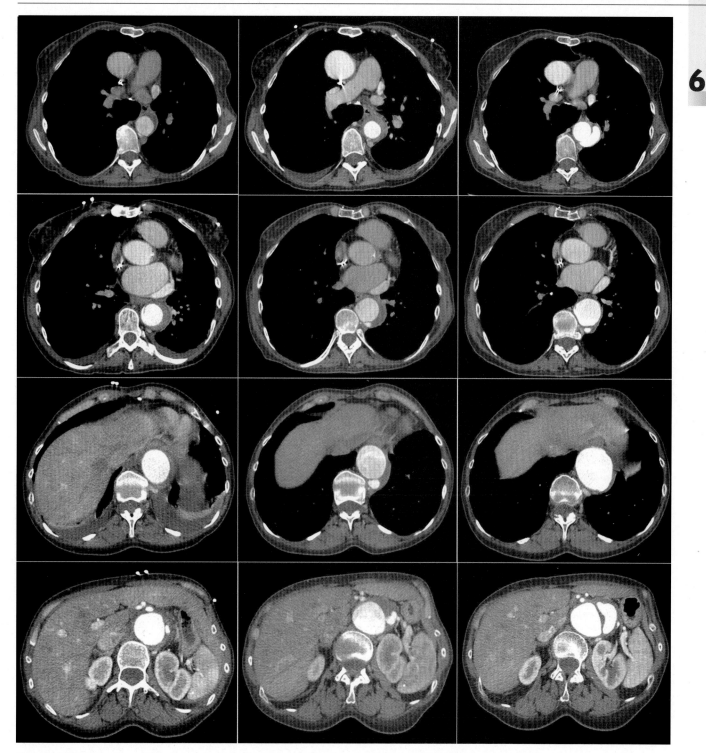

Figure 6-4. Contrast-enhanced CT scans at the time of presentation with an acute distal intramural hematoma (LEFT COLUMN), 3 weeks later (MIDDLE COLUMN), and 3 months later (RIGHT COLUMN). There has been development and progressive dilation of a false lumen–aneurysm in the descending aorta and also of the aneurysmal abdominal aorta.

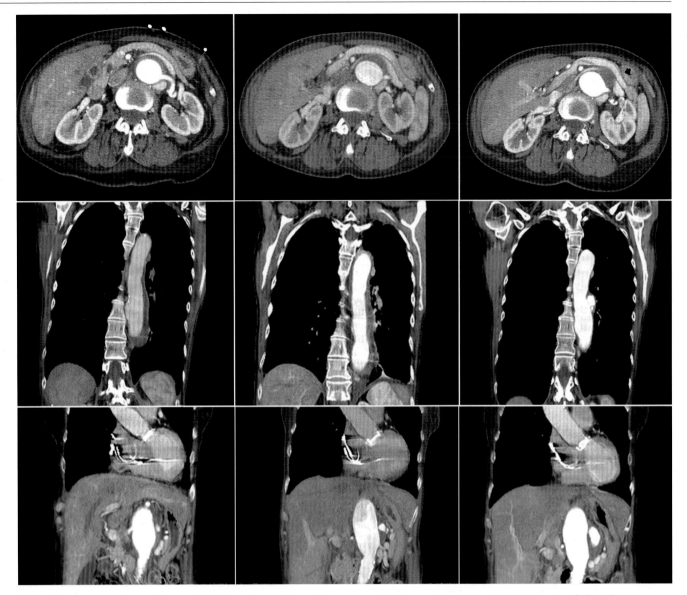

Figure 6-5. Contrast-enhanced CT scans at the time of presentation with an acute distal intramural hematoma (LEFT COLUMN), 3 weeks later (MIDDLE COLUMN), and 3 months later (RIGHT COLUMN). There has been development and progressive dilation of a false lumen–aneurysm in the descending aorta and also of the aneurysmal abdominal aorta.

is undertaken in up to 20% to 25% of patients within 4 to 5 years. The decision to reoperate invariably faces an older patient and may usually be confronted with greater comorbidities. For this reason, reoperation rates do not exactly reflect the need for reoperation because they are tempered by greater risk.

The role of interventional procedures on the distal aorta is increasing.

Consideration of family screening should be undertaken for patients who have a positive family history or who appear to have a hereditary connective tissue disorder, such as Marfan syndrome or Ehlers-Danlos syndrome.

CASE 1

History

▸ A 74-year-old man presented with sudden onset of severe chest pain.
▸ Proximal aortic dissection 7 years before: Bentall operation performed at that time.
▸ Anticoagulation supervised, but little follow-up of the aorta. BP variably controlled.

Physical Examination

▸ Frail looking
▸ No venous distention
▸ Normal mechanical valve sounds; no aortic insufficiency murmur; apex sustained

Clinical Impression

▸ Persistent false lumen in the descending aorta
▸ Dilation of the true and false lumens in the descending aorta
▸ False aneurysm at the proximal end of the Bentall composite graft

▸ The exact cause of the chest pain was unclear, as all of these features could have predated the chest pain, and there was no CT or transesophageal echocardiography (TEE) imaging from routine regular follow-up with which to compare the findings.

Management and Outcome

▸ BP control and beta-blockers
▸ Given the frail state of the patient and the uncertainty of the acuity of the findings, reoperation was not offered.
▸ Alive 3 years later

Comments

▸ Breakdown of the proximal insertion of the composite graft (Bentall procedure)
▸ False aneurysm expansion may or may not have explained the development of acute symptoms.
▸ Interpretation of the imaging at presentation is difficult without availability of prior (baseline) imaging findings.
▸ Survivors of first operations for type A AAD are inevitably older and more frail when they are evaluated later.

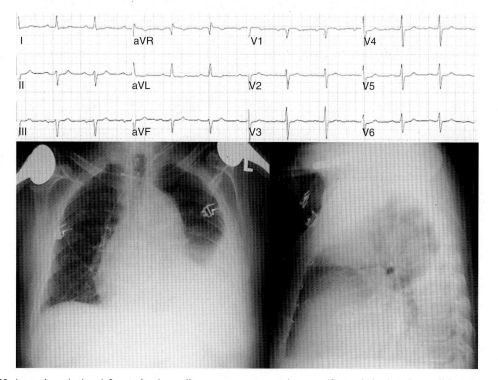

Figure 6-6. TOP, ECG shows sinus rhythm, left anterior descending coronary artery, and nonspecific repolarization abnormalities. BOTTOM, Posteroanterior and lateral chest radiographs. The aortic valve replacement is obscured on the posteroanterior film by the superimposition of its shadow on that of the heart and spine. The aortic contour is abnormal, and the arch and descending aorta appear enlarged. There is a left pleural effusion.

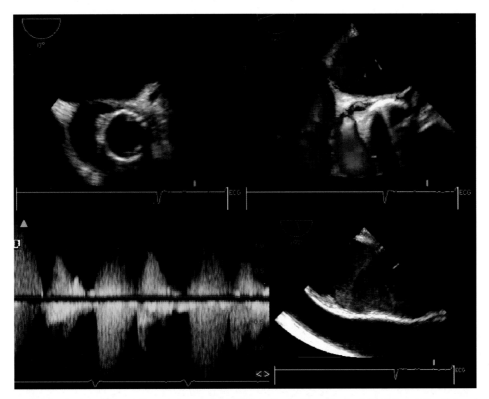

Figure 6-7. TEE. TOP LEFT, Short-axis view of the aortic root shows a fluid-filled cavity, to the patient's right of the aortic valve replacement, that contains flow. TOP RIGHT, Short-axis view of the aortic root with color Doppler mapping shows flow into and out of the cavity, communicating at the sewing ring level with the left ventricular outflow tract. BOTTOM LEFT, Spectral display of pulsed wave Doppler imaging of the neck of the cavity shows reciprocating to-and-fro flow into and out of the periaortic fluid-filled cavity—false aneurysm type of flow. BOTTOM RIGHT, Longitudinal view of the descending aorta. There is persistence of the false lumen. The true lumen is dilated and with slow flow (spontaneous contrast). There is no flow within the false lumen.

CASE 2

History

▸ 78-year-old woman with sudden onset of severe chest pain
▸ Proximal aortic dissection 8 years before; tube graft inserted in the root–ascending aorta, aortic valve spared

Physical Examination

▸ BP 180/95 mm Hg
▸ Severe COPD; frail appearing
▸ Aortic insufficiency and mitral regurgitation murmurs; apex enlarged

Management and Outcome

▸ Clinical impression was that of a false aneurysm at the proximal sewing margin of the tube graft.
▸ Conservative management, given the COPD and age of the patient
▸ Alive 2 years later

Comments

▸ False aneurysm at the proximal margin of the tube graft
▸ The actual cause of the acute symptoms at the later presentation is unclear.
▸ Persistence of a false lumen in the upper and mid descending aorta
▸ Significant comorbidities in late survivors of initially successful surgery for repair of AAD

6

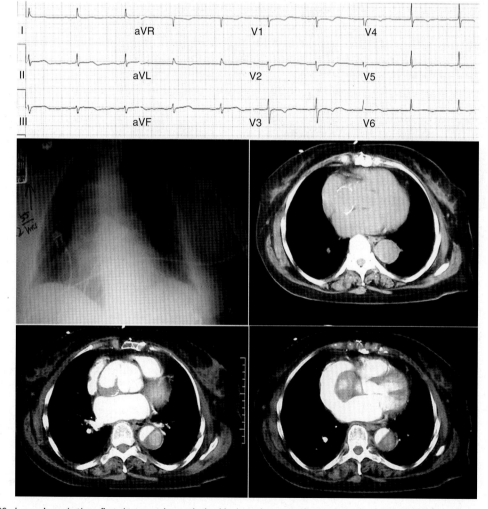

Figure 6-8. TOP, ECG shows sinus rhythm, first-degree atrioventricular block, and nonspecific repolarization abnormalities. MIDDLE LEFT, Chest radiograph rotated projection shows a prominent ascending aorta and no signs of pulmonary edema. MIDDLE RIGHT, Non–contrast-enhanced axial CT image. Abnormal calcification is seen faintly within the descending aorta and also within the heart. The site of calcification within the heart is unclear. BOTTOM, Contrast-enhanced axial CT images show a partially thrombosed false lumen on the descending aorta, abnormal cavity with possible thrombus arising off the right side of the aortic root, abnormal soft tissue mass near the crux of the heart, and no pleural effusion.

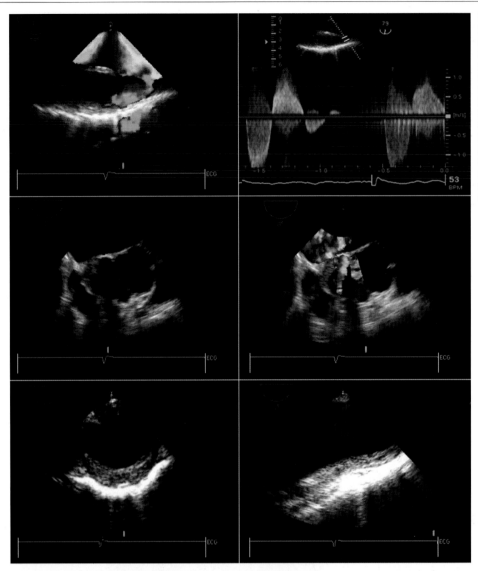

Figure 6-9. TEE. TOP LEFT, There is an intimal flap in the descending aorta, with portioning of flow. There is also an entry tear into the false lumen on the right side of the image. TOP RIGHT, Pulsed Doppler study at the intimal tear shows reciprocating flow into and out of the tear through the intimal flap into the false lumen. MIDDLE, Horizontal plane view of the aortic root shows a fluid-filled and thrombus-lined cavity at the aortic root level under the proximal margin of the tube graft. There is flow within the cavity. BOTTOM, Distal thoracic aorta in cross-sectional (LEFT) and longitudinal (RIGHT) views: the false lumen is thrombosed.

CASE 3

History

▸ 77-year-old man presenting with severe nonischemic chest pains and shortness of breath for 2 weeks
▸ Past medical history is significant for hypertension and type A dissection 7 years previously in another city; Bentall composite graft repair at that time. Other than warfarin management, lost to follow-up since. INR at admission, 1.8.

Physical Examination

▸ BP 190/90 mm Hg, HR 60 bpm, RR 16/min
▸ No venous distention or edema
▸ Clear mechanical valve clicks; no aortic insufficiency murmur
▸ Pulses increased
▸ Reduced air entry at bases; no adventitious sounds

Evolution

▸ Most imaging observations were common after composite graft insertion for type A dissection, and they were not convincingly acute and responsible for the symptoms and pleural effusions.

   ▸ The finding of a persistent distal false lumen is common and not likely to be acute.

   ▸ The distal false lumen was not severely dilated, and no false aneurysm had developed or ruptured.
   ▸ The mechanical valve functioned well, and the appearance of the tube graft was usual.
   ▸ The soft tissue around the ascending aorta was ambiguous; but as the tube graft appeared normal, rupture was considered unlikely.
   ▸ Biomarkers and results of ischemic testing were normal.
▸ The chest pains subsided spontaneously.
▸ The pleural effusions were serous, not sanguineous.
▸ One side tested positive for malignant cells, which were subsequently established as metastatic from an abdominal source.
▸ The cause of the acute presentation was unclear.

Comments

▸ Difficult real-life scenario: evaluation of a patient with a prior aortic repair, given the lack of baseline imaging with which to compare present findings.
▸ Consideration of most late complications of AAD and surgical repair was sustained, but no specific complication could be identified.
▸ Persistent and prolonged observation and testing established the cause of the pleural effusions, but the source of the chest pains remained unproven.

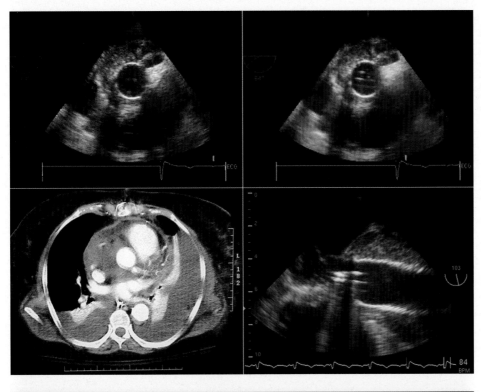

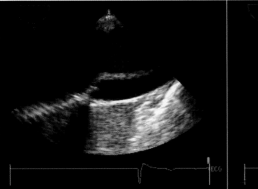

Figure 6-10. TEE. TOP LEFT, View of the aortic root at the level of the tube graft. The implantation of the left coronary artery is seen. TOP RIGHT, The bileaflet occluders rise into the plane of imaging in systole. There is a large amount of thrombus around the tube graft. The Dacron tube graft is apparent by its woven texture. BOTTOM LEFT, Contrast-enhanced CT scan shows bilateral pleural effusions. The very proximal part of the implanted left coronary artery is visible. Soft tissue around the ascending aorta. BOTTOM RIGHT, Longitudinal view of the ascending aortic tube graft also shows a large amount of surrounding thrombus. The aortic valve replacement occluders are again open.

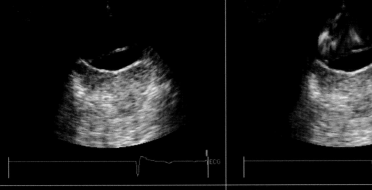

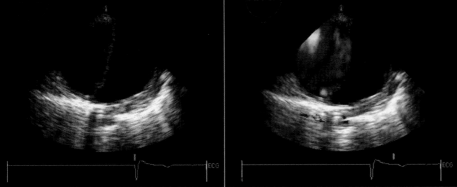

Figure 6-11. TEE. TOP LEFT, View of the distal aspect of the tube graft. The far end of the tube graft, in the midportion of the arch, is where the false lumen begins. The intimal flap and outer wall had been sewn together at the distal end of the tube graft. TOP RIGHT, Although there is still a false lumen, there is little flow in it in this segment. MIDDLE, Descending thoracic aorta in cross section. The intimal flap is well seen, and there is complete partitioning of flow, without detected flow in the false lumen. BOTTOM, Same pattern. Occluders of the aortic valve replacement are open in this systolic phase.

References

1. Genoni M, Paul M, Jenni R, et al: Chronic beta-blocker therapy improves outcome and reduces treatment costs in chronic type B aortic dissection. Eur J Cardiothorac Surg 2001;19:606-610.

2. Fann JI, Smith JA, Miller DC, et al: Surgical management of aortic dissection during a 30-year period. Circulation 1995;92(Suppl):II113-II121.

3. Sueyoshi E, Sakamoto I, Hayashi K, et al: Growth rate of aortic diameter in patients with type B aortic dissection during the chronic phase. Circulation 2004;110(Suppl 1):II256.

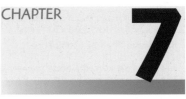

7

Aortic Complications of Catheterization, Surgery, and Instrumentation

KEY POINTS

▸ Surgical and catheter manipulation of the aorta may result in early or late injury to the aorta, including dissection.

▸ Cardiac surgical manipulation of the aorta carries particular risk of causing disruption to the ascending aorta (at the sites of cross-clamping, afferent cannula insertion, and aortotomy of AVR cases).

▸ Patients undergoing angiography who develop AAD are obviously far more likely to have coronary artery disease than are most other AAD patients—an important comorbidity that AAD patients are otherwise usually fortunate to be without.

Wires, catheters, and devices can penetrate into the wall of the aorta, particularly if it is diseased or if excessive manipulation occurs. Retrograde cannulation is the usual scenario. Greater tortuosity of the aorta and greater irregularity of the inner surface increase the risk of entrance of a wire, catheter, or device into the wall, initiating dissection or rupture. Cross-clamping, cannula insertion, and incision of the wall of the aorta can damage the wall and lead to disruption. External manipulation of the aorta can lead to embolization of preexisting thrombus overlying aortic plaque. Introduction of the afferent bypass cannula through the aortic wall to return pressurized blood can readily lead to dissection or other forms of disruption if the cannula does not pass into the lumen, but rather pushes into the lumen an overlying plaque, and pressurized afferent blood pressurizes a medial blood collection that initiates a dissection.

The International Registry of Aortic Dissection reports that 5% of acute aortic dissection (AAD) cases are iatrogenic.[1] Of iatrogenic type A dissections, 69% resulted from cardiac surgery, 27% from coronary angiography or percutaneous coronary intervention, and 4% from other causes (such as renal percutaneous transluminal coronary angioplasty). Of iatrogenic type B dissections, 12% resulted from cardiac surgery and 87% from coronary angiography or percutaneous coronary intervention.

Patients with iatrogenic AADs are much more likely to have myocardial ischemia (36% versus 5%; $P < .001$) or myocardial infarction (15% versus 3%; $P < .001$) than are patients with noniatrogenic AADs.[1] The mortality of iatrogenic dissection is higher than that of noniatrogenic dissection (35% versus 24%).[1]

AORTIC COMPLICATIONS OF CATHETER-BASED INTERVENTIONS

Aortic complications of catheter-based interventions include dissection of the thoracic or abdominal aorta, rupture or perforation of the aorta, embolization of thrombus (from complex atheromatous disease, thoracic or abdominal aneurysms, or embolization of atheromatous particles), and thrombosis of the aorta by intraaortic balloon counterpulsation catheters.

AORTIC COMPLICATIONS OF CARDIAC SURGERY

Aortic complications of cardiac surgery include (1) dissections and false aneurysms of the thoracic aorta, (2) embolization of thrombus or atheromatous material by surgical manipulation, and (3) breaking of a calcified (porcelain) ascending aorta by cross-clamping.[2] Dissections of the thoracic aorta may arise from the afferent cannula site, the cross-clamp site, the valvulotomy or sewing margin of an aortic valve replacement (AVR), or the anastomosis of a saphenous graft. False aneurysm of the thoracic aorta may occur at the afferent cannula site, at the cross-clamp site, at the valvulotomy or sewing margin of an AVR, or at the anastomosis of a saphenous graft.

CASE 1

History and Physical Examination

- 40-year-old man with acute coronary syndrome
- Positive anterior wall perfusion defect
- No notable family history and no apparent risk factors
- Normal physical examination findings and body habitus

Evolution

- Angioplasty was technically straightforward and successful, but the patient became distressed half an hour later.
- No angina or ST changes on the electrocardiogram to support stent thrombosis
- No rub, normal neck veins, making tamponade unlikely
- Urgent bedside transthoracic echocardiography (TTE) confirmed normal left ventricular function and only a very small pericardial effusion—poor and limited windows
- Worsening distress and BP slowly falling, 100/60 → 85/50 → 70/40
- Vague chest pain, prominent abdominal pain and tenderness, altered mental status
- Possibilities entertained included retroperitoneal hemorrhage, aortic dissection, and stroke.

Clinical Impression, Management, and Outcome

- Clinical impression was that of shock from aortic dissection with left pleural rupture and probably intrapericardial rupture as well.
- Abdominal pain was due to bladder distention only. There was no evidence of retroperitoneal bleeding.
- Volume and vasopressors were maximized, and urgent surgery was arranged.
- Bentall procedure (AVR composite graft) was performed.
- Uneventful outcome

Comments

- Sudden and unexpected deterioration in patients with coronary artery disease (CAD) after a procedure not explained by ischemia or bleeding prompts consideration of aortic dissection.
- The presentation was treacherous, given the lack of prominent chest pain and early—if not immediate—external rupture.
- In this case, bedside TTE was helpful only with excluding acute infarction. Computed tomography (CT) was invaluable to address the multiple concerns of retroperitoneal hemorrhage, aortic injury, and intracerebral hemorrhage.

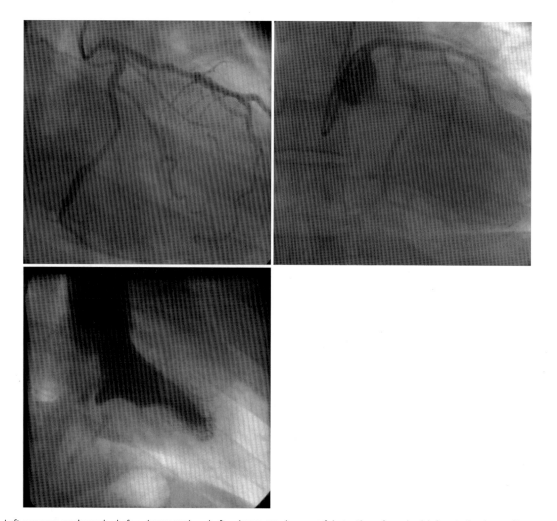

Figure 7-1. Left coronary angiography before (UPPER LEFT) and after (UPPER RIGHT) successful stenting of proximal left anterior descending coronary artery stenosis. LOWER LEFT, Contrast ventriculogram reveals dilation of the ascending aorta and lack of clear sinus of Valsalva architecture. No intimal flap is present.

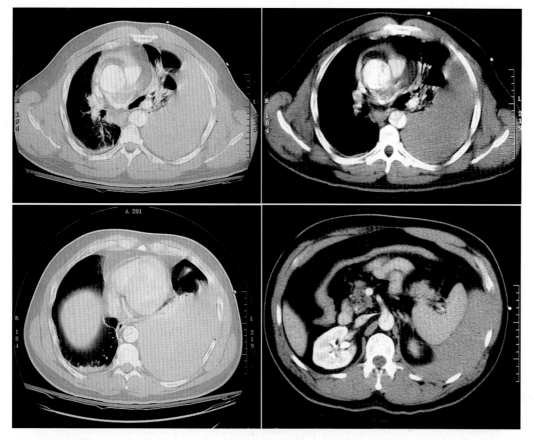

Figure 7-2. Contrast-enhanced axial CT scans. TOP, The ascending aorta is enlarged. There is an intimal flap in the descending aorta. There is a probable intimal flap in the ascending aorta. There is a large left pleural effusion and a pericardial effusion surrounding the great vessels. BOTTOM LEFT, There is an intimal flap in the descending aorta and a large pleural effusion. BOTTOM RIGHT, The superior mesenteric artery arises from the false lumen.

CASE 2

History

▶ Class III angina, positive noninvasive testing, underwent cardiac catheterization
▶ CAD risk factor: smoking
▶ Claudication at 3 blocks, no cardiovascular disease
▶ Difficulty in getting past the iliac arteries, severe back pain during the procedure—strong suspicion of a catheter-induced dissection

Physical Examination

▶ BP 150/80 mm Hg, 210/95 mm Hg with agitation
▶ Lungs clear
▶ S_1, S_2 normal; +S_4; no aortic insufficiency (AI)
▶ Decreased femoral pulses, no ischemic changes

Evolution and Management

▶ Clinical impression was that of dissection or intramural hematoma of the aorta from retrograde passage of the catheter up the planes of tissue within the aortic wall, atherosclerotic aortic obstruction, and renal artery stenosis.
▶ Aortic injury was managed conservatively, and resolution was documented during a week.
▶ Optimal BP control with larger beta-blocker dose
▶ Coronary angiography was performed later through the radial artery: three-vessel CAD operated on uneventfully.
▶ Uneventful outcome

Comments

▶ Complete abdominal atherosclerotic occlusion of the aorta, unrecognized as the collateral flow was enough to allow only mild claudication
▶ Associated CAD and renal artery stenosis
▶ Hypertension from aortic occlusion and probably from the renal artery stenosis
▶ Resolution of the intramural hematoma during 1 week, clinically and seen on serial testing
▶ Subsequent angiograms performed by radial access

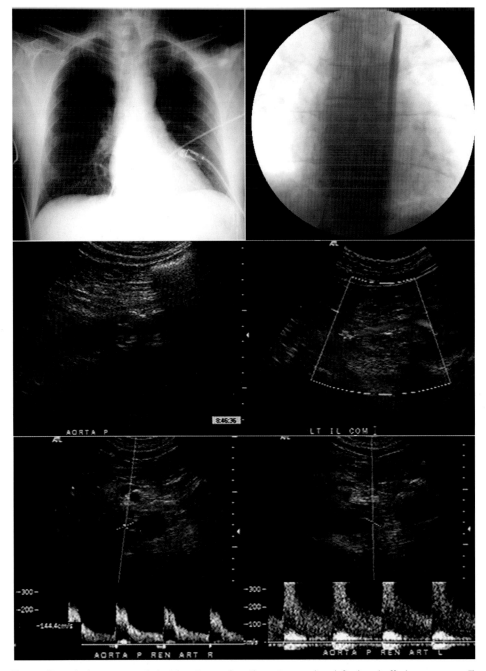

Figure 7-3. TOP LEFT, Chest radiograph shows a normal-sized heart, normal aortic contour, and no left pleural effusion. TOP RIGHT, Fluoroscopy during the catheterization procedure that injured the aorta. Contrast dye has been hand injected and fills a long discrete plane within the medial wall of the descending aorta. The dye did not wash out. MIDDLE, There is no flow detected in the lower abdominal aorta by ultrasonography. There is a very large inferior mesenteric collateral that supplied the iliac system. BOTTOM LEFT, Renal artery Doppler recording shows normal right renal artery flow. BOTTOM RIGHT, Severe flow acceleration in the ostium of the left renal artery consistent with stenosis, which may have underlain the hypertension.

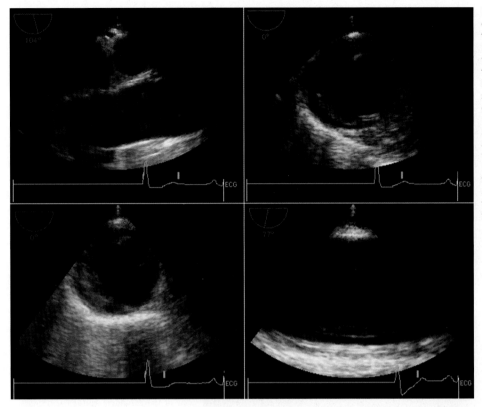

Figure 7-4. Transesophageal echocardiography. TOP LEFT, Longitudinal view of the ascending aorta. Other than mild dilation, the aorta is normal and without an intimal flap or mural thickening. No pericardial effusion. TOP RIGHT, Mid descending aorta in cross section. There is a crescentic thickening of the medial half of the aortic wall with prominent echolucency, suggesting fresh blood. BOTTOM LEFT, Distal thoracic aorta again has a crescentic mural thickening, with a uniform appearance. BOTTOM RIGHT, Longitudinal view of the descending thoracic aorta shows thickening of the aortic wall and a long stripe of echolucent thickening. The appearance is that of an intramural hematoma.

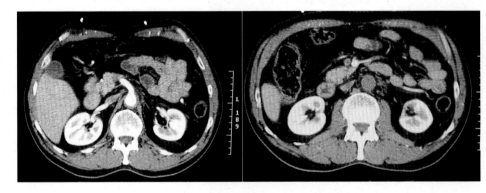

Figure 7-5. Contrast-enhanced axial CT scans. The appearance of the abdominal aorta at the level of the superior mesenteric artery is unremarkable. More distally, the aorta is occluded. Large mesenteric collateral vessels are present.

CASE 3

History and Physical Examination

▸ A 63-year-old man developed sudden severe chest pains 10 days before.
▸ Prior medical history is significant for AVR for aortic stenosis 5 years before and hypertension.
▸ BP 190/100 mm Hg, HR 90 bpm
▸ No venous distention
▸ No AI murmur, no rub
▸ Normal valve clicks, normal pulses, no crepitations

Evolution and Management

▸ Clinical impression was that of a post-AVR dissection of a dilated ascending aorta, limited to the aortic root and ascending aorta.

▸ It was confirmed at surgery.
▸ Tube graft insertion in the ascending aorta was performed, with uneventful outcome.

Comments

▸ Post-AVR dissection of the aortic root
▸ The preoperative ascending aorta dimension was only 49 mm.
▸ The aortic valve morphology preoperatively was bicuspid.
▸ No echocardiography was performed postoperatively; therefore, the issue of progressive postoperative dilation was not resolvable.

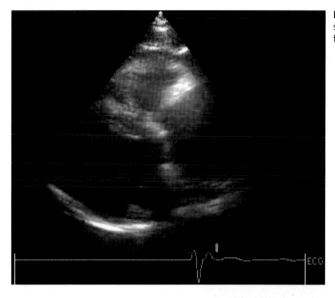

Figure 7-6. Transthoracic echocardiographic parasternal long-axis view showing dilated aortic root and ascending aorta. There is no definite intimal flap.

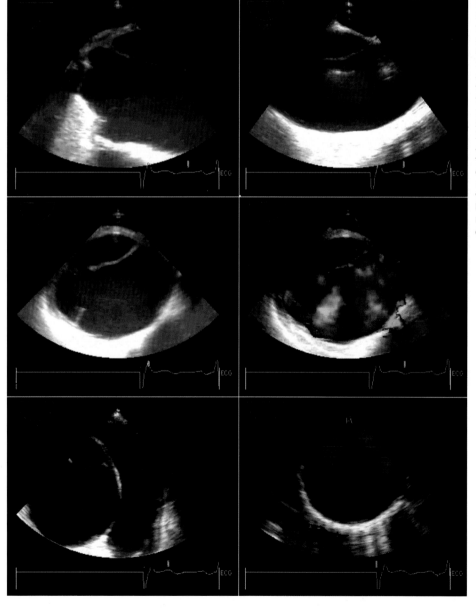

Figure 7-7. Transesophageal echocardiography. TOP LEFT, Longitudinal view of the ascending aorta. Normal appearance to the bileaflet AVR. Dilated ascending aorta. Intimal flap posteriorly down to the level of the aortic annulus and AVR sewing ring. TOP RIGHT, Long-axis view of the ascending aorta. The intimal flap ends at the level of the right pulmonary artery. MIDDLE LEFT, Cross-sectional view of the ascending aorta. Intimal flap and intimal tear in the ascending aorta. MIDDLE RIGHT, The intimal flap partitions flow. Some flow is seen entering the false lumen through the tear. BOTTOM LEFT, The dilated ascending aorta with an intimal flap and tear is seen at the level of the main pulmonary artery. BOTTOM RIGHT, Normal appearance and flow in the descending aorta.

CASE 4

History and Physical Examination

▸ 76-year-old woman undergoing carotid stenting
▸ Prior medical history is significant for "inoperable" (nonintervenable) CAD; 12 years previously, a ruptured descending thoracic aneurysm with 3 weeks of bilateral leg paralysis, but eventually full recovery, unoperated on; high-grade carotid lesion; hypertension; and a 50-mm aneurysm of the ascending aorta.
▸ During stenting of the common carotid artery, a dissection of the carotid artery developed. A second stent was inserted in the more proximal portion of the common carotid, extending into the innominate artery, eliminating dye opacification of a false lumen beside the carotid artery. The intimal flap was seen to extend down into the brachiocephalic (innominate) artery, but the patient was without pain.
▸ That night, the patient developed pain in the high anterior chest.

Evolution and Management

▸ Clinical impression was that of a retrograde dissection of the carotid artery–innominate dissection into the proximal aortic arch and ascending aorta, down to the root.
▸ The AI antedated the dissection.
▸ The patient was believed to be a poor candidate for surgical repair because of COPD.
▸ The patient was managed conservatively. Antihypertensive medications were maximized.
▸ The patient remained stable.

Comments

▸ Extensive retrograde dissection into the ascending aorta and root
▸ The minimal contrast enhancement of the false lumen in the ascending aorta suggests little communication with the true lumen. This may have been the reason that there was no observed progression.

▸ The preexistent aneurysm of the aorta may have supplied substrate to the retrograde dissection of the aorta.
▸ The systolic hypertension in her case was easily understandable, given the obvious and extensive plaques conferring noncompliance and stiffness.
▸ The AI was determined to predate the dissection by obtaining prior medical records; the configuration of the aortic valve leaflets (tented as if from root dilation rather than with prolapse of leaflets from unseating from an adjacent false lumen) was consistent with chronicity.
▸ There was no evidence of a descending thoracic aneurysm. The complex calcification pattern seen in the minimally dilated descending thoracic aorta suggested somewhat a healed prior dissection that may have been responsible for the leg paralysis, presumed anterior spinal ischemia a decade ago.

Evolution

▸ The following year, the patient was seen and described class IV angina. She had been stable otherwise through the year.
▸ She was readmitted for evaluation of coronary disease and review of the status of her aorta.

Outcome

▸ The aorta did not offer findings that precluded coronary angiography, which was subsequently obtained and provided the forum to intervene successfully with stents to the left anterior descending and right coronary arteries.
▸ She was angina free after this.

Comments

▸ Complete healing of the stent-induced aortic dissection within 1 year
▸ Probable complete healing of the presumed former distal dissection a decade before
▸ The coronary disease had been inaccurately deemed inoperable.

Text continued on p. 152.

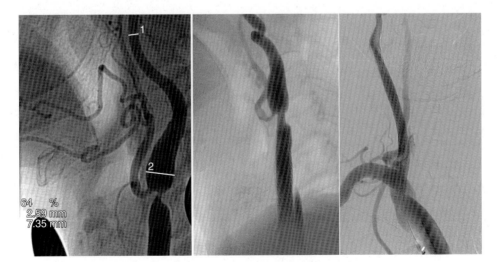

Figure 7-8. Angiographic images before and after right common carotid stenting. Before stenting (LEFT), there is a high-grade stenosis of the distal common carotid artery. After the first stent has been inserted, a false lumen has developed (MIDDLE). An intimal flap can be seen to extend down into the brachiocephalic (innominate) artery (RIGHT).

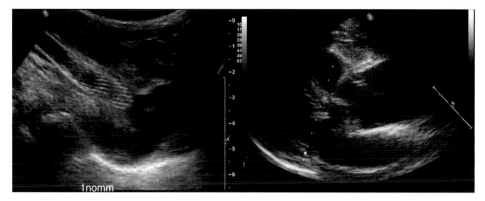

Figure 7-9. LEFT, Vascular ultrasound examination after carotid stenting. There is a mobile flap proximal to the stent, within the innominate artery. The most distal extent of the flap is unclear, but the most proximal extent is not. RIGHT, Parasternal long-axis view. There is a dimly seen flap within the aortic root down to the right sinotubular junction. There was moderate AI from the root dilation, not from the dissection (as the aortic leaflets are tented, not prolapsing).

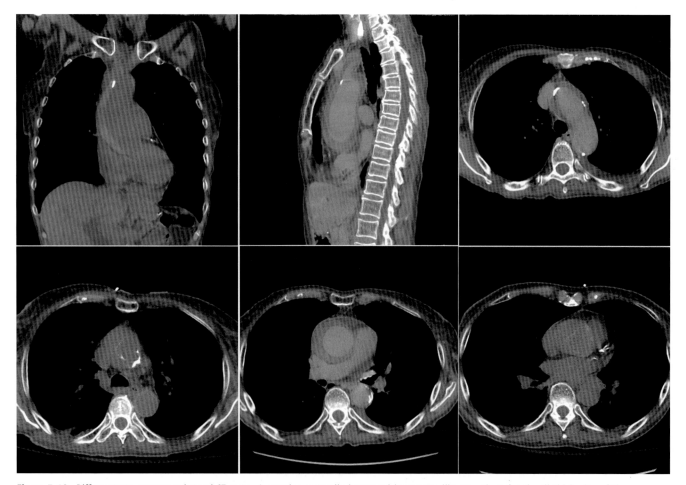

Figure 7-10. Different non–contrast-enhanced CT scans. A complex, generally intramural hematoma–like smooth-surfaced wall thickening of the ascending aorta and root is present, and there is intimal calcium displacement at a number of sites. There is coronary calcification and complex calcification in the descending aorta, which does not appear to have significant wall thickening.

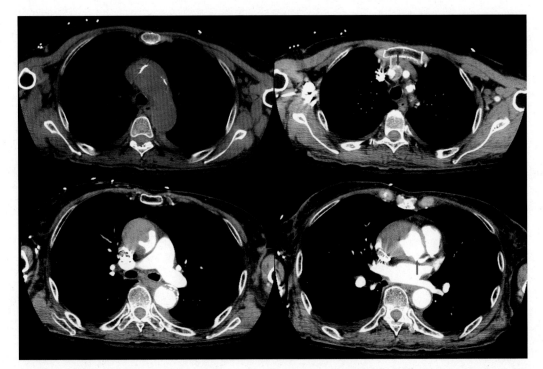

Figure 7-11. TOP LEFT, Non–contrast-enhanced axial CT scan shows obvious displacement of the intimal calcification into the lumen of the arch, indicating dissection of intramural hematoma. TOP RIGHT, Contrast-enhanced axial CT scan at the level of the arch branch vessels shows a prominent streaking artifact from the contrast material in the right subclavian vein. The innominate artery has a contrast-enhancing true lumen *(yellow arrow)* and a less contrast-enhancing (larger) false lumen *(red arrow)*. BOTTOM LEFT, Contrast-enhanced axial CT scan shows a very large false lumen within the ascending aorta, with a very convoluted intimal face. The descending aorta is heavily atheromatous with extensive intimal calcification and overlying thrombus. BOTTOM RIGHT, Contrast-enhanced axial CT scan shows that the false lumen extends to within 1 cm of the left main coronary artery ostium *(red arrow)*.

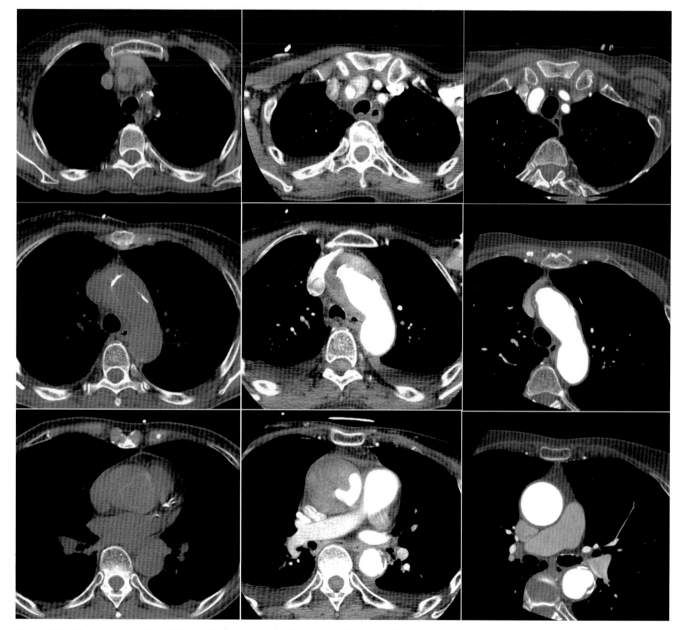

Figure 7-12. CT scans at the time of the aortic dissection complicating carotid stenting (LEFT AND MIDDLE COLUMNS) and 1 year later (RIGHT COLUMN). There has been complete resolution of the marked wall thickening of the ascending aorta and brachiocephalic artery. There are no false aneurysms. The intimal calcification is no longer displaced by wall thickening.

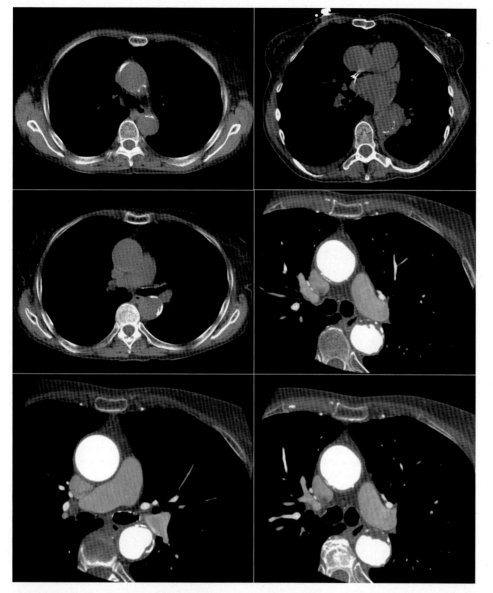

Figure 7-13. Non–contrast-enhanced and contrast-enhanced CT scans reveal a number of patterns of calcification. TOP LEFT, The pattern of the calcification in the ascending and descending aorta is usual for intimal calcification. TOP RIGHT, The pattern of calcification in the descending aorta is usual for displacement of intimal calcification due to mural thickening. MIDDLE LEFT, The pattern of calcification is complex as it occurs at two different layers. This may represent displaced intimal calcification on the more luminal aspect and calcification of a former false lumen on the outer aspect. MIDDLE RIGHT AND BOTTOM, Contrast dye delineates soft tissue over what otherwise would have been assumed to be usual intimal calcification in the descending aorta. The few flecks of calcification in the ascending aorta are usual in appearance for intimal calcification. The more outside location of the calcification may imply either thrombus overlying calcified intimal plaque or organization of a former, now healed, distal dissection, with calcification of the former outer wall of the false lumen.

CASE 5

History and Physical Examination

▸ 70-year-old man admitted with severe chest pains
▸ Prior medical history is significant for an aortocoronary bypass (ACB) 8 years before and hypertension.
▸ Initial myocardial biomarkers (×3) were normal.

Comments

▸ Although the cause of the chest pain was initially unclear, serial testing established that the cause was an acute coronary syndrome (biomarkers rose 5 × normal).

▸ The thrombosed false aneurysm off the ascending aorta was presumed to be a sequela of previous ACB.
▸ The cause of the false lumen extending from the ascending aorta was presumed to be ACB cross-clamp related.

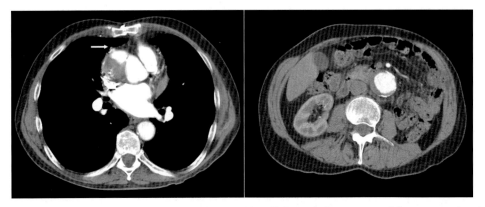

Figure 7-14. Contrast-enhanced axial CT scans. LEFT, There is a complex extension off the ascending aorta, partially contrast enhancing, partially not. There is an intimal disruption between the true lumen and the contrast-enhancing false lumen. The right coronary ostium appears off the false lumen *(arrow)*. RIGHT, There is a medium-sized abdominal aortic aneurysm containing some mural thrombus.

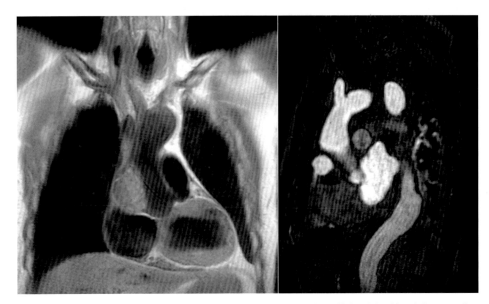

Figure 7-15. LEFT, Coronal spin echo magnetic resonance image shows an egg-sized abnormality off the right side of the ascending aorta, appearing to be thrombus. RIGHT, Gadolinium contrast–enhanced aortography. The right coronary ostium extends off a cavity separate from the ascending aorta.

CASE 6

History and Physical Examination

▸ A 25-year-old man with aortic stenosis developed recurrent exertional syncope.

▸ Physical findings were consistent with severe aortic stenosis (pulsus parvus et tardus, sustained apex, late-peaking murmur, and S_4).

▸ His aortic valve area was 0.6 cm², and the mean gradient was 72 mm Hg.

▸ The aortic valve was bicuspid, and there was dilation of the ascending aorta.

▸ He underwent aortic valve replacement because of symptomatic severe aortic stenosis.

▸ He was discharged home in 6 days and was well for 2 weeks before he developed severe chest pain and presyncope.

▸ On physical examination, he was overtly shocky, with dull agitation, cold extremities, and livido.

▸ BP 75/– mm Hg, HR 150 bpm, RR 24/min

▸ The venous pressures were prominently distended, and the mechanical heart sounds were distant.

Clinical Impression, Management, and Outcome

▸ Bicuspid valve–related aortopathy (dilation)

▸ Post-AVR dissection and rupture into the pericardial space, mediastinum, and left pleural space

▸ The patient underwent emergent surgery to replace the aortic root and ascending aorta with a tube graft and survived. The intimal tear was at the level of the cross-clamping for the AVR.

Comments

▸ Bicuspid valve–related aortopathy

▸ AAD caused by aortopathy and recent cross-clamping

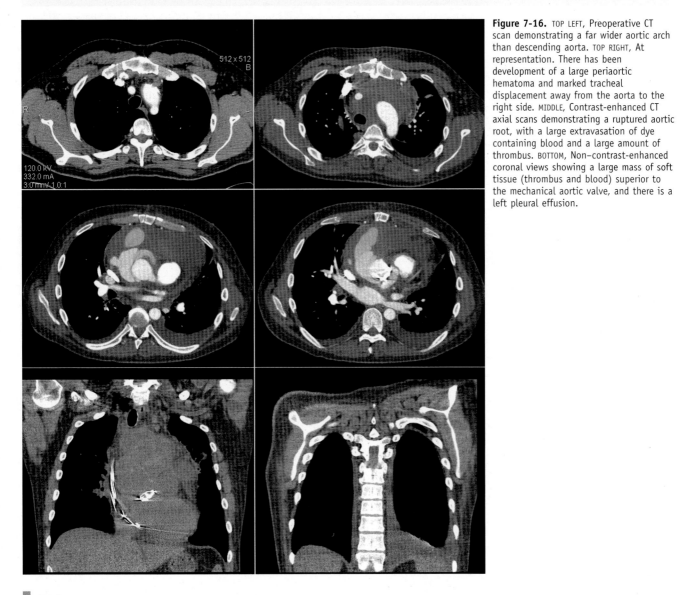

Figure 7-16. TOP LEFT, Preoperative CT scan demonstrating a far wider aortic arch than descending aorta. TOP RIGHT, At representation. There has been development of a large periaortic hematoma and marked tracheal displacement away from the aorta to the right side. MIDDLE, Contrast-enhanced CT axial scans demonstrating a ruptured aortic root, with a large extravasation of dye containing blood and a large amount of thrombus. BOTTOM, Non–contrast-enhanced coronal views showing a large mass of soft tissue (thrombus and blood) superior to the mechanical aortic valve, and there is a left pleural effusion.

References

1. Januzzi JL, Sabatine MS, Eagle KA, et al: Iatrogenic aortic dissection. Am J Cardiol 2002;89:623-626.

2. Sullivan KL, Steiner RM, Smullens SN, et al: Pseudoaneurysm of the ascending aorta following cardiac surgery. Chest 1988;93:138-143.

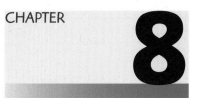
Aortic Atheromatous Disease: Plaques, Debris, and Obstruction

Atherosclerosis is a generalized process that affects all arterial vasculature, including the aorta. What is seen on a millimeter scale in the coronaries is seen on a centimeter scale in the aorta. Atheromatous plaques in the aorta may occasionally be bulky enough to narrow the aortic lumen or to obstruct it (which is more common in the smaller abdominal aorta) but are more relevant as markers of generalized atheromatous disease risk (coronary artery disease [CAD] risk and stroke) and as markers and mediators of greater instrumentation risks (aortocoronary bypass; aortic, renal artery, left-sided heart catheterization; intra-aortic balloon pump). Rarely, atheromatous plaques may incite acute thrombosis of the aorta or allow embolization of overlying thrombus, debris, or cholesterol-laden content.

Aortic atheroma extent correlates with global atheroma extent and events within other arterial beds. Aortic atheroma also causes clinical events within the distribution of the aorta itself, being responsible for thrombosis of the aorta and embolization distally of debris, thrombus, and cholesterol through the aorta.

Aortic atherosclerosis begins as an intimal and subintimal process of migration of lipid between endothelial cells into the subintimal space, producing soft plaques that enlarge and become increasingly complex during decades. The process does not stay limited to the intimal space but will extend into the media when plaques become advanced.

Aortic atherosclerosis begins early in life (Fig. 8-1).[1] In children, yellow, circumscribed fatty streaks of lipid are already present, usually located above the aortic valve and in the ductal area of the aorta. In adolescents, there is progression into fatty streaks, extending around the ostia of branches. In young adults, fatty streaks become partially fibrotic and gray (fibrotic plaques) with more complex and heterogeneous plaque composition typical of atherosclerosis. In older adults, further plaque complexity (calcification, ulceration, and thrombosis) and volume increase in plaques occur.

For unknown reasons, the greatest extent of atherosclerosis tends to be in the abdominal aorta, below the renal arteries. Postulated reasons include local hemodynamic stresses, the thinness of the wall, and the lack of local vasa vasorum. The site of second greatest involvement is the proximal descending aorta and distal floor of the arch. The ascending aorta is the least affected by atherosclerosis, except in diabetes mellitus and type III hyperlipoproteinemia.

AORTIC INTIMAL ATHEROSCLEROTIC CALCIFICATION

Aortic atherosclerotic calcification, a form of complication of atherosclerosis, increases with each decade of advancing age, until it is present in the majority of patients in their 80s (Fig. 8-2). Calcification is superbly imaged by non–contrast-enhanced computed tomography (CT) scanning, but it may also be detected by

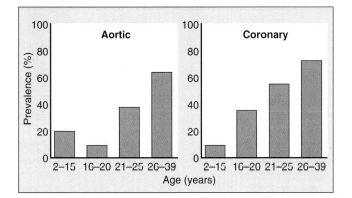

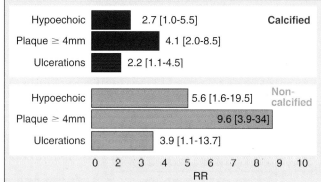

Figure 8-1. Aortic atherosclerosis begins early in life and progresses, as shown by this study of 204 autopsies of traumatic deaths, aged 2 to 39 years. (From Berenson GS, Srinivasan SR, Bao W, et al: Association between multiple cardiovascular risk factors and atherosclerosis in children and young adults: the Bogalusa Heart Study. N Engl J Med 1998;338:1650-1656. Copyright © [2001] Massachusetts Medical Society. All rights reserved.)

Figure 8-2. Noncalcified aortic atheromas are associated with greater stroke risk, as shown by this study of 334 patients with cardiovascular accident observed by transesophageal echocardiography for 2 to 4 years. RR, relative risk. (From Cohen A, Tzourio C, Bertrand B, et al: Aortic plaque morphology and vascular events: a follow-up study in patients with ischemic stroke. FAPS Investigators. French Study of Aortic Plaques in Stroke. Circulation 1997;96:3838-3841.)

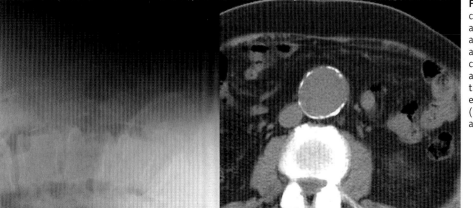

Figure 8-3. Plain radiographic and non–contrast-enhanced CT visualization of aortic atherosclerosis (abdominal aortic aneurysm). LEFT, A lateral shoot-through abdominal radiograph reveals prelumbar calcification outlining an obvious abdominal aortic aneurysm. RIGHT, In the same patient, CT (without contrast enhancement) demonstrates extensive (near-circumferential) calcification of the abdominal aortic aneurysm.

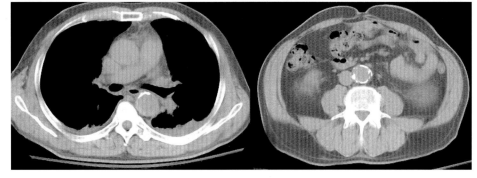

Figure 8-4. Non–contrast-enhanced axial CT scans. LEFT, Intimal calcification of the thoracic aorta between the 10-o'clock and 12-o'clock positions. There is a faint crescentic thickening of the wall of the aorta between the 3-o'clock and 10-o'clock positions—an intramural hematoma. The hematoma is less likely to accumulate in aortic wall that is deeply calcified, as in this image. RIGHT, Intimal calcification of the abdominal aorta. Note the complexity of the calcification and the heterogeneity of calcium within plaque.

plain radiography (chest radiography and prelumbar radiography) if the projection of the calcification is away from other (radiopaque) structures (Figs. 8-3 to 8-7). The posteroanterior chest radiograph commonly detects intimal calcification at the distal aortic arch (knob); this site within the aorta is commonly atherosclerotic, and it projects clearly of the spine.

There is a twofold increase in cardiovascular death if atherosclerotic calcification of the aorta is present before 65 years of age. Some studies have shown up to a sevenfold increase in mortality with aortic calcification at younger ages.[2]

It has been suggested that atheromas of the aorta be graded because they are commonly imaged, and risk (CAD, stroke) approximates their extent, except in the elderly.[3,4] In the strongest series, aortic atheroma as predictor of CAD risk had a sensitivity of 90%, specificity of 90%, positive predictive value of 95%, and negative predictive value of 82%. In patients older than 70 years, aortic atheroma was not a predictor of CAD (seen in 12 of 13 patients with CAD and 9 of 10 patients without CAD). Lack of aortic atheroma correlates with lack of angiographic CAD.[5] Aortic atheroma extent correlates with risk of stroke with aortocoronary

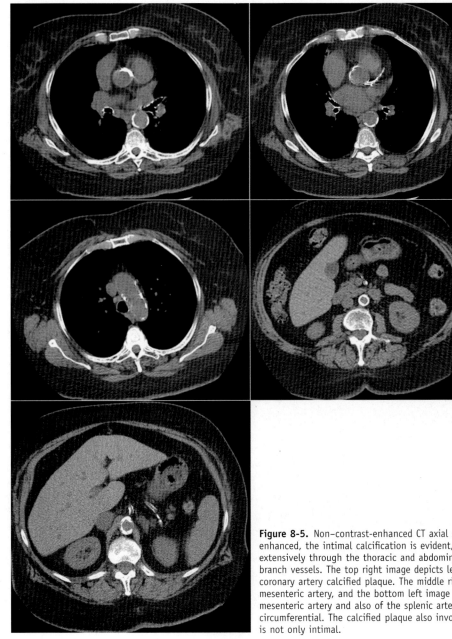

Figure 8-5. Non–contrast-enhanced CT axial scans. Because the lumen is not contrast enhanced, the intimal calcification is evident, if not prominent. There are calcified plaques extensively through the thoracic and abdominal aorta. There is also extensive calcification of branch vessels. The top right image depicts left main coronary and left anterior descending coronary artery calcified plaque. The middle right image demonstrates calcium of the superior mesenteric artery, and the bottom left image demonstrates extensive calcium of the superior mesenteric artery and also of the splenic artery. In many places, the calcium is thick or nearly circumferential. The calcified plaque also involves much of the thickness of the aortic wall and is not only intimal.

bypass; of 268 patients undergoing aortocoronary bypass, stroke occurred in 11.6% of those with arch plaques of more than 5 mm.[6]

Although aortic atherosclerosis occurs in tandem with CAD, to date there have been no large randomized prospective trials based on presence, absence, or extent of aortic atheromatous disease that directly evaluated any intervention and associated clinical endpoints. Identification, though, of aortic atheroma in a patient hitherto unknown to have atherosclerosis would reasonably prompt implementation of general measures of secondary prevention and consideration of the higher risks of aortic instrumentation if overlying thrombus is seen.

A TEE grading of aortic atheroma has been proposed[3]:

- Grade 1: normal intima
- Grade 2: minimal plaque
- Grade 3: raised irregular plaque <5 mm
- Grade 4: complex protruding plaque ≥5 mm, with ulceration or calcific density

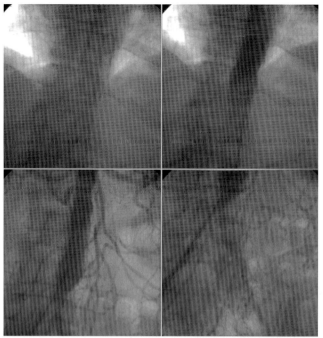

Figure 8-6. Fluoroscopy/aortography. There are thick and irregular calcified plaques along the walls of the abdominal aorta. Train track calcification of the splenic artery (seen on the left side) in the same patient as in Figure 8-5. There is a small abdominal aortic aneurysm as well.

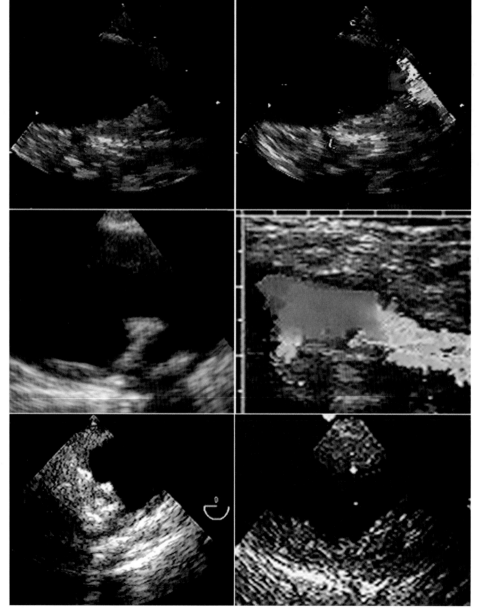

Figure 8-7. Ultrasonography and transesophageal echocardiography (TEE) images of aortic atherosclerosis. TOP, TEE longitudinal views of the mid descending aorta reveal thick plaque on both walls that intrudes on the lumen. Color Doppler flow mapping demonstrates turbulence from flow acceleration. There was a 50 mm Hg gradient. MIDDLE LEFT, TEE view of a steep shelf-like plaque rigidly sticking into the lumen of the aorta. Although it caused turbulence, there was no gradient. MIDDLE RIGHT, Abdominal ultrasound image of the lower abdominal aorta. There is thick plaque on the right side of the image and flow acceleration of turbulence caused by the narrowing plaque. BOTTOM LEFT, TEE cross-sectional view of the mid descending aorta. There is voluminous plaque, with calcium, but there appears to be Glagovian remodeling of the artery to preserve lumen. BOTTOM RIGHT, TEE longitudinal view of the thoracic aorta. There is thick plaque along both walls.

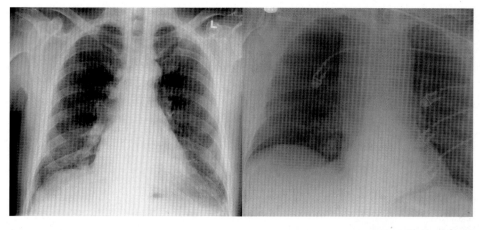

Figure 8-8. LEFT, A well-delineated calcified intimal plaque is present in the distal arch, a common site for aortic atherosclerosis. RIGHT, Calcified aortic intimal atheroma is a marker of intimal location. On the posteroanterior chest radiograph, a distance >0.5 or >1.0 cm between intimal calcification and the outside wall of the aorta is an older but often useful sign of thickening within the wall of the aorta consistent with acute dissection (or intramural hematoma, as in this case).

ATHEROSCLEROTIC OBSTRUCTION OF THE AORTA

Obstruction of the proximal or ostial portion of the branches of the aorta (left main coronary, right coronary, great arch vessels, renal and splanchnic vessels) is a far more common clinical occurrence than is obstruction of the aorta itself.

The usual site of atherosclerotic obstruction is the aortoiliac bifurcation because it is the narrowest portion of the aorta, and it is the site most prone to atherosclerosis. Obstruction of the aorta itself seldom occurs elsewhere. As the atherosclerosis is not limited to the aorta, there is considerable associated mortality from CAD, cerebrovascular disease, and renovascular disease.

Atherosclerotic obstruction in the aortoiliac bifurcation is far more common in men, usually in their sixth decade of life, with several CAD risk factors, particularly smoking. René Leriche described lower aortic obstruction, and hence it is termed Leriche's syndrome; lumbar, buttock, and thigh claudication and impotence are usual. Although the lesion of atherosclerotic obstruction of the aorta is clinically fairly stable, severe and limiting symptoms of claudication should prompt consideration of surgical revascularization by the most feasible and tolerable means.

Abdominal Coarctation (Middle Aorta Syndrome)

Abdominal coarctation, also known as the middle aorta syndrome, is a rare but surgically correctable cause of severe hypertension and results in hypertension by several mechanisms. It may result from either congenital coarctation or healed (scarred) aortitis. If it is congenital, it may be associated with hypoplasia of abdominal branch vessels, hence the frequent occurrence of renovascular disease and hypertension. Lumbar or umbilical bruit, hypertension, and reduced femoral pulses are usual.

Causes of Acute Obstruction of the Distal Aorta

- Thrombosis
- Embolization of a large bulk of thrombus

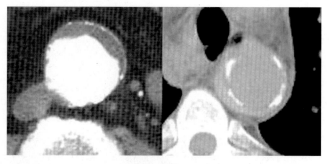

Figure 8-9. Calcified aortic intimal atheroma is a marker of intimal location. LEFT, Contrast-enhanced CT scan shows an abdominal aortic aneurysm with anterior thickening that is clearly a mural thrombus as intimal calcification is obvious, localizing the intima. RIGHT, Non–contrast-enhanced CT scan. Thoracic aorta with wall thickening due to an intramural hematoma as the luminal displacement of the intima is demarcated by the intimal calcification.

- From the heart: atrial level, from atrial fibrillation; ventricular level, from an aneurysm or infarction
- From thrombosis of the more proximal aorta
- Acute dissection
- Trauma

Acute lower extremity ischemia typically results in the five p's: pain, pallor, pulselessness, paresthesia, and paralysis. Treatment is directed to sustain the viability of the extremities, to address the cause, and to attend to complications.

CALCIFIED AORTIC INTIMAL ATHEROMA IS A MARKER OF INTIMAL LOCATION

Intimal atheroma, if it is calcified, is visible by abdominal and chest radiography, TEE, and CT scanning (Figs. 8-8 and 8-9). On occasion, recognition of intimal calcification assists in resolving uncertainties concerning imaging of pathologic changes of the aorta, as the calcification marks the intimal location. Luminal displacement of calcification is a reliable marker of a *mural* process, such as dissection or intramural hematoma. Conversely, mural thrombus *overlies* intimal calcification.

CASE 1

History

▸ A 44-year-old male smoker with dyslipidemia presented with a transient ischemic attack (TIA) episode.

▸ A prior angiogram prompted by atypical symptoms and ambiguous perfusion imaging had identified borderline significant single-vessel (circumflex) CAD.

▸ Examination findings normal; ECG normal (rhythm sinus)

No source of the embolism was detected. TEE was requested to evaluate cryptogenic sources.

Comments

▸ Generalized atherosclerosis involving the coronary tree and aorta, occurring in similar (mild) proportions—limited aortic atherosclerosis associated with limited CAD

▸ No ulcers or thrombi seen complicating the aortic atherosclerosis

▸ The source of the TIA remained undetermined.

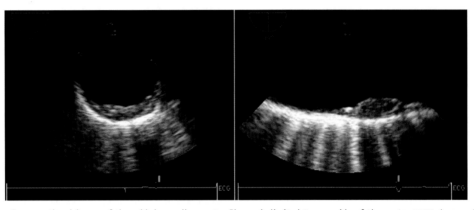

Figure 8-10. TEE. LEFT, Cross-sectional image of the mid descending aorta. Plaque is limited to one side of the aorta. RIGHT, Long-axis view of the mid descending aorta. There is a well-defined plaque with heterogeneous appearance, but other areas of the aortic intima are without plaque or even intimal thickening.

CASE 2

History

▸ 73-year-old man with class III angina

▸ Former heavy smoker with chronic hypertension and newly diagnosed type 2 diabetes mellitus

▸ Recent coronary angiography identified three-vessel disease with poor anatomy for revascularization.

▸ Presented in atrial fibrillation of unknown duration

▸ TEE was requested to assess for any left atrial appendage clot as part of an early cardioversion strategy.

Comments

▸ Advanced coronary disease associated with extensive atheromatous plaque in both the ascending (less well visualized) and descending (better visualized) aorta

▸ Generalized severe atherosclerosis involving the coronary tree and aorta, occurring in similar proportions

▸ No ulcers or thrombi seen complicating the aortic atherosclerosis

▸ Uneventful electrical cardioversion

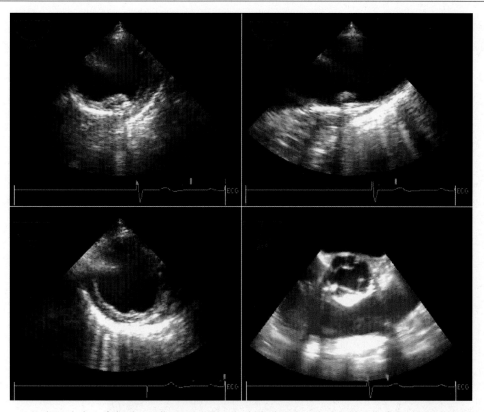

Figure 8-11. TEE. TOP LEFT, Horizontal view of the descending aorta. There is thick plaque on the lateral wall of the descending aorta. TOP RIGHT, Horizontal view of the arch. There is thick plaque on the anterior wall of the distal arch. BOTTOM LEFT, Horizontal view of the descending aorta again shows a thick plaque on the lateral wall. BOTTOM RIGHT, Aortic valve in cross section. There is aortic valve sclerosis, typical among patients with extensive aortic atherosclerosis.

CASE 3

History

▸ 66-year-old woman undergoing femoral-popliteal bypass for stable lower limb ischemia
▸ Patient was hypertensive and a smoker
▸ Bruits heard over the carotid and femoral arteries

Comments

▸ Extensive atherosclerosis of the aorta associated with extensive peripheral vascular disease
▸ Part of the hypertension was caused by the thoracic aortic narrowing (subsequent cardiac catheterization identified a 40 mm Hg gradient), and part by rapid pulse wave conduction of the heavily atherosclerotic (stiff) aorta.

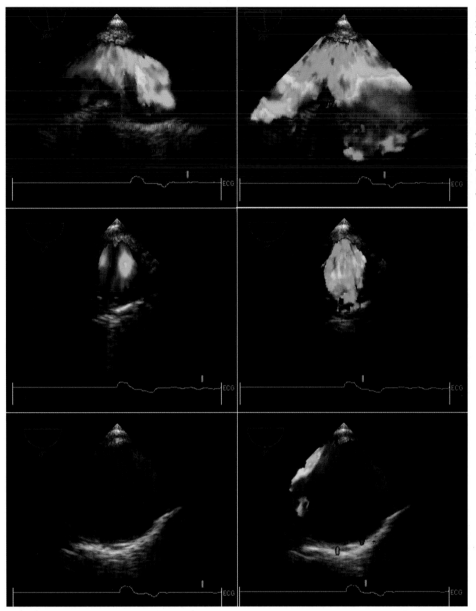

Figure 8-12. LEFT IMAGES: Diastole. RIGHT IMAGES, Systole. TOP, Longitudinal views of the mid descending aorta. MIDDLE, Cross-sectional views of the mid descending aorta at the site of greatest narrowing. There is circumferential plaque that narrows the lumen of the aorta, with a slight waist. In systole, there is flow acceleration across the site of greatest narrowing, but there is no diastolic flow acceleration, consistent with only mild stenosis. BOTTOM, Cross-sectional view of the more distal aorta. The lumen is larger, and the accelerated systolic jet from the more proximal mild stenosis is dissipating along the medial wall.

CASE 4

History

▶ A 49-year-old woman underwent magnetic resonance (MR) imaging as part of a hypertension work-up. Presence of some low back pain and inconclusive MR images generated suspicion of an intramural hematoma of the aorta, and the patient was transferred for further evaluation.

▶ Prior medical history was significant for more than 7 years of hypertension (4 years of resistant hypertension) and two prior hypertensive crises.

▶ Work-up for secondary causes of hypertension was negative.

▶ Renal function was worsened, but no renovascular disease was identified.

▶ Unexplained transient anemia

Physical Examination

▶ BP up to 295/77 mm Hg, HR 70 bpm (regular)
▶ No edema, no jugular vein distention
▶ Sustained, mildly enlarged and displaced apex
▶ S_1 normal, A_2/S_2 accentuated; S_4 present
▶ No murmurs

Management and Evolution

▶ Patient underwent surgical excision of the mass through a left thoracotomy.
▶ Surgery was uneventful, other than embolization of a fragment that was seen during intraoperative TEE.
▶ There were no sequelae to the embolism.
▶ The histology was of nonspecific calcific thrombus. No signs of aortitis were seen.

▸ There was an associated mutation of the common prothrombin mutation.

▸ Postoperatively, the blood pressure has normalized, the renal function has remained normal, and the claudication has improved.

▸ Lower extremity duplex scanning identified left >> right superficial femoral artery stenosis.

Comments

▸ Hypertension was due to aortic obstruction by the mass.

▸ The mass may have been a calcified thrombus associated with the thrombin mutation, possibly initiated by an atherosclerotic plaque.

▸ MR imaging did not prominently visualize the calcific mass.

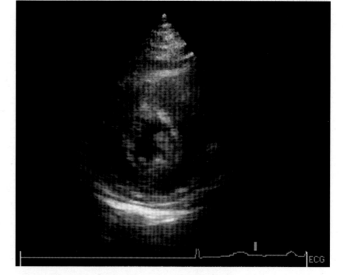

Figure 8-13. Although the ECG (TOP) does not indicate left ventricular hypertrophy, there is severe concentric hypertrophy, consistent with chronic hypertension (BOTTOM). ECG sensitivity for left ventricular hypertrophy is only 50%.

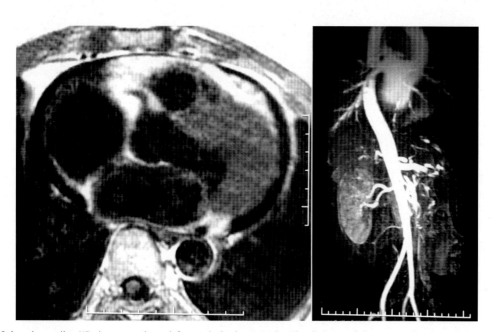

Figure 8-14. LEFT, Spin echo cardiac MR shows prominent left ventricular hypertrophy. The diameter of the retrocardiac aorta is normal. Abnormality versus artifact within the retrocardiac aorta. MR is insensitive to calcium and poorly depicted the heavily calcified lesion. RIGHT, MR angiography of the lower aorta and renal arteries. Normal aorta in the visualized portions. The lesion was in the portion of the aorta immediately superior to the imaged segment. No renal artery stenosis.

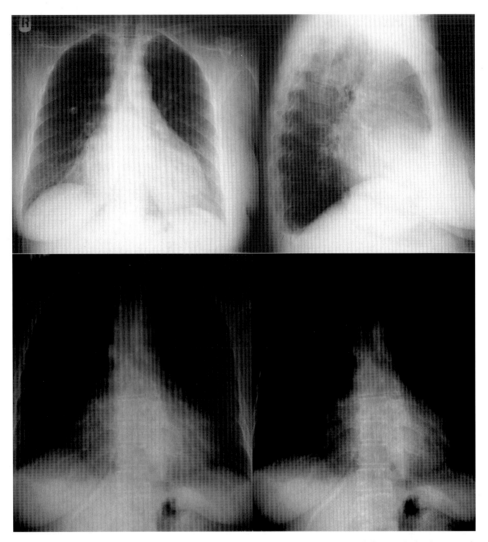

Figure 8-15. Chest radiographs. TOP, Posteroanterior and lateral films. There is mild cardiomegaly due to left ventricular hypertrophy and left atrial enlargement. With standard penetration, no aortic calcification, enlargement, or abnormality is detectable. BOTTOM, Increased penetration views: retrocardiac calcification is seen lateral to the vertebral column. The heart shadow had obscured the calcification on the posteroanterior view, and the vertebral column had obscured the calcification on the lateral view.

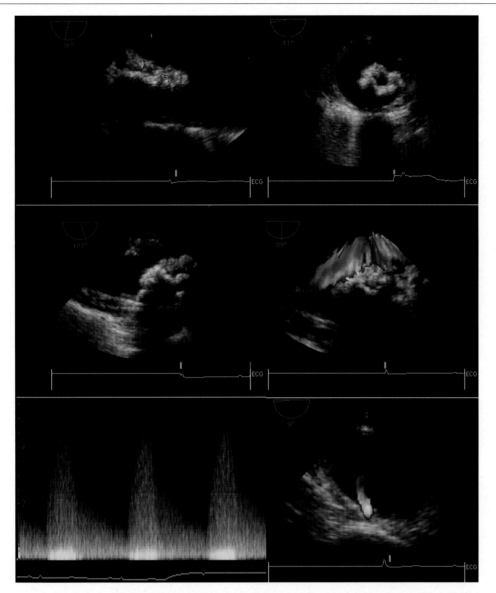

Figure 8-16. TEE. TOP LEFT, Longitudinal view of the midportion of the descending retrocardiac aorta shows a large, rigid shelf of plaque protruding into the aorta. TOP RIGHT, Cross-sectional view at the upper end of the lesion visualizes the mass within the lumen. The wall of the aorta elsewhere has a normal appearance. MIDDLE, At the lower end of the lesion, the mass is bulkier and occupying a large proportion of the lumen. BOTTOM LEFT, Spectral Doppler display of flow across the lesion. There is severe flow acceleration through the narrowest portion of the lesion. There is both a systolic and diastolic gradient, typical of severe coarctation-like pathophysiology. The peak systolic gradient is approximately 135 mm Hg. BOTTOM RIGHT, Color Doppler flow mapping distal to the lesion. There is flow returning into the lumen distal to the lesion, consistent with collateralization and chronicity of the obstructive lesion.

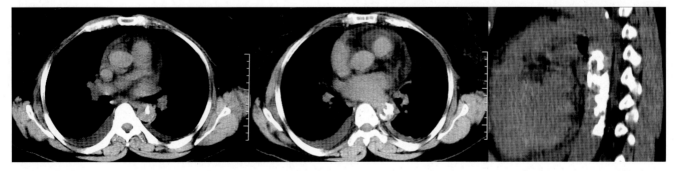

Figure 8-17. Non–contrast-enhanced CT scans. LEFT AND MIDDLE, There is a calcified mass within the retrocardiac aorta that is narrower superiorly and bulkier beneath the top portion. There are small pleural effusions. There are no other masses seen. RIGHT, As shown on the sagittal image, nearly the entire height of the retrocardiac aorta contains a complex and irregular calcified mass.

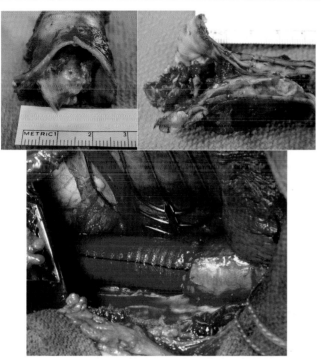

Figure 8-18. TOP, Surgical specimen. The upper end of the coral-like mass within the resected aorta is shown. BOTTOM, Dacron interposition tube graft replacing the involved segment of the descending aorta.

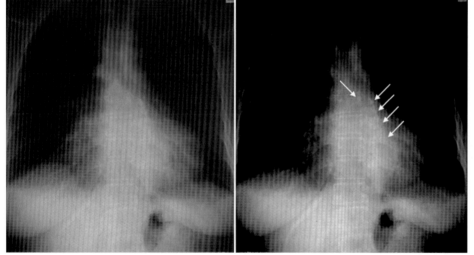

Figure 8-19. LEFT, Original chest radiograph offers little conclusive evidence on the abnormalities of the aorta. RIGHT, Original chest radiograph with overpenetration shows a probable calcific mass behind the heart, not over the spine.

CASE 5

History

- A 53-year-old man with known history of CAD and peripheral vascular disease presented with crushing severe ischemic-type chest pains.
- Prior remote surgical mitral commissurotomy
- The patient has hypertension and dyslipidemia, has no diabetes, and is a heavy smoker.

Physical Examination

- Distressed, BP 80/45 mm Hg, HR 90 bpm (regular)
- Venous distention, no edema
- Distant heart sounds, gallop present
- No murmurs
- Reduced air entry, no crepitations
- Cool extremities, altered mentation

Management and Evolution

- After initial improvement, the patient abruptly developed blue-mottled cold legs and buttocks.
- Ultrasound examination identified massive thrombosis within the distal aorta and iliac and femoral arteries and no flow.
- The patient underwent emergent surgery that found extensive thrombus in both iliac and femoral systems.
- Fogarty balloon extraction of a large burden of clot improved perfusion, apparent as the legs warmed up.

▸ Extensive rhabdomyolysis occurred with CK >200,000 U.
▸ Anuria persisted, presumably because of renal ischemia from clot ± atheroma within the aorta ± myoglobinemia and myoglobinuria.
▸ Progressive cardiogenic shock occurred, and the patient died after 26 hours.

Comments

▸ Acute aortic obstruction from thrombosis of an atherosclerotic aorta, caused by the intra-aortic balloon counterpulsation.
▸ The metabolic consequences of the lower extremity ischemia were unmanageable.

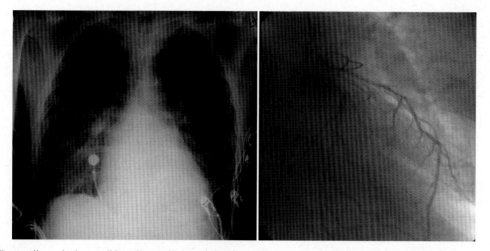

Figure 8-20. LEFT, Chest radiograph shows mild cardiomegaly, hyperinflation (presumably due to COPD), interstitial pulmonary edema (atypical pattern due to concurrent COPD), and intra-aortic balloon tip at distal arch. RIGHT, There is diffuse disease of the left coronary system.

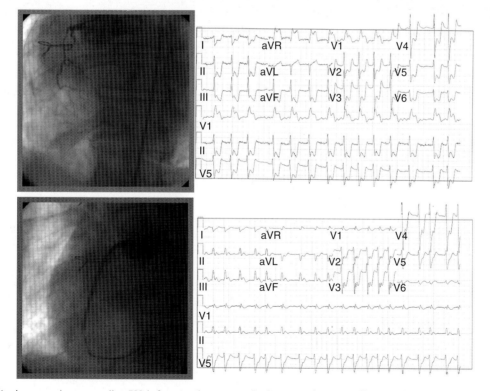

Figure 8-21. TOP, Angiogram and corresponding ECG before stenting. BOTTOM, Angiogram and corresponding ECG after stenting of an occluded right coronary artery.

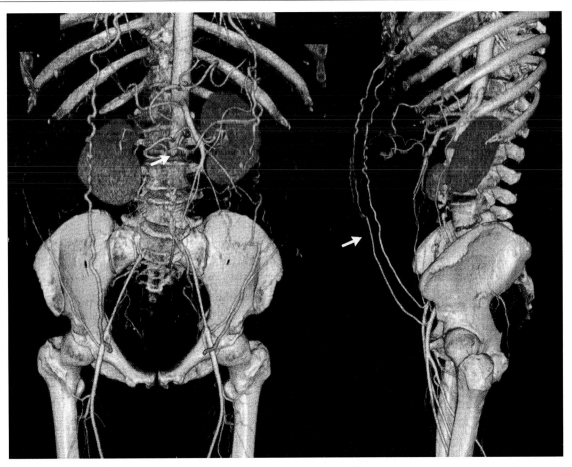

Figure 8-22. Computer tomographic angiography of a 55-year-old female smoker with dyslipidemia shows complete occlusion of the infrarenal abdominal aorta (LEFT, *arrow*). A lateral view shows collateral blood flow from both internal thoracic arteries through subcutaneous epigastric abdominal vessels to the external iliac arteries (RIGHT, *arrow*). (From Hirsch AT, Miedema MD: Infrarenal aortic occlusion. N Engl J Med 2008;359:7735.)

References

1. Berenson GS, Srinivasan SR, Bao W, et al: Association between multiple cardiovascular risk factors and atherosclerosis in children and young adults: the Bogalusa Heart Study. N Engl J Med 1998;338:1650-1656.
2. Faxon DP, Creager MA, Smith SC Jr, et al: Atherosclerotic Vascular Disease Conference: Executive summary: Atherosclerotic Vascular Disease Conference proceeding for healthcare professionals from a special writing group of the American Heart Association. Circulation 2004;109:2595-2604.
3. Vaduganathan P, Ewton A, Nagueh SF, et al: Pathologic correlates of aortic plaques, thrombi and mobile aortic debris imaged in vivo with transesophageal echocardiography. J Am Coll Cardiol 1997;30:357-363.
4. Cohen A, Tzourio C, Bertrand B, et al: Aortic plaque morphology and vascular events: a follow-up study in patients with ischemic stroke. FAPS Investigators. French Study of Aortic Plaques in Stroke. Circulation 1997;96:3838-3841.
5. Parthenakis F, Skalidis E, Simantirakis E, et al: Absence of atherosclerotic lesions in the thoracic aorta indicates absence of significant coronary artery disease. Am J Cardiol 1996;77:1118-1121.
6. Stern A, Tunick PA, Culliford AT, et al: Protruding aortic arch atheromas: risk of stroke during heart surgery with and without aortic arch endarterectomy. Am Heart J 1999;138(pt 1):746-752.

Aortic Atheromatous Disease: Thrombosis, Thromboembolism, and Atheroembolism

KEY POINTS

▸ Embolization of either thrombus or atheromatous particles may occur from the aorta.

▸ Atheroma of the ascending aorta and arch may be responsible for stroke; atheroma of the descending aorta may be a marker for generalized atherosclerosis (responsible for stroke).

▸ Plaque burden of the aorta correlates with probability of CAD (>4-mm plaques are 90% sensitive and specific for significant CAD).

▸ Approximately half of patients with mobile debris in the aorta experience emboli with catheterization.

▸ The optimal treatment of atherosclerosis complicated by aortic thrombus is unproven. Anticoagulation is more logical for thromboembolism than for atheroembolism, but distinguishing between the two is difficult.

Much of the literature on aortic thrombosis and embolism is derived from transesophageal echocardiography (TEE) studies seeking to identify the source of embolism or stroke and from studies of patients undergoing cardiac surgery who underwent intraoperative TEE. As such, most of the literature cites TEE findings. TEE is able to depict aortic thrombus and some aspects of plaque morphology, but severely atheromatous aorta (especially if it is heavily calcified) is difficult to image by TEE. The upper ascending aorta and arch are often obscured in part by the tracheal air column. Large thrombi, thrombi with independent motion, and especially protruding thrombi are the most readily imaged by TEE (Fig. 9-1). Distinction of thrombus from plaque may be challenging by TEE, and the ability to detail plaque composition is poor. Mobile elements are generally assumed to be thrombi (Fig. 9-2) but may also be plaque fibrous caps.

Contrast-enhanced computed tomography (CT) is able to image aortic wall thrombus and is certainly the best test to identify calcified atheroma. Again, large, mobile, and protruding thrombi are most easily imaged. Unless the acquisition is electrocardiography (ECG) gated, any mobility of thrombus will only blur its margins and reduce its depiction.

Distinguishing an atheroma from the wall, or more specifically the boundary of intimal disease from the wall itself, is difficult by any imaging modality, especially when advanced atherosclerosis invades into the wall, extending beneath the intima.

Aortic plaques may remain simple or may be complicated with rupture, thrombosis, or embolization of overlying thrombus and embolization of atheromatous plaque debris or content—cholesterol embolism. Embolization of thrombus and also of cholesterol content has been described into nearly every arterial bed supplied by the aorta—coronary, cerebral, renal, mesenteric, and extremities.

Emboli to the brain are the most likely emboli to be recognized and originate from the ascending aorta or arch. As emboli to the brain are the most likely emboli to be recognized and as stroke investigation regularly involves TEE imaging, most studies addressing aortic emboli have observationally followed up patients for recurrent stroke and correlated outcome with TEE findings.

Emboli propagation is flow dependent—they propagate distally to their source. Emboli originating from atheromatous disease of the proximal descending aorta may cause renal, mesenteric, or lower extremity ischemia. Emboli originating from atheromatous disease of the abdominal aorta will cause lower extremity ischemia.

Large plaque burden, mobility, arch lesion location, and instrumentation increase risk of embolization and are associated with recurrent stroke. Among a series of 48 patients with aortic atheroma who underwent cardiac catheterization through the groin, the presence of mobile aortic thrombi was substantially associated with embolization risk: 15% had an embolic event

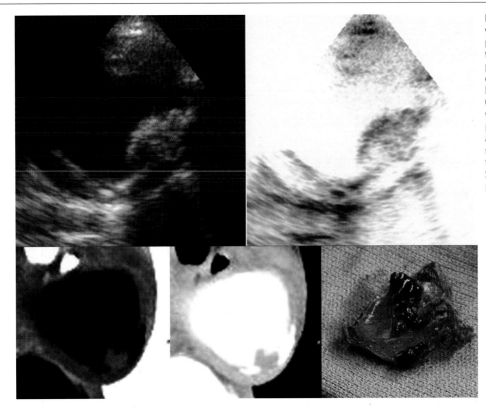

Figure 9-1. TOP LEFT, TEE cross-sectional view of the descending aorta. There is a protruding thrombus on the lateral wall of the aorta. There appears to be calcified plaque beside the thrombus at the 6-o'clock position. TOP RIGHT, TEE image with black and white inverted. BOTTOM LEFT, Contrast-enhanced axial CT scan (black-white inverted) shows a thrombus protruding from the lateral wall of the aorta. BOTTOM MIDDLE, Contrast-enhanced CT scan. There is calcium in the plaque beside the protruding thrombus. BOTTOM RIGHT, Surgical specimen shows a thrombus protruding from calcified plaque.

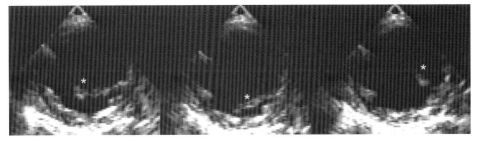

Figure 9-2. TEE short-axis views of the descending aorta. There is a very mobile length of soft tissue "windmilling" in the lumen (denoted by asterisks). The material may represent thrombus or a partially disintegrated atheromatous plaque. The wall of the aorta is circumferentially atheromatous.

(43% of those with mobile thrombi, 7% of those without mobile thrombi).[1]

Observationally, among stroke patients, aortic plaque thickness of more than 4 mm is associated with a 1-year recurrent stroke rate of 12% and a recurrent stroke–peripheral embolus rate of 33%. Several factors have been associated with increased risk: absence of calcification (2× increased risk); mobility (9×); aorto-coronary bypass (12% or 6×); and location (arch versus descending location has a 13% or 10× increased risk).[2]

The Stroke Prevention in Atrial Fibrillation study of 382 patients with high-risk atrial fibrillation (>75 years, hypertension, previous stroke) found that 35% had complex plaque on TEE (mobile, ulcerated, ≥4 mm).[3] Stroke risk per year was 12% to 20% in patients with an identified plaque, whereas it was only 1.2% in patients with no significant plaque, whether or not the patient was receiving aspirin or warfarin therapy.

The French Study of Aortic Plaques in Stroke found that increasing plaque thickness increases risk of stroke, and a cutoff of 4 mm was strongly associated with greater relative risk (RR): <1 mm: RR 1.0; 1 to 3.9 mm: RR 3.9; ≥4 mm: RR 13.8 (Fig. 9-3).[4]

The location of plaques is likely to have a causal relation to stroke. Descending plaques carry a relative risk of only 1.5, whereas arch plaques have a relative risk of 13.8. Progression of aortic arch atheroma as imaged by TEE is associated with a significantly greater incidence of vascular events.[5]

The SPARC (Stroke Prevention: Assessment of Risk in a Community) study, a prospective population-based longitudinal TEE-based study, did not confirm that the presence of simple or complex (≥4 mm or mobile debris) plaques in the descending aorta is predictive of future cardiac or cerebrovascular events.[6] The utility of aortic plaque as a marker may be limited to patients with established coronary artery disease (CAD) or with prior stroke and may not be independent of detailed cardiovascular risk factor assessment including age, prior infarction, or a history of atrial fibrillation.

Pedunculation of thrombus or debris is associated with embolization (Fig. 9-4). Karalis and associates[7] analyzed 556 patients by TEE, of whom 36 had intra-aortic atherosclerotic debris. Of the 15 patients who underwent invasive procedures, 4 (27%) were temporally related.

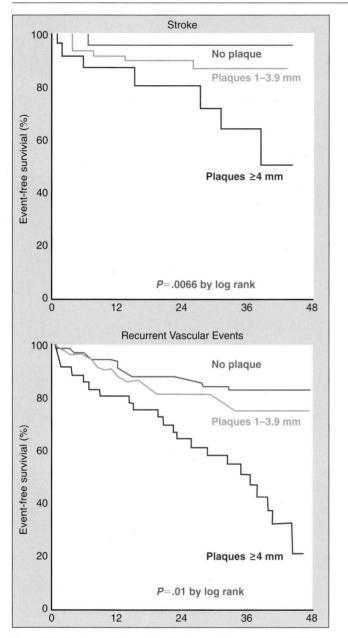

Figure 9-3. The French Study of Aortic Plaques in Stroke analyzed 331 patients, 60 years of age or older, with ischemic stroke. Proximal to left subclavian artery plaques were observed by TEE for a total of 788 patient-years. TOP PANEL, After adjustments for carotid stenosis, atrial fibrillation, peripheral vascular disease, and other risk factors, plaques ≥4 mm carried a 3.8 relative risk of recurrent stroke [1.8-7.8; *P* < 0012]. BOTTOM PANEL, Plaques ≥4 mm carried a 3.5 relative risk of recurrent vascular events (recurrent stroke, myocardial infarction, arterial emboli, and vascular death) [2.1-5.9; *P* < 001]. (From The French Study of Aortic Plaques in Stroke Group: Atherosclerotic disease of the aortic arch as a risk factor for recurrent ischemic stroke. N Engl J Med 1996;334:1216-1221. Copyright © [2001] Massachusetts Medical Society. All rights reserved.)

AORTIC THROMBOEMBOLISM

Embolized thrombus from the aorta may vary in size from micrometers to centimeters. The larger the thrombus, the larger the vessel obstructed, and the more classic findings of pulse deficits, pain, pallor, paresthesia, and purple color. TEE studies demonstrate that the larger and more mobile the thrombus, the greater

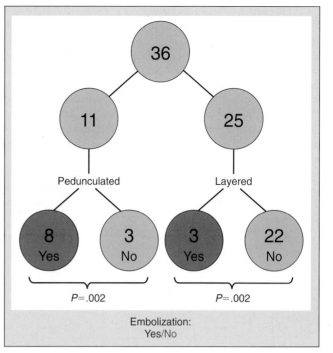

Figure 9-4. Pedunculation of thrombus or debris is associated with embolization. (From Karalis DG, Chandrasekaran K, Victor MF, et al: Recognition and embolic potential of intraaortic atherosclerotic debris. J Am Coll Cardiol 1991;17:73-78.)

the risk of embolization. Aortic mural thrombus should be considered a potential source of thromboembolism in the absence of a cardiac source of embolism (absence of atrial fibrillation, absence of intracavitary thrombus).

AORTIC ATHEROEMBOLISM

Aortic wall atheroembolism may occur spontaneously, but it is more commonly seen after catheterization or manipulation of the aorta or after use of anticoagulants. No acute *pulse* deficits occur, as the emboli are so small as to obstruct only the distal, very small arteries—distal to where pulses are palpated.

The clinical picture is variable, depending on the arterial beds that are embolized and the severity of the embolization. Typically, blue toes or livido reticularis develops. Mesenteric and renal artery ischemia and infarction may dominate the clinical picture. Eosinophilia may occur. There is substantial associated mortality.

The presence of aortic atheroma is associated with increased vascular risk: recurrent stroke, with stroke during aortocoronary bypass, embolization from instrumentation, and CAD.

In a series of 268 patients undergoing aortocoronary bypass, stroke occurred in 11.6% of those with *arch* plaques of more than 5 mm.[8] The presence of aortic atheroma predicts the presence of CAD (sensitivity, 90%; specificity, 90%; positive predictive value, 95%; negative predictive value, 82%),[9] although this correlation appears to be age dependent. In older patients (>70 years), aortic atheroma was not a predictor of CAD (seen in 12 of 13 patients with CAD and 9 of 10 patients without CAD).[10]

The optimal treatment regimen of aortic thrombosis is not established, but risks of anticoagulation in some series outweigh the benefits (Figs. 9-5 to 9-7).[11,12] There have been no large randomized trials to prove or to disprove the use of anticoagulation (or aspirin) in the context of aortic atheromatosis. Arguments can be made in favor of anticoagulation of presumed thrombus, but anticoagulation is also recognized to result in thromboembolism and atheroembolism. In a series of 78 patients, 38 patients received heparin or warfarin (nonrandomized), and 4 of them experienced atheroemboli (blue toes and renal insufficiency, increased transient ischemic attacks [TIAs], or both). Of the 40 patients who did not receive anticoagulants, none had embolic phenomena. Another patient underwent superior mesenteric artery embolectomy after streptokinase for an arch thrombus that was no longer present on repeated TEE.[13]

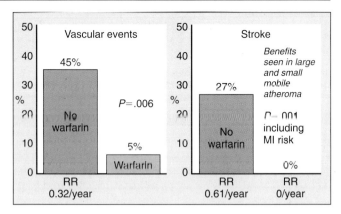

Figure 9-6. Therapeutic effect of warfarin on mobile aortic atheroma. MI, myocardial infarction; RR, relative risk. (From Dressler FA, Craig WR, Castello R, Labovitz AJ: Mobile aortic atheroma and systemic emboli: efficacy of anticoagulation and influence of plaque morphology on recurrent stroke. J Am Coll Cardiol 1998;31:134-138. Copyright Elsevier, 1998.)

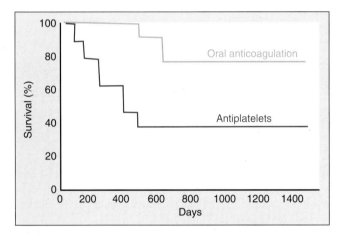

Figure 9-5. Efficacy of anticoagulation on mobile aortic atheroma in a nonrandomized study that analyzed 31 patients with systemic emboli and mobile aortic atheroma. (From Dressler FA, Craig WR, Castello R, Labovitz AJ: Mobile aortic atheroma and systemic emboli: efficacy of anticoagulation and influence of plaque morphology on recurrent stroke. J Am Coll Cardiol 1998;31:134-138.)

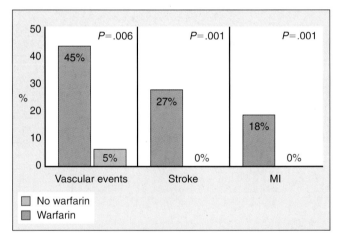

Figure 9-7. Association of treatment and clinical effect. Aortic atheroma was found in 12% of all TEE and 27.5% of all TEE performed for stroke ($P < .001$). The worse the atheroma, the greater the event rate, and the presence of debris was associated with more events (RR 7.1; $P < .001$). MI, myocardial infarction. (From Ferrari E, Vidal R, Chevallier T, Baudouy M: Atherosclerosis of the thoracic aorta and aortic debris as a marker of poor prognosis: benefit of oral anticoagulants. J Am Coll Cardiol 1999;33:1317-1322. Copyright Elsevier, 1999.)

CASE 1

History and Physical Examination

▸ 75-year-old man with a TIA
▸ Hypertensive
▸ No carotid bruits
▸ Normal cardiac examination findings; sinus rhythm
▸ TEE requested to identify subtle sources of stroke

Evolution and Management

▸ Clinical impression was that of a complex atheromatous disease of the aorta with ulceration and thrombus of the descending aorta, thus not plausibly responsible for the TIA. No such lesions were seen in the ascending aorta or arch.

▸ Management included aggressive general risk factor modification, especially of hypertension, which was probably the cause of the TIA.
▸ Warfarin use was attempted, but bleeding occurred, obviating its use.
▸ Uneventful outcome

Comments

▸ Incidental finding of mobile thrombus or atherosclerotic debris complicating complex atheromatous disease of the aorta
▸ No clear explanation for the TIA emerged. The abnormal findings in the descending aorta, although associated with disease of the more proximal aorta, do not prove it.

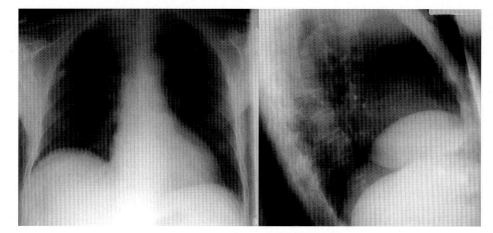

Figure 9-8. Chest radiograph shows a calcified intimal plaque at the aortic knob (distal arch) level.

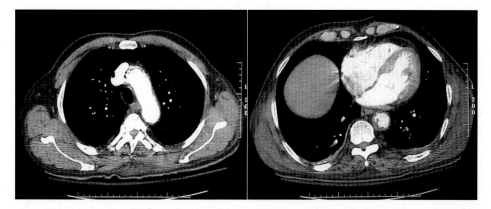

Figure 9-9. Contrast-enhanced CT scans. The anterior ascending aorta is calcified. The retrocardiac mid descending aorta has extensive, thick, and irregular plaque. Without real-time or cine imaging, motion of a thrombus or debris cannot be ascertained. On TEE, the protruding piece of tissue, thrombus or atherosclerotic debris, was seen to be mobile.

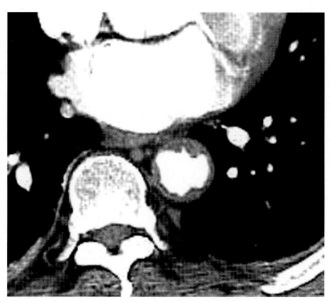

Figure 9-10. Contrast-enhanced CT scan. Irregular surfaced, crevassed plaque of the retrocardiac aorta. Distinguishing an ulcer from such irregularity is difficult.

CASE 2

History and Physical Examination

▸ 72-year-old man with acute lower extremity ischemia
▸ Limb salvage by surgery
▸ History of hypertension, dyslipidemia, and smoking
▸ No vascular bruits
▸ Normal cardiac examination findings

Evolution and Management

▸ Clinical impression was that of a thromboembolism from thoracic aortic plaque.
▸ Management was with heparin, then warfarin, followed by an aggressive general risk factor modification.
▸ Uneventful outcome

Comments

▸ Classic presentation of aortic embolism: ECG rendered cardiac source of thrombus embolism unlikely (other than left atrial myxoma or vegetations) as there was sinus rhythm and no evidence of prior or acute myocardial infarction, and there was no history of claudication to suggest iliofemoral thrombosis. Therefore, by exclusion, embolism of thrombus from aortic atheroma and embolism of mural thrombus from aortic aneurysm or false aneurysm were real possibilities.
▸ Impressive and complete response to anticoagulation verified by follow-up TEE
▸ The location of the thrombus in the arch made embolization to the brain a possibility, which fortunately never occurred or recurred.

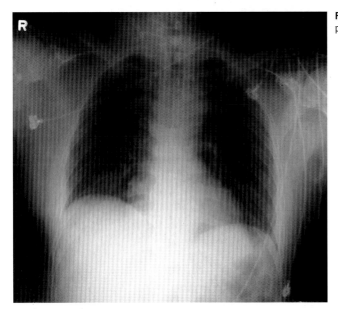

Figure 9-11. Chest radiograph shows a normal cardiac silhouette, mildly prominent "knob," and no calcification of the aorta.

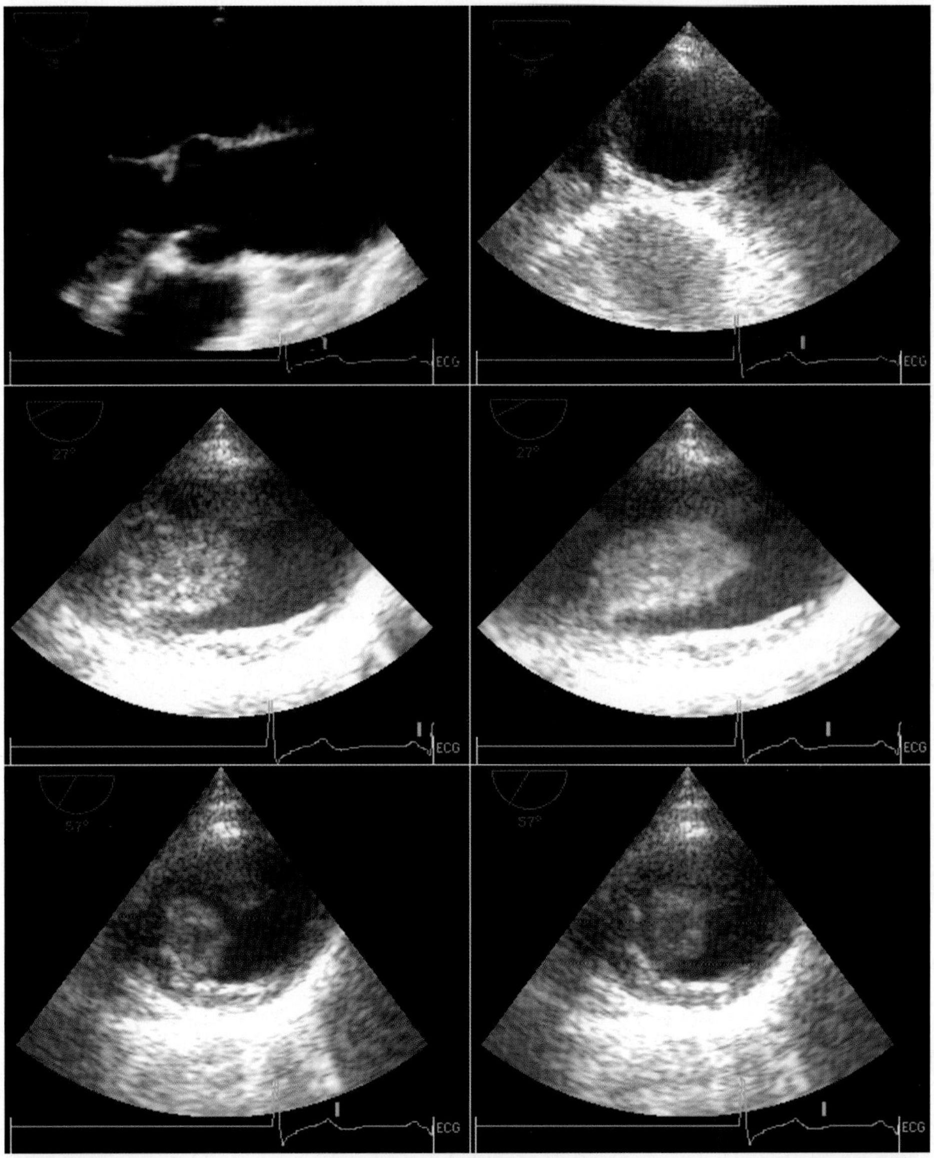

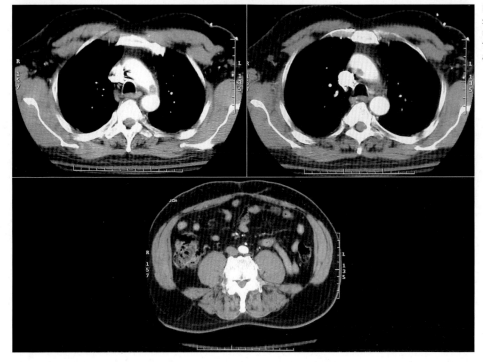

Figure 9-12. TEE. TOP LEFT, Longitudinal view of the ascending aorta is normal. TOP RIGHT, Cross-sectional view of the mid descending aorta. There is mild atherosclerotic intimal thickening only. MIDDLE, The aortic arch in longitudinal axis. BOTTOM, The aortic arch in cross section. There is a large mobile thrombus overlying a plaque on the anterior aortic arch. There is a smaller posterior thrombus.

Figure 9-13. Contrast-enhanced CT axial scans of the aortic arch. There is noncalcified soft tissue (presumed thrombus) overlying the distal aortic arch and the anterior arch.

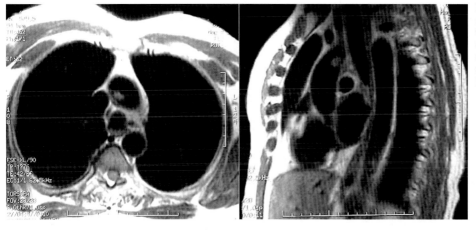

Figure 9-14. Spin echo magnetic resonance images. LEFT, Axial view beneath the aortic arch. A thrombus is present overlying the posterior wall of the ascending aorta. RIGHT, Sagittal view. The same thrombus is again seen overlying the posterior wall of the ascending aorta.

CASE 3

History and Physical Examination

▸ 68-year-old woman with cardiogenic shock due to an acute inferior infarction
▸ Previously hypertensive
▸ No murmurs or bruits

Comments

▸ Mobile thrombus
▸ Potentially, the low-flow state of cardiogenic shock may have allowed thrombosis to occur, or the thrombus may have antedated the infarction.
▸ Intra-aortic balloon counterpulsation use was avoided.

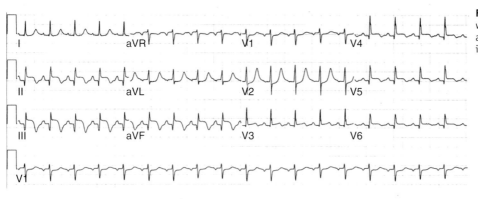

Figure 9-15. ECG shows inferolateral Q waves, ST elevation consistent with recent and evolving infarction. Signs of posterior infarction as well.

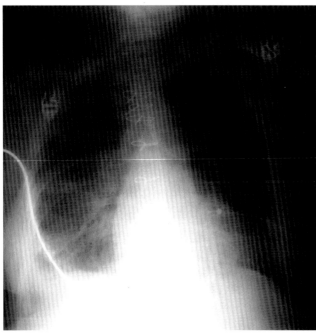

Figure 9-16. Chest radiograph shows sternal wires, endotracheal tube, interstitial edema, and borderline cardiomegaly.

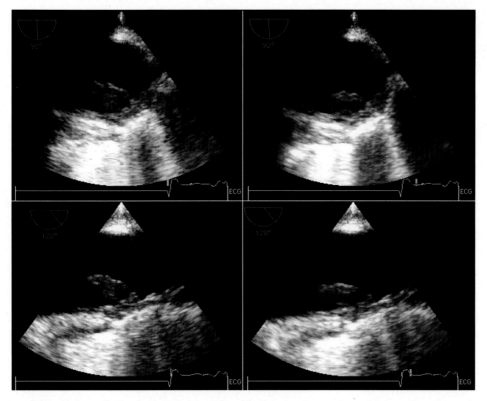

Figure 9-17. TEE images of the mid descending aorta. A 2- to 3-cm-tall mobile thrombus is present, overlying an atheromatous plaque. The right images are systolic and demonstrate the thrombus being pressed forward by the stroke volume.

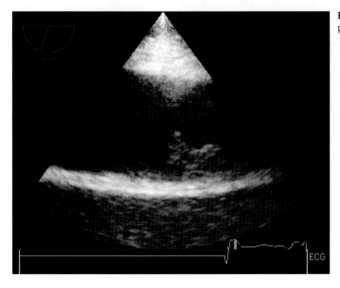

Figure 9-18. TEE image of the lower descending aorta. Irregular and protruding atheromatous plaque is present, without apparent thrombus.

CASE 4

History

▸ 68-year-old woman with hypertensive crisis and acute pulmonary edema
▸ Past medical history is significant for chronic hypertension, chronic renal insufficiency, claudication (2 blocks), cirrhosis; former smoker

Physical Examination

▸ BP 240/130 mm Hg, HR 110 bpm, severely dyspneic
▸ Bruits over carotids, femorals, abdominal aorta, flanks
▸ 2/6 SEM at base, query aortic insufficiency murmur, sustained forceful apex
▸ Crepitations bilaterally

Management and Evolution

▸ No ECG evolution
▸ Negligible troponin rise
▸ Echocardiography demonstrated nonsevere aortic stenosis.
▸ Catheterization demonstrated borderline three-vessel disease, but it was inoperable because of widespread distal disease.
▸ Hypertensive crisis and acute diastolic heart failure were presumed to be the principal cause of the left-sided heart failure.
▸ Renovascular etiology was sought, given the chronic hypertension, chronic renal insufficiency, flank bruits, and widespread vasculopathy.

Outcome

▸ After renal artery stenting, hypertensive crisis, anuria, and acute pulmonary edema ensued.
▸ 2-mm punctate blue spots appeared on the soles of the feet and the toes—presumed atheroemboli from the aortic instrumentation for the coronary and renal arteriograms had occurred and had showered the kidney and the lower extremities.
▸ Abdominal pains and ileus developed. Black, bloody stools were passed. Emboli into the splanchnic and mesenteric arteries were presumed to have also occurred.
▸ Death occurred within a few days as a result of multiorgan failure, bowel infarction, lower gastrointestinal bleed presumed secondary to the bowel infarction, and sepsis.

Comments

▸ Heavily atheromatous aorta in a vasculopathic patient with renal artery stenosis
▸ Acute pulmonary edema may have been secondary to a combination of renal artery stenosis (acute hypertension), hypertensive (left ventricular hypertrophy) heart disease, aortic stenosis, and CAD.
▸ Massive embolization of emboli from the aortic instrumentation fatally infarcted the remaining kidney, the intestines, and the lower extremities.

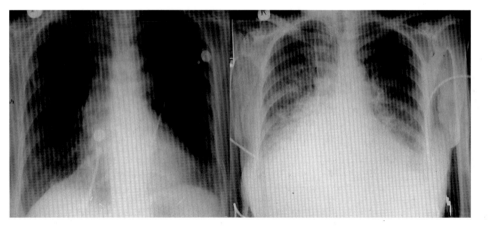

Figure 9-19. Chest radiographs. LEFT, Previous chest radiograph for comparison. There is borderline cardiomegaly and lung hyperinflation. RIGHT, Chest radiograph at presentation. There is interstitial pulmonary edema. The loss of lung volume is consistent with pulmonary edema.

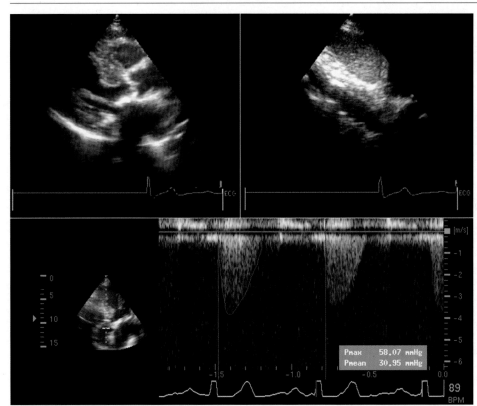

Figure 9-20. Transthoracic echocardiography. TOP LEFT, There is severe concentric left ventricular hypertrophy. Systolic function was normal. The aortic valve is calcific, and its motion was reduced. TOP RIGHT, Atherosclerosis of the abdominal aorta. BOTTOM, There is a 31 mm Hg mean gradient across the aortic valve, suggestive of moderate aortic stenosis.

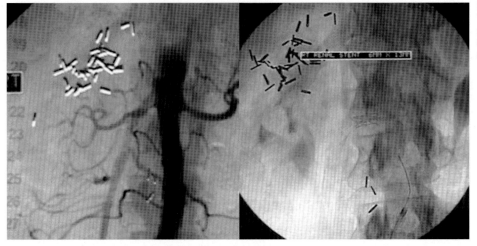

Figure 9-21. Abdominal aortography. LEFT, There is a tight ostial right renal artery stenosis. RIGHT, After right renal artery stenting. Much difficulty had been encountered in wiring of the lesion.

CASE 5

History

▸ A 78-year-old woman presented with refractory myocardial ischemia after anterior ST elevation myocardial infarction.
▸ Past medical history is significant for chronic hypertension, claudication (2 blocks); former smoker.

Physical Examination

▸ BP 150/90 mm Hg, HR 90 bpm
▸ No bruits
▸ No murmurs; enlarged apex
▸ No crepitations

Evolution and Outcome

▸ Underwent emergent percutaneous coronary intervention to left anterior descending coronary artery with excellent angiographic result
▸ Developed abdominal pains, then ileus that day, followed by metabolic acidosis
▸ Punctate blue lesions evident on toes and soles
▸ Anuria followed by death

Comments

▸ Heavily atheromatous aorta in an unrecognized vasculopathy
▸ Massive and fatal embolization of emboli from the aortic instrumentation infarcted the kidneys, the intestines, and the lower extremities. Intractable metabolic acidosis ensued.

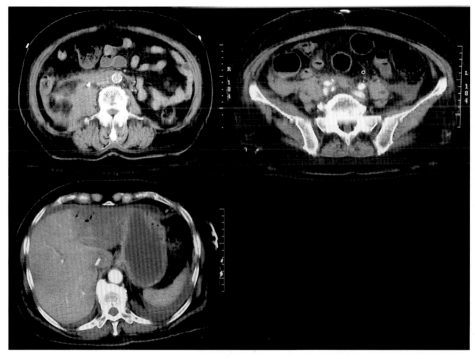

Figure 9-22. Contrast-enhanced axial CT scans. There is severe calcific atherosclerosis of the abdominal aorta with nearly circumferential calcification. No abdominal aortic aneurysm is present. Air-fluid levels are present in dilated bowel. The bowel wall is thickened, consistent with edema. There is possible air in the wall of the bowel. All are features consistent with bowel infarction. The lower image reveals air in the portal system as well.

References

1. Karalis DG, Quinn V, Victor MF, et al: Risk of catheter-related emboli in patients with atherosclerotic debris in the thoracic aorta. Am Heart J 1996;131:1149-1155.
2. Tunick PA, Kronzon I: Atheromas of the thoracic aorta: clinical and therapeutic update. J Am Coll Cardiol 2000;35:545-554.
3. The Stroke Prevention in Atrial Fibrillation Investigators Committee on Echocardiography: Transesophageal echocardiographic correlates of thromboembolism in high-risk patients with nonvalvular atrial fibrillation. Ann Intern Med 1998;128:639-647.
4. Atherosclerotic disease of the aortic arch as a risk factor for recurrent ischemic stroke. The French Study of Aortic Plaques in Stroke Group. N Engl J Med 1996;334:1216-1221.
5. Sen S, Hinderliter A, Sen PK, et al: Aortic arch atheroma progression and recurrent vascular events in patients with stroke or transient ischemic attack. Circulation 2007;116:928-935.
6. Meissner I, Khandheria BK, Sheps SG, et al: Atherosclerosis of the aorta: risk factor, risk marker, or innocent bystander? A prospective population-based transesophageal echocardiography study. J Am Coll Cardiol 2004;44:1018-1024.
7. Karalis DG, Chandrasekaran K, Victor MF, et al: Recognition and embolic potential of intraaortic atherosclerotic debris. J Am Coll Cardiol 1991;17:73-78.
8. Stern A, Tunick PA, Culliford AT, et al: Protruding aortic arch atheromas: risk of stroke during heart surgery with and without aortic arch endarterectomy. Am Heart J 1999;138(pt 1):746-752.
9. Fazio GP, Redberg RF, Winslow T, Schiller NB: Transesophageal echocardiographically detected atherosclerotic aortic plaque is a marker for coronary artery disease. J Am Coll Cardiol 1993;21:144-150.
10. Matsumura Y, Takata J, Yabe T, et al: Atherosclerotic aortic plaque detected by transesophageal echocardiography: its significance and limitation as a marker for coronary artery disease in the elderly. Chest 1997;112:81-86.
11. Dressler FA, Craig WR, Castello R, Labovitz AJ: Mobile aortic atheroma and systemic emboli: efficacy of anticoagulation and influence of plaque morphology on recurrent stroke. J Am Coll Cardiol 1998;31:134-138.
12. Ferrari E, Vidal R, Chevallier T, Baudouy M: Atherosclerosis of the thoracic aorta and aortic debris as a marker of poor prognosis: benefit of oral anticoagulants. J Am Coll Cardiol 1999;33:1317-1322.
13. Koren MJ, Bryant B, Hilton TC: Atherosclerotic disease of the aortic arch and the risk of ischemic stroke. N Engl J Med 1995;332:1237-1238.

10

Aortic Atheromatous Disease: Ulcers and Penetrating Aortic Ulcers

KEY POINTS

▸ Advanced atherosclerosis of the aorta may lead to ulceration and penetrating ulceration of the aorta. Ulceration is associated with thromboembolism and atheroembolism; penetrating ulceration is associated with dissection and rupture of the aorta.

▸ The natural history of ulcers and penetrating ulcers is not well understood. The estimated risk of rupture of symptomatic ulcers is 40%.

▸ Penetrating ulcers are usually detected in the evaluation of a suspected aortic dissection but may be found in evaluation of nonischemic chest pains.

▸ Imaging of penetrating ulcers is possible but requires persistence and often requires multiple modalities to achieve confidence.

▸ Use of multiple imaging modalities to establish the presence of a penetrating ulcer seems reasonable.

▸ The optimal management of these lesions is unknown.

Advanced atherosclerotic plaques may be complicated with overlying thrombus or with disintegration of underlying plaque, leaving ulcers (Fig. 10-1). A minority of ulcers are so deep that they penetrate into the wall of the aorta, as the atheromatous process may damage the media. As the boundary of intimal planes and mural planes of the aorta are not distinguishable by imaging, distinguishing an ulcer of a plaque from a penetrating ulcer through a plaque is difficult unless the penetration is frankly obvious. Plaques can be very thick, and therefore an ulcer, although deep, may not actually penetrate into the wall of the aorta and risk rupture or dissection.

True penetrating ulcers may initiate intramural hematoma by establishing continuity of the arterial lumen with mural tissue planes (Fig. 10-2). Intramural hematoma associated with true penetrating ulcer has a worse outcome because the intramural hematoma has a persistent and sometimes progressive inciting cause. A penetrating ulcer may lead to frank rupture of the aorta. The natural history of penetrating ulcer has not been well characterized.

IMAGING OF ULCERS AND PENETRATING AORTIC ULCERS

Ulcers and penetrating ulcers of the aorta can be visualized by modalities that offer clear depiction of the blood pool, such as aortography, contrast-enhanced computed tomography (CT), gadolinium contrast–enhanced magnetic resonance (MR) angiography, and transesophageal echocardiography (TEE) (Fig. 10-3). The larger and the deeper the penetrating ulcer, the more likely it is to be detected by any means. Challenges are rife in the assessment of suspected penetrating ulcers of the aorta:

• Atherosclerotic ulcers tend to be multiple; distinguishing the culprit from the others may not be straightforward.
• Establishing the distinction of an ulcer from a penetrating ulcer: ulcers are far more common. Delineation of the depth of the ulcer, and just what it is extending into, is often an

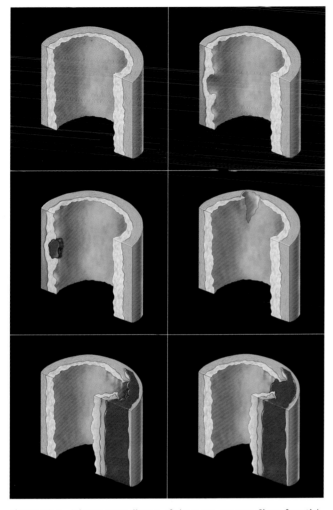

Figure 10-1. Atheromatous disease of the aorta. TOP LEFT, Circumferential atheromatous plaque, with irregular surface but without well-formed ulcers. TOP RIGHT, Circumferentially atheromatous aorta with one well-formed ulcer extending into plaque but not into the wall proper. MIDDLE LEFT, Circumferentially atheromatous aorta with one well-formed ulcer extending into plaque, not complicated by penetration but complicated by overlying thrombus. MIDDLE RIGHT, Circumferentially atheromatous aorta with one well-formed ulcer extending (penetrating) into the wall. BOTTOM LEFT, Circumferentially atheromatous aorta with one well-formed ulcer penetrating into the wall and complicated by intramural hemorrhage. BOTTOM RIGHT, Circumferentially atheromatous aorta with one well-formed ulcer penetrating into the wall, complicated by intramural hemorrhage and protrusion of thrombus.

imaging challenge that exceeds the spatial resolution of current imaging modalities.

- A substantial proportion of the data on ulcers and penetrating ulcers derives from TEE studies, but contrast-enhanced CT is more widely used in the assessment of the aorta.
- Thrombus overlying the ulcer may obscure it.
- Most imaging studies have been small observational series, usually retrospective, single-center studies, without comparison of different imaging modalities.

Ulcerated aortic atheroma is associated with increased stroke risk. Ulceration greater than 2 mm is seen in 39% of patients with stroke but in only 7% of patients without stroke. However, this may simply associate stroke with more extensive generalized atherosclerosis.[1]

The presentations of penetrating ulcers are numerous and may resemble that of an aortic dissection: sudden severe chest (or back) pain, without myocardial ischemic markers. The background of extensive atherosclerosis that results in ulcers and penetrating ulcers often is associated with significant coronary disease in such patients.

A series of 12 patients with penetrating ulcers among 94 patients with aortic diseases undergoing TEE revealed that all were hypertensive and all had presented with chest pain or back pain; the mean age was 65 years (56 to 79 years). The initially suspected diagnosis was aortic dissection in most (9 of 12) cases. Two of the 12 died of rupture of the aorta.[2] Most penetrating ulcers were located in the descending aorta (8 of 12), although some were in the arch (2 of 12) or ascending aorta (2 of 12). TEE identified 10 of 12, including 4 with limited dissection.[2]

MANAGEMENT OF PENETRATING ULCERS OF THE AORTA

The optimal management is unknown because the natural history is poorly understood. Traditional management, if there was clinical suspicion of threatening rupture of the aorta, was control of blood pressure and surgical excision of the involved portion of the aorta. This often proved difficult to effect safely and with success, as the aorta in such cases is typically extensively diseased and unforgiving to work with. Endovascular covered stents have been used successfully in small series to cover the ulcer and to seal it off (Fig. 10-4).

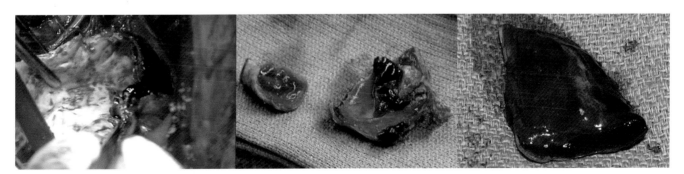

Figure 10-2. Surgical specimens. LEFT, Gelatinous thrombus filling the ulcerated atheromatous plaque and extending into an intramural hematoma within the wall. MIDDLE, Penetrating aortic ulcer. Heavily fibrotic and calcified aortic atheromatous pieces of aortic wall with overlying thrombus. RIGHT, Intramural hematoma associated with the penetrating atheromatous ulcer.

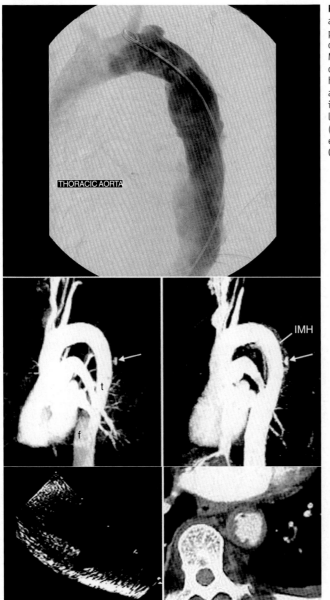

Figure 10-3. Imaging of aortic ulcers and penetrating ulcers. TOP, Contrast aortography. The ulcers that are seen in a tangential projection are distinct, particularly the one immediately distal to the left subclavian artery takeoff on the outside curvature of the aorta. MIDDLE, Gadolinium contrast–enhanced MR aortography. A button-like ulcer is clearly projected tangentially to the outside curvature of the aorta. There is also evidence of associated intramural hematoma (IMH). BOTTOM LEFT, TEE two-dimensional view of a deep ulcer into a thick atheromatous plaque. It is unclear as to whether the ulcer penetrates into the wall. BOTTOM RIGHT, Contrast-enhanced axial CT scan shows a button-like ulcer at the 11-o'clock position in the mid descending thoracic aorta. (Middle images from Mohiaddin RH, McCrohon J, Francis JM, et al: Contrast-enhanced magnetic resonance angiogram of penetrating aortic ulcer. Circulation 2001;103:E18-E19.)

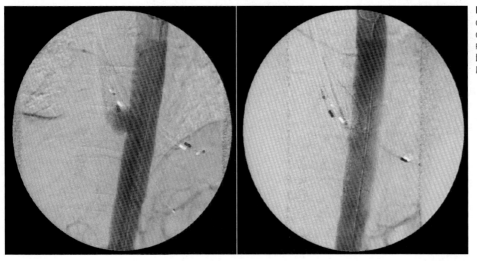

Figure 10-4. Aortography. LEFT, There is a deep ulcer of the descending thoracic aorta delineated to the medial side of the aorta. RIGHT, After covered stenting, the ulcer has been excluded. (Courtesy of Mark Peterson, MD, Toronto, Canada.)

CASE 1

History and Physical Examination

▸ 78-year-old man with a transient ischemic attack (TIA)
▸ Hypertensive, smoker, type 2 diabetes
▸ No arterial bruits or palpable abdominal aortic aneurysm
▸ BP 165/70 mm Hg, HR 80 bpm (sinus rhythm)

Clinical Diagnosis

▸ Complex atheromatous disease of the aorta
▸ Incidentally identified ulcer into the plaque, but not convincingly into the wall; therefore, it is not believed to be penetrating.
▸ The cause of the TIA remained speculative, even if there was severe atheromatous disease of the aorta present, which could have released a thrombus.

Management

▸ More aggressive general risk factor management
▸ Warfarin was debated but avoided, given the lack of strong evidence and the gait unsteadiness of the patient.

Comments

▸ Extensive complex atheromatous disease of the aorta, with calcification (as seen on the CT scan) and ulceration of bulky plaques (as seen on the TEE)
▸ The thickly plaque-encircled aorta demonstrated its impaired compliance by a huge pulse pressure of 100 mm Hg.

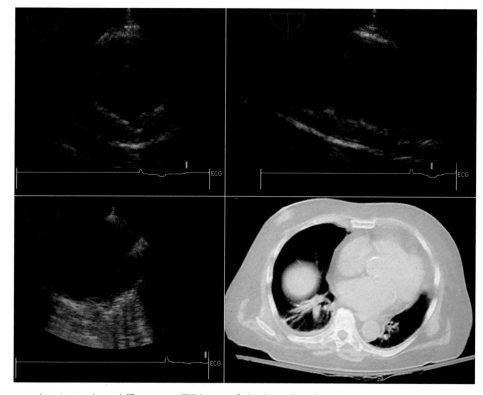

Figure 10-5. TEE images and contrast-enhanced CT scan. TOP, TEE images of the descending thoracic aorta reveal severe atherosclerotic thickening with prominent surface irregularity. BOTTOM LEFT, There is an ulcer with an overhanging shelf at the 4-o'clock position. BOTTOM RIGHT, The CT scan demonstrates atherosclerotic calcification of the aortic root but not of the descending aorta, despite the bulky atherosclerosis seen on TEE.

CASE 2

History and Physical Examination

▸ A 64-year-old man presented with a 30-second episode of sudden and excruciating chest pain.
▸ Heavy smoker
▸ No claudication or angina
▸ BP 115/70 mm Hg despite history of hypertension and no medications
▸ Normal peripheral pulse volumes; bilateral femoral bruits

Evolution and Management

▸ Atheromatous penetrating ulcer of the aorta with rupture and leakage into the pleural space
▸ Poor surgical candidate for a thoracotomy to address the descending aorta, given the COPD (and possible significant coronary artery disease)

▸ Preintervention beta-blockade to reduce BP surges and myocardial ischemia
▸ Endograft insertion to seal off the leaking ulcer
▸ Uneventful outcome

Comments

▸ Sudden onset of severe chest pain prompts consideration of acute aortic syndromes (dissection, intramural hematoma, and aneurysm and rupture).
▸ The penetrating ulcer caused an intramural hematoma, which had leaked outside the aorta.
▸ Advanced atheromatous disease of the aorta includes ulceration and thrombosis.
▸ BP of 115/70 at presentation in a patient with known hypertension required an explanation, which was that the aorta had leaked significantly.

10

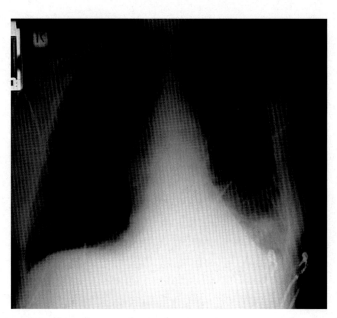

Figure 10-6. Chest radiograph shows hyperinflated lung fields consistent with obstructive lung disease. Hilar overlay sign due to enlargement of the ascending aorta is present. No calcification of the aorta is evident. Grossly normal heart size. There is a left pleural effusion ± left lower lobe atelectasis.

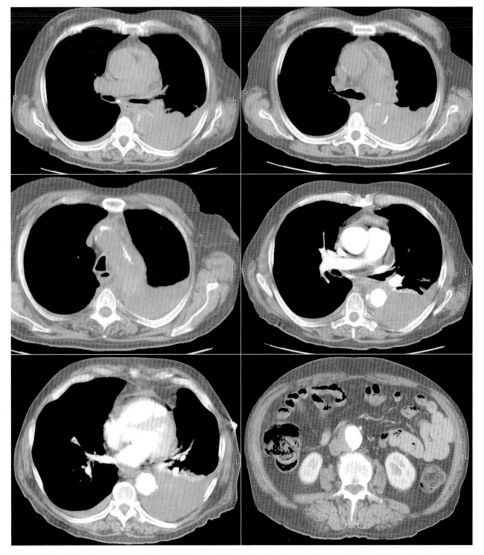

Figure 10-7. Non–contrast-enhanced and contrast-enhanced CT scans. Non–contrast-enhanced scans demonstrate extensive intimal calcification of the arch and the ascending and descending aorta. There is a left pleural effusion. TOP, Intimal displacement and crescentic wall thickening medially. MIDDLE RIGHT, An ulcer is seen extending into the crescentic mural thickening that, being smooth-walled, suggests an intramural hematoma. BOTTOM LEFT, There is an irregularity of the atherosclerotic surface of the aorta and intimal calcification at the 3-o'clock position. BOTTOM RIGHT, The image reveals an abdominal aortic aneurysm with mural thrombus.

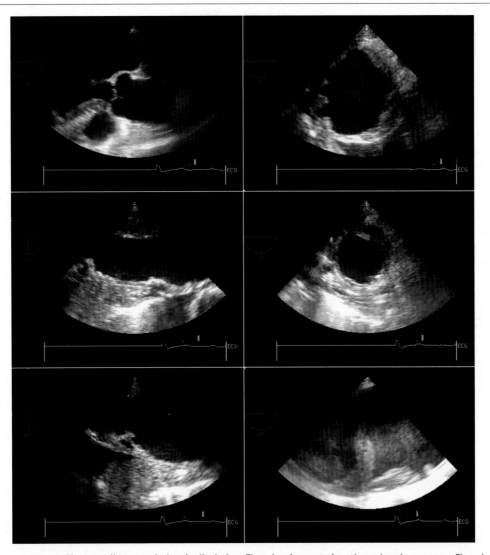

Figure 10-8. TEE images. TOP LEFT, The ascending aorta in longitudinal view. There is minor anterior atherosclerosis. TOP RIGHT, There is extensive circumferential atherosclerosis. Distinguishing the atherosclerosis from mural thickening is difficult. MIDDLE, Again, atherosclerotic thickening is seen, but the homogeneous, more lucent thickening of the near (medial) wall is consistent with intramural hematoma. BOTTOM LEFT, Lower thoracic aorta in longitudinal axis: severe atherosclerotic irregularities. There is a pleural effusion. BOTTOM RIGHT, Pleural effusion with specular echoes, consistent with blood.

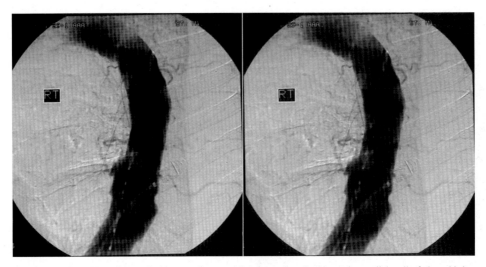

Figure 10-9. Aortography shows diffuse intimal irregularities consistent with atherosclerosis. Along the medial wall of the mid descending thoracic aorta, there is extension of contrast material, consistent with the suspected button-like penetrating ulcer seen on CT scanning.

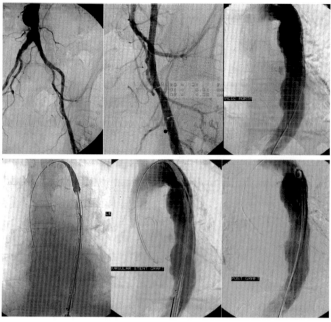

Figure 10-10. Endograft insertion. UPPER LEFT TWO IMAGES, Access. There is an abdominal aortic aneurysm, but no iliac stenoses or aneurysms. The caliber of the femoral and iliac arteries was smaller than the introducer sheath for the intended endograft. This necessitated surgical access to the vessels above the inguinal ligament. OTHER IMAGES, Insertion of the endograft to cover the ulcer along the medial wall. Note the exclusion to the ulcer seen on the final image compared with the middle left image.

CASE 3

History

▸ A 74-year-old man presented with sudden-onset severe back pain.
▸ Hypertensive, receiving monotherapy
▸ No known coronary artery disease, peripheral vascular disease, or cardiovascular disease

Physical Examination

▸ BP 220/115 mm Hg
▸ No pulse deficits, no murmur of aortic insufficiency
▸ No findings of tamponade

Evolution and Management

▸ BP controlled with labetalol
▸ As BP was controlled, the pain subsided.
▸ Referral to surgery for repair of the descending aorta

Comments

▸ Penetrating atheromatous ulcer initiating intramural hematoma
▸ Sudden onset of pain from the intramural hematoma or from the rupture
▸ Diagnosis of intramural hematoma was made by TEE and CT; TEE suggested rupture, CT was convincing.
▸ TEE and CT showed the protruding thrombus; neither showed the penetrating ulcer convincingly.
▸ As the thrombus filled in the ulcer that had initiated the intramural hematoma, imaging did not depict the penetration of the ulcer into the wall.
▸ The intramural hematoma was less thick under the penetrating ulcer than elsewhere.
▸ Surgery was complicated by stroke.

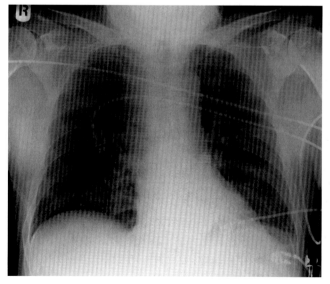

Figure 10-11. Chest radiograph shows a widened mediastinum with an ambiguous aortic contour. Normal cardiopericardial silhouette. No left-sided heart failure. No left pleural effusion.

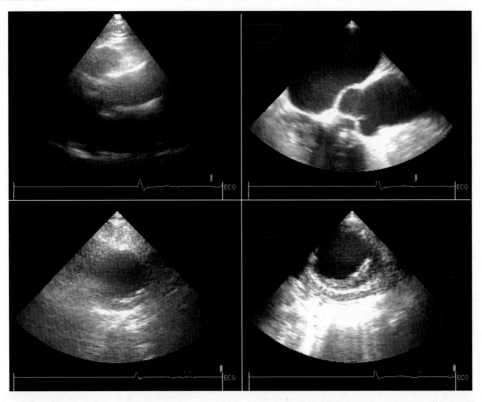

Figure 10-12. LEFT IMAGES, Transthoracic echocardiography. RIGHT IMAGES, Transesophageal echocardiography. TOP ROW, Ascending aorta. BOTTOM ROW, Mid descending aorta. (The transthoracic view was obtained from a posterior chest view.) There is no intimal flap in either portion of the aorta. There is homogeneous crescentic thickening of the wall of the mid descending thoracic aorta consistent with intramural hematoma. There also appears to be an adventitial hematoma.

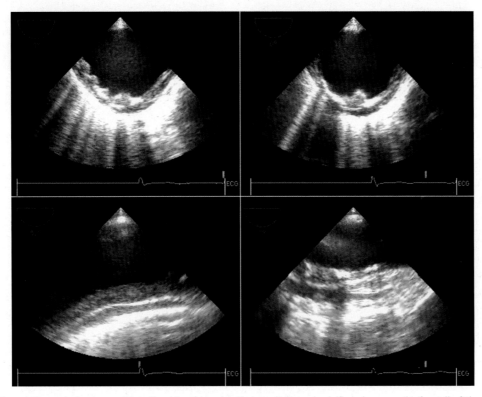

Figure 10-13. TOP, Descending aorta in cross section. There is atherosclerotic irregularity and calcified plaque on the far wall of the aorta. There appears to be thrombus protruding from the plaque into the lumen. BOTTOM, Longitudinal views. The homogeneous mural thickening of the far wall extends through the sectors of imaging. There is adventitial hematoma seen as lucent thickening on the outside wall of the aorta.

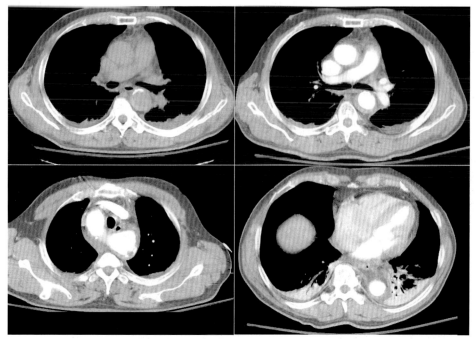

Figure 10-14. TOP, Non–contrast-enhanced and contrast-enhanced axial images at approximately the same level. Intimal calcification is present on the anterior wall. On both the non–contrast-enhanced and contrast-enhanced axial images, crescentic thickening of the medial wall of the aorta is present. On the non–contrast-enhanced axial image, there is a hint of intimal displacement (as a confirmatory sign of mural thickening). BOTTOM LEFT, Contrast-enhanced view at the aortic arch level. Thrombus is protruding from the calcified plaque on the lateral wall of the aorta, as it had been seen on TEE. BOTTOM RIGHT, The thickening of the aortic wall is again seen, but also variable-appearance streaking among adjacent tissue planes and an adjacent pleural effusion consistent with rupture.

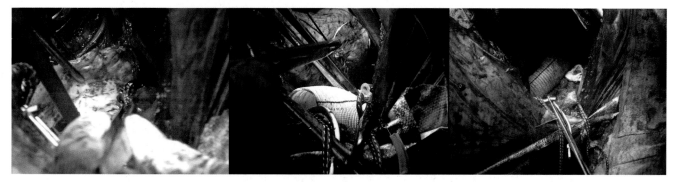

Figure 10-15. Surgical findings and procedure. LEFT, Protruding thrombus arising from a penetrating atherosclerotic ulcer of the proximal descending aorta. There is associated intramural hematoma seen as clotted blood in the wall of the aorta. MIDDLE AND RIGHT, Insertion of a Dacron interposition graft at the location of the penetrating ulcer that initiated the intramural hematoma.

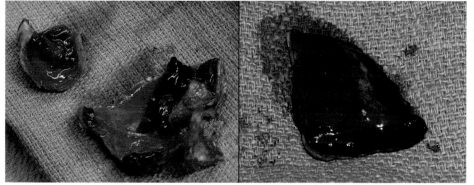

Figure 10-16. Surgical specimens. LEFT, Atherosclerotic plaque and overlying thrombus. RIGHT, Intramural hematoma of the wall of the descending aorta.

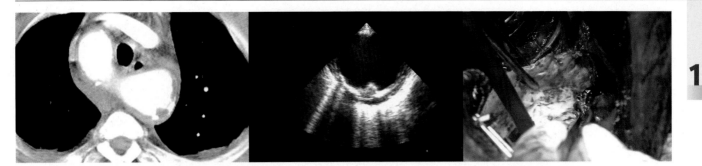

Figure 10-17. CT and TEE images corresponding to the surgical finding of protruding thrombus filling a penetrating ulcer.

CASE 4

History

▸ A 90-year-old man presented with sudden-onset chest and back pain.
▸ Contrast-enhanced CT of chest at community hospital described a distal aortic dissection with pericardial fluid.
▸ Transferred for evaluation
▸ Past medical history is significant for hypertension for 6 years; receiving monotherapy.
▸ No known coronary artery disease, peripheral vascular disease, or cardiovascular disease

Physical Examination

▸ BP 105/70 mm Hg
▸ No pulse deficits, no murmur of aortic insufficiency
▸ No findings of tamponade
▸ Reduced air entry in left side of chest

Clinical Impression

▸ Not hypertensive, as a known hypertensive patient would normally be when in pain.
▸ Left-sided chest bedside findings suggest a large pleural effusion.

Evolution and Outcome

▸ No dissection flap
▸ Atheromatous aorta (irregular intima and calcifications)
▸ Probable intramural hematoma
▸ Either a penetrating ulcer into the wall, causing an intramural hematoma, or rupture of the intramural hematoma, disrupting the wall

▸ Findings consistent with rupture: streaking of soft tissues around the aorta and a large and otherwise unexplained pleural effusion
▸ Lack of hypertension can be explained by the findings consistent with rupture.
▸ Abrupt asystole developed, and resuscitation was started.
▸ Refractory asystole and unsuccessful resuscitation

Comments

▸ Penetrating atheromatous ulcer initiated intramural hematoma, with early rupture into the tissues around the aorta and into the left pleural space.
▸ Sudden onset of pain is likely to be from the intramural hematoma or from the rupture.
▸ Diagnosis was evident from the CT scan, although it was not recognized. The only issue that CT was confusing about was whether there was pericardial fluid. The pleural effusion had in fact extended so far around the heart that it masqueraded as a pericardial effusion.
▸ All of the pathologic process was in the distal arch–proximal descending aorta. The ascending aorta had not been involved, and there were no proximal complications, such as pericardial fluid.
▸ Endovascular aortic repair (covered stent) to close off the penetrating ulcer had been intended, but the patient expired within 10 minutes of arrival.
▸ Mild hypotension at arrival was ominous for rupture, as a hypertensive patient with either an intramural hematoma or acute aortic dissection should otherwise be frankly hypertensive.
▸ Prior hypertension had been isolated systolic, consistent with a stiff (due to severe atheromatosis) aorta.

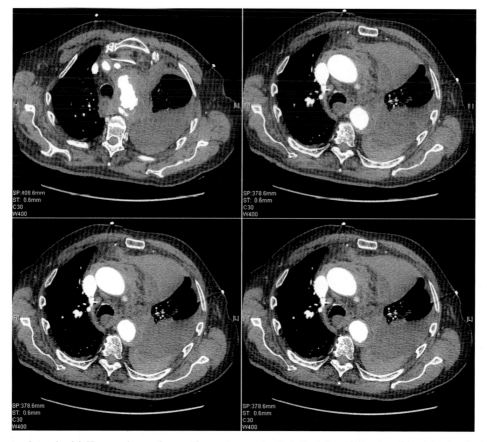

Figure 10-18. Contrast-enhanced axial CT scans show a shaggy atheromatous aorta. No intimal flap. Thickening of the lateral wall of the arch and of the descending aorta. The posterior aspect of the arch has a complex appearance—contrast dye is seen behind irregular soft tissue as blood in the wall of the aorta versus overhanging atheromatous shelf. There is a large left pleural effusion consistent with rupture. Streaking appearance of soft tissues anterior, lateral, and posterior to the ascending aorta and a large anterior and posterior pleural effusion. Tracheal displacement due to the large effusion.

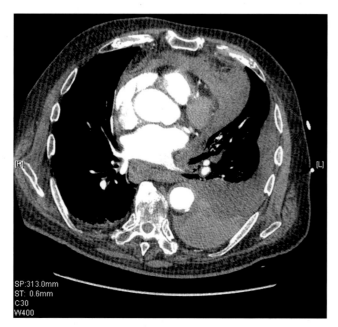

Figure 10-19. Contrast-enhanced CT scan. No intimal flap. Intimal calcification of the descending aorta and coronary arteries. Left pleural effusion. Possible pericardial effusion versus anterior pleural effusion.

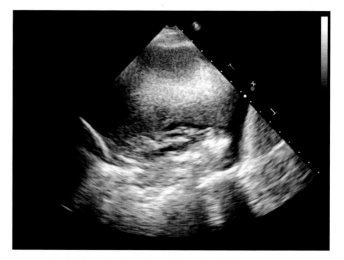

Figure 10-20. Transthoracic echocardiography, left chest view. Large pleural effusion filling the pleural cavity with gelatinous specular echoes, strongly suggestive of blood and confirmed by pleural tap.

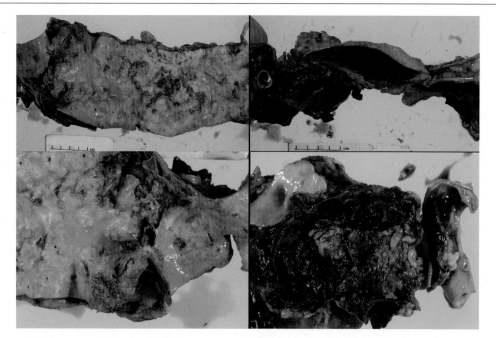

Figure 10-21. Autopsy findings. TOP LEFT, Markedly atheromatous aorta with a complex surface and obvious calcific intimal areas. Deep recess into the aorta among the most atheromatous areas. TOP RIGHT, Intramural hematoma in the wall of the distal arch and proximal descending aorta. Blood streaking into soft tissues around the aorta. BOTTOM LEFT, Ulcer-like crater among intimal plaques in the distal arch. Penetrating ulcer. BOTTOM RIGHT, Blood exterior to the aortic arch extending along tissue planes and within fat.

References

1. Stone DA, Hawke MW, LaMonte M, et al: Ulcerated atherosclerotic plaques in the thoracic aorta are associated with cryptogenic stroke: a multiplane transesophageal echocardiographic study. Am Heart J 1995;130:105-108.

2. Vilacosta I, San Román JA, Aragoncillo P, et al: Penetrating atherosclerotic aortic ulcer: documentation by transesophageal echocardiography. J Am Coll Cardiol 1998;32:83-89.

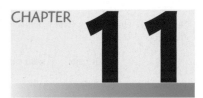

Thoracic Aortic Aneurysms

Whereas abdominal aortic aneurysms are generally very similar, thoracic aortic aneurysms, defined as more than 50% increase in aortic diameter, involve many permutations of location, length, morphology, branch vessel involvement, and complications. The true incidence of aneurysms of the thoracic aorta is unknown because of underdetection, but it is estimated to be 60 to 100/million. The mean age at diagnosis is 59 to 69 years. There is male gender predominance, with a male:female ratio of 2:1. The arch segment is less commonly involved (10%) and the ascending aorta is slightly more frequently involved than is the descending segment (40%).

The range of anatomic appearance begets the use of morphologic descriptive terms. The term *tubular* is used to describe a long length of aorta with all parts dilated similarly. The term *fusiform* describes a tapered beginning and end to the spindle-shaped dilated segment, with circumferential dilation. *Saccular* aneurysm describes a localized, shorter, round dilation. *Thoracoabdominal* aneurysm describes an aneurysm extending across the diaphragm.

These terms have more utility for recognition and planning of intervention than they do for establishing etiology. Many aneurysms are so complex, atypical, or extensive that they are not well described by any single term. The aneurysmal aorta is nearly inevitably also an elongated aorta; therefore, unfolding of the normally tighter curvature of the arch and tortuosity are almost invariable in the context of aortic aneurysm. Pseudocoarctation may occur at sites where there is some fixation to the aorta (isthmus and diaphragm).

Potential complications of aortic aneurysm include rupture into an adjacent space (pericardial space, mediastinum, left pleural space, or retroperitoneum), into a cardiac cavity (fistula), into an adjacent vessel (pulmonary artery or inferior vena cava), or into another space (trachea); dissection; embolism of thrombus; compression of an adjacent structure, such as bronchus, bone, or

recurrent laryngeal nerve; and distortion of the aortic valve and secondary aortic insufficiency (sinus of Valsalva aneurysms, aortic root aneurysms, annuloaortic ectasia).

The natural history of aortic aneurysm is influenced by aneurysm size (diameter), rate of expansion, location, complications (aortic insufficiency, rupture, dissection, thrombosis), associated factors (bicuspid aortic valves, concurrent hypertension, smoking, COPD), and underlying causes (Marfan syndrome, Ehlers-Danlos syndrome, infection, inflammation, or atherosclerosis). The yearly complication rate is influenced by thoracic aneurysm diameter (Table 11-1).[1]

Assessment of aneurysm size by different modalities (echocardiography, transesophageal echocardiography [TEE], computed tomography [CT], magnetic resonance imaging [MRI]) may yield intertest differences. There is invariably some degree of interobserver and intraobserver variation for each modality of testing, as evidenced by a reduction in size on follow-up testing. Sizing of aneurysms with respect to operative threshold applies only to asymptomatic aneurysms, not to symptomatic aneurysms.[1]

Aneurysms grow progressively at an approximate average overall rate of +1.2 mm/year. Larger aneurysms expand faster than smaller ones, the descending aorta expands faster (0.19 cm/year) than the ascending aorta (0.07 cm/year), and the abdominal aorta expands the fastest (3.9 ± 3.2 mm/year).[2,3] Therefore, it is only an issue of time before aneurysms achieve a size of clinical risk. Larger aneurysms experience faster rate of expansion. Should the patient not die of other causes in the intervening period, the patient will eventually die of the aneurysm.[1]

In 2007, the validity of the 55-mm threshold for establishing unacceptable risk of acute aortic dissection of the ascending aorta was challenged; among nearly 600 cases of acute aortic dissection, the majority occurred with ascending aortic dimensions of less than 55 mm.[4] Because of a higher risk of rupture for any

Table 11-1. Complication Rate is Influenced by Thoracic Aneurysm Diameter

	>3.5 cm	>4.0 cm	>5.0 cm	>6.0 cm
Rupture	0.0%	0.3%	1.7%	3.6%
Dissection	2.2%	1.5%	2.5%	3.7%
Death	5.9%	4.6%	4.8%	10.8%
Any of above	7.2%	5.3%	6.5%	14.1%

From Elefteriades JA: Thoracic aortic aneurysm: current approach to surgical timing. ACC Curr J Rev 2002;11:82-88, with permission from Elsevier.

Table 11-2. Threshold to Surgical Intervention is Lower in Patients with Marfan Syndrome

Location of Aneurysm	Patients without Marfan Syndrome	Patients with Marfan Syndrome
Ascending aorta	>5.5 cm[1]	>5.0 cm[1]
	>5.0-5.5 cm[4]	>4.5 cm[4]
Arch	>5.5-6.0 cm[4]	
Descending aorta	>6.5 cm[1]	>6.0 cm[1]
Thoracoabdominal	>5.0-6.0[4]	

Superscript numbers refer to references listed at the end of the chapter.

size of the aorta in Marfan syndrome, a lower threshold to surgical intervention is used (Table 11-2).

Although most aneurysms are commonly said to be due to atherosclerosis, coexistence versus causality remains unresolved, and the case for atherosclerosis as causative remains unproven. Risk factors for coronary artery disease are similarly risk factors for aneurysms, especially abdominal aortic aneurysm (AAA). The large majority of AAAs occur in the infrarenal site, which has predilection for atherosclerosis. In general, atherosclerosis risk factors account for little variability of aortic dimension, after the influence of major variables such as age, body surface area, and gender are excluded. Other than in familial cases of aneurysms, which often occur at younger ages, there is often concurrence of atherosclerotic disease of the coronary, cerebral, and renal arteries and aortic aneurysms, complicating the management of such cases.[5]

ETIOLOGY OF THORACIC AORTIC ANEURYSMS

Congenital and hereditary causes of thoracic aortic aneurysms are manifold. Aortic aneurysms are frequently associated with bicuspid valves and most commonly involve the ascending aorta above the sinotubular junction; they can sometimes involve the root as well but typically spare the arch. Marfan syndrome and related hereditary connective tissue disorders typically involve the aortic root and ascending aorta, but any segment of the aorta may become involved.

Acquired causes of thoracic aortic aneurysms involve hypertension, atherosclerosis, inflammatory diseases, and infections. Hypertension generally dilates and elongates the entire aorta but may be complicated by a frank aneurysm anywhere.

Atherosclerosis-associated aneurysms are most common in the descending aorta. Inflammatory diseases have a known association with aortic conditions. Aortic root inflammation and later dilation complicate many arthropathies (e.g., ankylosing spondylitis). Giant cell arteritis and Takayasu's arteritis may initiate aneurysms of any part of the thoracic aorta. Infections (staphylococcal, salmonella, syphilis, tuberculosis, mycotic) are also known causes of aortic diseases. Typically, syphilis involves the aortic root and ascending aorta.

ANEURYSMS OF THE AORTIC ROOT

Aneurysms of the aortic root include aneurysms of the sinus of Valsalva, annuloaortic ectasia, bicuspid valve–associated aneurysms, and post-stenotic aneurysms as well as those occurring as part of a more extensive aneurysm.

Aneurysms of the Sinus of Valsalva

Sinus of Valsalva aneurysms may be isolated (usually the right sinus, sometimes the noncoronary sinus, and very rarely the left sinus) or may be associated with dilation of the entire root and ascending aorta.

Congenital failure of fusion of the aortic media to the aortic valve annulus is held to be the cause, leading to aneurysmal dilation through the area of weakness. Sinus of Valsalva aneurysms may be complicated and present with aortic insufficiency, rupture and fistulization into the right ventricle (right sinus) or right atrium (noncoronary sinus), rupture into the pericardial space beneath the pulmonary artery (left sinus), right-sided heart obstruction (if large), and heart block from pressure on the septum.

Diagnosis can be readily obtained noninvasively, usually by echocardiography, but CT, MRI, and aortography may all depict sinus of Valsalva aneurysms.

Surgery for large aneurysms and for ones complicated by significant aortic insufficiency, fistulization, or right-sided heart obstruction is tailored to the specific anatomic involvement and is generally successful.

Annuloaortic Ectasia

Annuloaortic ectasia is a characteristic (but neither specific nor sole) lesion of Marfan syndrome, comprising dilation of the sinuses of Valsalva, effacement of the sinotubular junction, and dilation of the aortic root and ascending aorta that ends by the innominate artery. Terms commonly used to describe the morphologic appearance of the aorta in annuloaortic ectasia include Florence flask, onion bulb, and pear shaped (Figs. 11-1 to 11-3).

Although it may be seen in association with classic Marfan syndrome, most cases are seen in patients without any clear marfanoid features.

Presentations of annuloaortic ectasia include aortic insufficiency from aortic valve annular dilation or from poor cusp apposition due to dilated sinuses, rupture into adjacent cavities (fistula), dissection of the root, and obstruction of an adjacent lumen (rare).

11

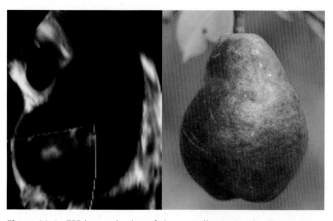

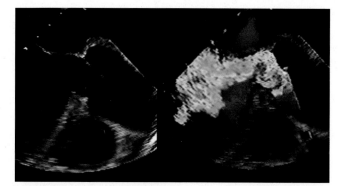

Figure 11-1. TEE long-axis view of the ascending aorta visualizes a pear-shaped aneurysm of the aortic root, characteristic of annuloaortic ectasia, with effacement of the sinotubular junction.

Figure 11-4. Annuloaortic ectasia causing severe aortic insufficiency. TEE long-axis views of the ascending aorta. Color Doppler flow mapping demonstrates flow into the left ventricle from the aneurysmal aortic root, filling most of the left ventricular outflow tract.

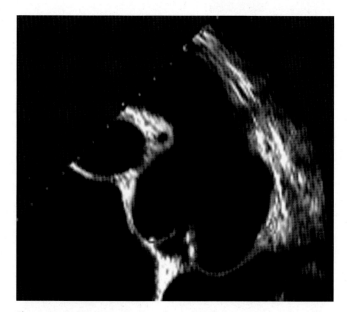

Figure 11-2. TEE long-axis view of an onion-like aneurysm of the aortic root (sinuses).

Degenerative changes of the aortic media seen on light microscopy may be found in many diseases of the aorta (congenital, heritable, acquired, aneurysmal, and dissection) and also with aortic aging.

The most florid cases involve prominent fragmentation of elastin fibers, replacement by collagen, and widespread interstitial infiltration (cysts with basophilic ground substance). The term *cystic medial necrosis* was formerly popular and often (erroneously) equated with Marfan syndrome; however, the term has fallen out of favor because there are neither cysts nor necrosis, and the entity is not specific for Marfan syndrome.

Noninvasive imaging (transthoracic echocardiography, TEE, MRI, and CT) as well as aortography can depict the typical aneurysmal lesion gross morphology of annuloaortic ectasia. Imaging modalities that can display the root and ascending aorta in their true long axis (which is off the sagittal plane) are the most useful. As availability of three-dimensional (3D) reconstruction by CT and also of MRI becomes more widespread, these will probably become the leading modalities to image the lesion of annuloaortic ectasia. However, for diagnosis of the complications such as aortic insufficiency, echocardiography and aortography retain a contributing role (Fig. 11-4).

Management is surgical once the aortic dimensions achieve surgical threshold or there is complication by severe aortic insufficiency, dissection, or rupture. Tube graft replacement of the root and ascending aorta, often with a composite graft that includes an aortic valve prosthesis, is the usual surgery. When possible, the aortic valve is spared replacement; but if it is severely deformed or insufficient, it is generally replaced.

ANEURYSMS OF THE ASCENDING AORTA

Aneurysms of the ascending aorta can be congenital or acquired disorders that weaken the aortic media. Congenital causes can be associated with bicuspid aortic valve or hereditary disorders, such as Marfan syndrome, Turner syndrome, Ehlers-Danlos syndrome, osteogenesis imperfecta, and polycystic kidney disease. Acquired disorders that can weaken the aortic media include hypertension, atherosclerosis, inflammatory diseases (Takayasu's arteritis, giant cell arteritis, rheumatoid arthritis, seronegative arthropathies), and infections such as syphilis (Fig. 11-5).

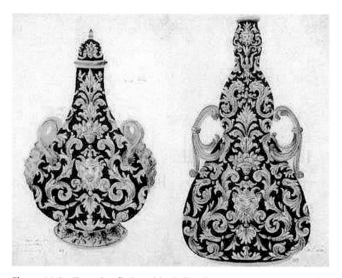

Figure 11-3. Florentine flasks, with similar shape to some aneurysms of the aortic root/ascending aorta.

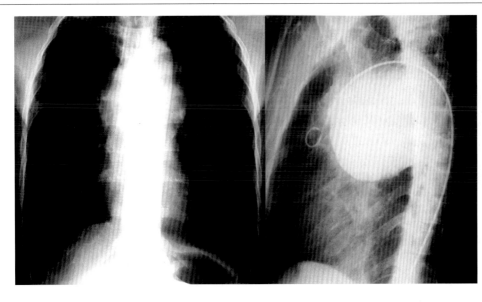

Figure 11-5. A 41-year-old Haitian man presented with 2 months of fatigue, respiratory distress on lying supine, and systolic ejection murmur. Remote history of venereal disease and soccer-related chest trauma. Chest radiograph was uniformly interpreted as bihilar adenopathy. Aortography conclusively identified a large aneurysm of the ascending aorta without aortic insufficiency. Given venereal disease history and VDRL positivity, the etiology was presumed to be syphilitic. The patient underwent uncomplicated surgical aortic repair.

Incidental diagnosis by an imaging modality and chest pain are the most common presentations. Chest pain may result from vertebral body erosion or rib erosion. Chest pain without erosion strongly suggests aneurysm expansion and increased risk of rupture. Aneurysms isolated to the ascending aorta are less likely to result in either aortic insufficiency (and therefore present with a murmur or congestive heart failure) or compression of mediastinal structures, such as the trachea and bronchi (cough or shortness of breath, or tracheal tug on physical examination), the recurrent laryngeal nerve (hoarseness), the esophagus (dysphagia), the superior vena cava (compression signs), the pulmonary artery (murmur), or the spine (back pain). Rupture into the pericardial space may be the initial manifestation. Dissection may occur.

Noninvasive imaging (transthoracic echocardiography, TEE, MRI, and CT) as well as aortography can depict the typical aneurysmal lesion of annuloaortic ectasia. The chest radiograph is reasonable in depicting aneurysms of the ascending aorta, but it is not specific enough, nor does it have the means to accurately measure dimension.

Imaging modalities that can display the root and ascending aorta in their true long axis (which is off the sagittal plane) are the most useful. As availability of 3D reconstruction by CT and also of MRI becomes more widespread, these will probably become the leading modalities to image the lesion of annuloaortic ectasia and most thoracic aneurysms.

Management is surgical once the aortic dimensions achieve surgical threshold (generally accepted as >5.5 cm with some patient individualization) or there is complication, assuming the patient is a surgical candidate (Fig. 11-6). Tube graft replacement of the ascending aorta is the usual surgery. Median sternotomy is performed to expose the aneurysmal ascending aorta, once total cardiopulmonary bypass and myocardial protection (cold cardioplegia) are achieved. Tube graft insertion is achieved with attention to the coronaries (which may need to be reimplanted).

Medical control of blood pressure is advisable, whether the patient is referred for surgery or observed.

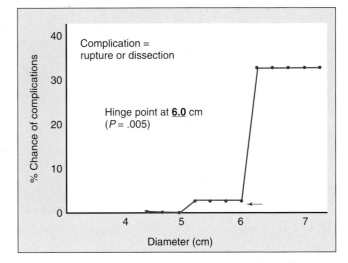

Figure 11-6. Ascending aortic aneurysm: size and risk of complications. As 6.0 cm represents the median value, the threshold is set less than the median to avoid complications. Surgical threshold for asymptomatic aneurysms based on size alone is >5.5 cm. (Data from Coady MA, Rizzo JA, Hammond GL, et al: What is the appropriate size criterion for resection of thoracic aortic aneurysms? J Thorac Cardiovasc Surg 1997;113:476-491; and Elefteriades JA: Thoracic aortic aneurysm: current approach to surgical timing. ACC Curr J Rev 2002;11:82-88.)

ANEURYSMS OF THE AORTIC ARCH

Aneurysms of the aortic arch, being removed from the heart proper, rarely cause cardiac complications; being in the vicinity of the arch vessels, major airways, and recurrent laryngeal nerve, complaints referable to these structures are more common. Presentations may be due to compression of structures as described before; erosion of vertebrae; expansion; or rupture into the

11

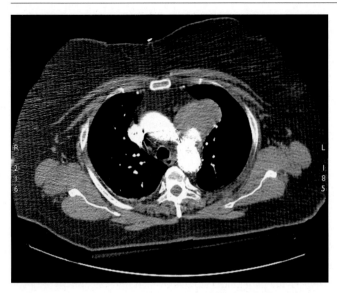

Figure 11-7. A saccular arch aneurysm, largely filled with thrombus, is seen arising off the left anterior aspect of the aortic arch. This had occurred in a 68-year-old woman with long-standing systemic lupus erythematosus. It was successfully excluded by endovascular repair. (Courtesy of Mark Peterson, MD, Toronto, Canada.)

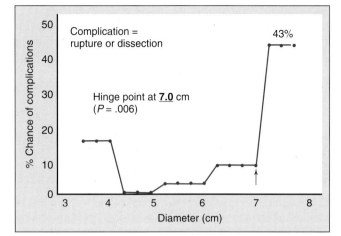

Figure 11-8. Descending aortic aneurysm: size and risk of complications. As 7.0 cm represents the median value, the threshold is set less than the median to avoid complications. Surgical threshold for asymptomatic aneurysms based on size alone is >6.5 cm. (Data from Coady MA, Rizzo JA, Hammond GL, et al: What is the appropriate size criterion for resection of thoracic aortic aneurysms? J Thorac Cardiovasc Surg 1997;113:476-491; and Elefteriades JA: Thoracic aortic aneurysm: current approach to surgical timing. ACC Curr J Rev 2002;11:82-88.)

mediastinum, pleural spaces, esophagus (hematemesis), or tracheobronchial tree (hemoptysis). The prognosis is approximately 50% to 75% mortality at 5 years, with half of the deaths from rupture.

Diagnosis is readily established by CT, MRI, or aortography. Transthoracic echocardiography is too limited to be sufficiently accurate, and TEE suffers from the inability to image the upper ascending aorta and proximal arch to interposed air in the trachea as well as the branch vessels. As branch vessel involvement and other mediastinal structures are relevant, CT and MRI are superior for their ability to image the thorax in detail.

Surgery is the standard treatment of arch aneurysms that are symptomatic and of surgical size. Surgery is performed through median sternotomy, with total cardiopulmonary bypass and cold cardioplegia cardiac arrest. Retrograde perfusion of the brain through the superior vena cava appears to increase brain protection. In some cases, hypothermic circulatory arrest with brain protection is necessary to achieve a bloodless field. Most surgeons use cardiopulmonary bypass with varying degrees of hypothermia and low flow or circulatory arrest. Synthetic tube graft insertion is performed, usually with the arch branch vessels left on an island of aortic wall that is sewn into a matching-sized hole cut out from the tube graft. Endovascular repair is increasingly performed with success (Fig. 11-7).

ANEURYSMS OF THE DESCENDING THORACIC AORTA

The incidence of aneurysms of the descending aorta is increasing. Aneurysms of the descending aorta are generally asymptomatic until expansion or rupture occurs. The 5-year survival of patients with untreated aneurysms of the descending aorta is only 9% to 13%. They are located distal to the heart and, depending on their

position, variably distal to mediastinal structures. Some aneurysms of the descending aorta will cause compression of mediastinal structures, if they are located superiorly. In morphologic appearance, they may be tubular, fusiform, or saccular.

Aneurysms of the descending aorta are often detected incidentally, although they are more likely to cause symptoms than are aneurysms of the ascending aorta by compressing mediastinal structures and causing hoarseness, dyspnea, dysphagia, or hemoptysis or by eroding adjacent vertebrae. Aneurysms of the descending aorta are less common than the AAAs (4 to 12/1000 versus 20 to 50/1000).

The greater surgical risks (both morbidity and mortality) of operating on aneurysms of the descending aorta versus AAA have resulted in increasing interest in medical and nonsurgical and percutaneous management (Fig. 11-8).[6]

Noninvasive modalities (CT, MRI, TEE) generally suffice for diagnosis of aneurysms of the descending aorta. Management for small and asymptomatic aneurysms constitutes blood pressure control, preferably beta-blockade, and follow-up. Management of symptomatic aneurysms or aneurysms of surgical size (>6.5 cm) is surgical repair of the aorta, if the patient is a surgical candidate.

Surgery is performed through left thoracotomy, with no cardiopulmonary bypass or partial (atrial-femoral or femoral-femoral) bypass or shunts during cross-clamping, careful attention to the spinal arteries, and tube graft insertion. Surgical mortality ranges from 10% to 15% in good surgical candidates.

Saccular Aneurysms of the Descending Thoracic Aorta

Saccular aneurysms of the descending thoracic aorta may be caused by atherosclerosis (penetration of an ulcer) or chronic dissection, or they may be syphilitic. They carry a risk of rupture, embolization of thrombus, and compression of adjacent structures. Diagnosis is readily achieved by CT, MRI, or TEE. The standard treatment is surgical repair if the aneurysm is rupturing, if it is symptomatic, or if it is large. Surgery consists of excision of the involved segment and interposition of a tube graft through left thoracotomy. Stent grafts have been successfully employed.

THORACIC ENDOVASCULAR AORTIC REPAIR (TEVAR)

Endovascular therapy for thoracic aneurysms as well as for penetrating ulcers and dissections is increasingly performed (Fig. 11-9).[7] Short-term results appear acceptable, but intermediate- and long-term results are not well established. As one segment of stent graft costs at least $5000 and most patients receive two graft segments for thoracic repair, financial issues limit availability at many centers.[8] Specialized centers have achieved excellent results with 4% in-hospital mortality in high-risk cases.[9] A review of series of endograft closure of aneurysms of the descending aorta described procedural mortality of 0% to 4%, technical success of more than 98%, 30-day aneurysm thrombosis of 90% to 100%, paraplegia in 0% to 3%, late migration in 1% to 2%, and breakage in 10% to 30%.[6,10]

New-generation devices have lower endoleak rates than do older generation devices (15% versus 46%; $P < .001$). They appear to have lower vascular access complication rates (23% versus 42%; $P = .069$) and absence of endoleak, rupture, dissection, or reintervention rates in 73% at 1 year, 69% at 3 years, and 64% at 5 years.[11]

Centers specializing in TEVAR have published mortality rates as low as 2% for repair of complex thoracoabdominal cases by use of branched endografts.[12]

EXTENSIVE AORTIC ANEURYSMS

The term *thoracoabdominal aneurysm* is generally held to mean an aneurysm starting in the descending aorta and extending into the abdominal aorta (Fig. 11-10). Aneurysms that involve both the descending thoracic and the abdominal aorta confer a challenge to the patient and surgeon. When they become large (>6 to 7 cm) in good surgical candidates, surgery may be undertaken. The goal of the surgery—to replace the dilated segment in its entirety—requires a left thoracotomy extended to a midline abdominal incision that exposes the thoracic and abdominal portions of the aorta. Tube graft insertion of the affected segment is the usual treatment. The renal, celiac, and superior mesenteric arteries are attached to the graft directly or on sections of aortic wall. As would be expected, renal ischemia and insufficiency may occur. The operative mortality is 15% or higher.

Some patients have extensive aneurysms involving the entire length of the aorta or several different segments. A corollary of this is that identification of an aneurysm in one part of the aorta should lead to a reasonable search that will identify or exclude aneurysms elsewhere. Provided the patient is an acceptable operative candidate, staged repair of the aorta is the usual approach, with the more proximal sections being repaired before the distal sections (Fig. 11-11).

Many techniques have been employed; the two most common are a single tour de force operation using deep hypothermic circulatory arrest and sequential operations to insert sequential sections of tube grafts. For extensive thoracic aneurysms, the "elephant trunk" technique (insertion of a tube graft into the proximal descending aorta while the tube is left floating in the aorta to be sewn in distally later) is sometimes used. Com-

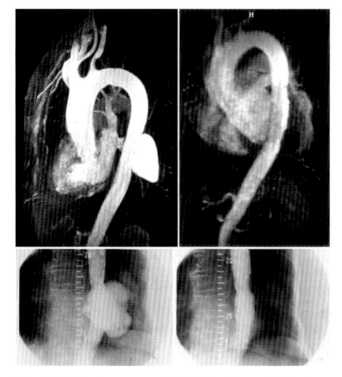

Figure 11-9. Percutaneous nonsurgical abolition of a saccular thoracic aneurysm in a 67-year-old woman with symptoms consistent with expanding aneurysm (pain, hoarseness). TOP LEFT, Gadolinium-enhanced MRA showing aneurysm larger than 5 cm. TOP RIGHT, Exclusion of the aneurysm by a stent graft with thrombosis of the lumen. BOTTOM LEFT, Aortogram showing the saccular lobulated aneurysm of the mid descending aorta. BOTTOM RIGHT, Exclusion of the aneurysm by a stent graft with thrombosis of the lumen. (From Lund GK, Diekmann C, Nienaber CA: Nonsurgical abolition of thoracic aortic aneurysm. Circulation 1999;99:E9.)

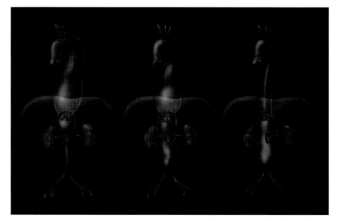

Figure 11-10. Variable lengths and locations of thoracoabdominal aortic aneurysms.

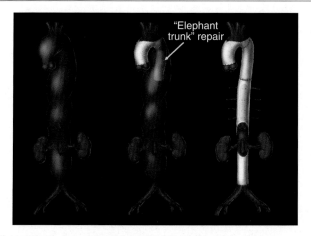

Figure 11-11. Staged surgical repair of thoracic aortic aneurysm.

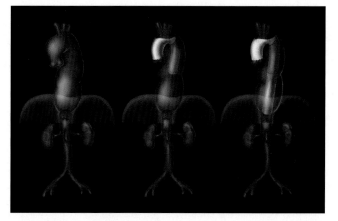

Figure 11-12. Combined surgical and stenting repair of thoracic aortic aneurysm.

pletion may be accomplished by surgical or stent techniques (Fig. 11-12).

In a large series of 1146 aortic operations performed between 1991 and 2000, 183 first- or second-stage operations for elephant trunk procedures performed in 117 patients observed the following mortality: 5.1% for first-stage operation; 3.6% between staged operations (75% were ruptures); and 6.2% for second-stage operation. Forty-three patients did not return for a second operation: 30% died in an average of 3 years and 30% as a result of rupture.[13]

CASE 1

History and Physical Examination

▸ 57-year-old woman with a thoracic aneurysm found incidentally on CT scanning (for abdominal surgery)
▸ Throbbing in the chest noted for 1 year, no chest pains
▸ No marfanoid elements to her history; no history of hypertension

Physical Examination

▸ BP 130/70 mm Hg, HR 60 bpm
▸ Pectus excavatum
▸ Systolic pulsation to the upper sternum; murmur of aortic insufficiency; apex not enlarged or displaced
▸ Peripheral pulse volumes and contours normal

Evolution and Outcome

▸ Clinical diagnosis was an aneurysm of the ascending aorta and arch, severe associated aortic insufficiency, and no dissection or clot (confirmed by surgery).
▸ A composite graft (mechanical aortic valve replacement + tube) was inserted through median sternotomy.

▸ The head and neck vessels were sewn onto the superior aspect of the graft as an island under circulatory arrest.
▸ Uneventful postoperative course; prescribed beta-blocker postoperatively

Comments

▸ Incidental and serendipitous finding of a large thoracic aneurysm in an otherwise healthy 57-year-old person
▸ Associated insufficiency of the aortic valve (unrepairable) necessitated composite replacement grafting (aortic valve replacement + tube graft).
▸ Circulatory arrest was needed to operate on the arch vessels.
▸ Although hypertension was a risk factor for enlargement, the cause of the aneurysm was unclear. Of note, the chest wall deformity was the only marfanoid characteristic and potentially the morphology of the aneurysm itself. The VDRL test result was negative, and there was no history of arthritis or vasculitis.
▸ Either the aneurysm of the ascending aorta against the sternum or the excavatum sternum or both were responsible for the symptom of 1-year of throbbing in the chest and the finding of systolic pulsation of the sternum.

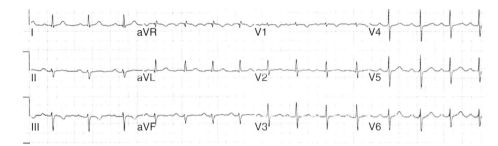

Figure 11-13. ECG shows no evidence of left ventricular hypertrophy and nonspecific repolarization abnormalities.

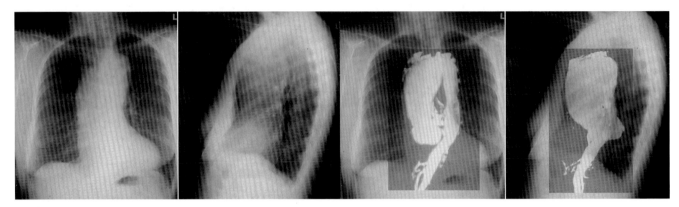

Figure 11-14. Chest radiographs and 3D CT overlay. There is dilation of the ascending aorta and arch, resulting in the right hilar overlay sign, and increased aortic and mediastinal width. The overlaid 3D CT images indicate the location of the various segments of the thoracic aorta on the posteroanterior and lateral chest radiographs. Normal cardiopericardial silhouette. Pectus excavatum.

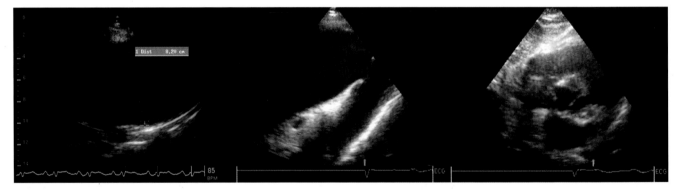

Figure 11-15. Transthoracic echocardiography. LEFT, Right parasternal view of the ascending aorta: 8.2 cm in diameter; no intimal flap present. MIDDLE, Suprasternal view shows the dilation of the ascending aorta as well as the normal-caliber descending aorta and slight kink at the distal arch. RIGHT, Short-axis view of the aortic valve, which is trileaflet.

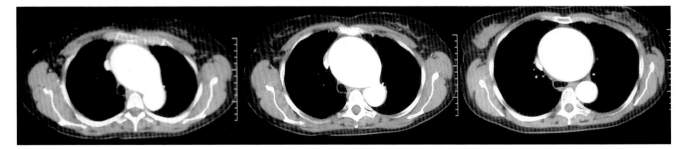

Figure 11-16. Contrast-enhanced axial CT scan from the arch to slightly inferiorly. The aneurysm involves the ascending aorta and the arch, not the descending aorta. There is no intimal flap. There is pseudocoarctation (folding of the floor of the distal arch), with the misleading appearance of coarctation being present.

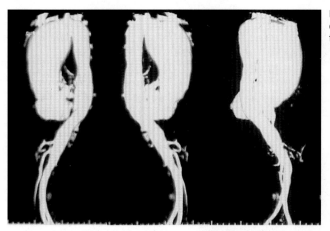

Figure 11-17. Contrast-enhanced CT scan: 3D reconstruction of the aorta demonstrating the aneurysm of the ascending portion and arch as well as the fold of the floor of the distal arch caused by the elongation of the aorta.

CASE 2

History

▸ 76-year-old man after abdominal aortic repair
▸ Past medical history is significant for recent repair of aortojejunal fistula.
▸ Aortobifemoral repair 9 years ago
▸ Bilateral iliac aneurysm repair 5 years before that
▸ Advanced COPD
▸ Coronary artery disease with prior myocardial infarction
▸ No recognized cerebrovascular disease
▸ Hypertension, smoker

Comments

▸ The entire aorta, if not the entire systemic arterial tree, was diseased in this patient (AAA, thoracic aneurysm, thoracic false aneurysm, iliofemoral aneurysms, coronary artery disease). The arterial disease was both aneurysmal and atherosclerotic.
▸ The small size of the presumed false aneurysm of the thoracic aorta (with, it is to be hoped, a fair prognosis), situated within such a diseased thoracic aorta of poor surgical quality, and particularly the advanced lung disease that still had the patient ventilated for the prior abdominal aortic repair discouraged surgical consideration.
▸ The mobile mural thrombus in the thoracic aorta precluded interventional consideration, as instrumentation within the thoracic aorta would have facilitated embolization, which seemed to be of risk anyway.

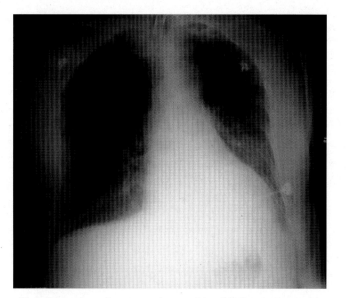

Figure 11-18. Chest radiograph shows mild cardiomegaly, tracheostomy tube, possible mild hilar overlay sign of ascending aortic dilation, normal arch diameter, no obvious aortic intimal calcification, and large lung fields.

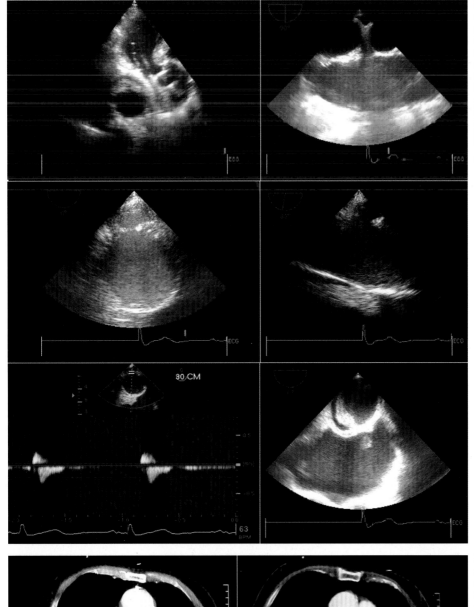

Figure 11-19. TOP LEFT, Apical 3-chamber view revealing an aneurysm of the descending aorta and mural thrombus. TOP RIGHT, TEE longitudinal view of the ascending aorta. The aorta is dilated, but without intimal flap or mural abnormality. MIDDLE, Cross-sectional (LEFT) and longitudinal (RIGHT) views of a small (1 cm) pouch in the near wall (medial side of the mid descending aorta). BOTTOM LEFT, Spectral flow profile of reciprocating flow into and out of the pouch. BOTTOM RIGHT, There is a blood-filled layer outside of the mural thrombus and a left pleural effusion.

Figure 11-20. Contrast-enhanced axial CT scans. There are large bilateral pleural effusions. The ascending aorta is dilated and with intimal calcification. The proximal descending thoracic aorta is not dilated but the mid and lower thoracic aorta are, as is the abdominal aorta. There is mural thrombus of the thoracoabdominal aneurysm. Intimal calcification is seen deep to the mural thrombus in the bottom right image. The top right image reveals a small pouch-like extravasation of dye into the wall medially (false aneurysm versus penetrating ulcer).

CASE 3

History and Physical Examination

▸ 78-year-old woman transferred with suspected aortic dissection
▸ Sudden-onset severe chest pain 4 hours before
▸ Previously hypertensive; no known coronary artery disease, cardiovascular disease, or peripheral vascular disease
▸ Normotensive on arrival; no aortic insufficiency murmur, rub, or pulse deficits

Evolution and Management

▸ Clinical diagnosis was a leaking thoracic false aneurysm (acute chest pain and probable mediastinal blood on TEE), severe aortic atherosclerosis, and no dissection of the aorta, as confirmed by surgery.
▸ Surgical management consisted of insertion of an interposition graft in the section of involved aorta through lateral thoracotomy.
▸ Uneventful outcome

Comments

▸ The etiology of the false aneurysm was unclear, but atheromatous penetrating ulcer was possible, given the extent of atherosclerosis. There was no history of trauma, and there were no findings of an old dissection.

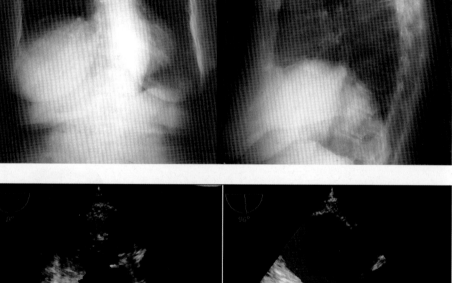

Figure 11-21. Chest radiograph shows borderline cardiomegaly, tortuous descending aorta, and the arch that is not dilated.

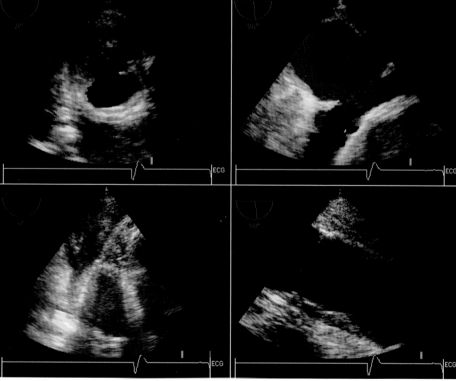

Figure 11-22. TEE. TOP LEFT, There is a large rounded chamber lateral to the mid descending aorta with thrombus occupying most of it. TOP RIGHT, Flow swirls around the lumen of the saccular chamber arising off of the mid descending thoracic aorta. BOTTOM LEFT, There is gelatinous material between the transducer and the heart, consistent with clotted blood. BOTTOM RIGHT, The lower thoracic aorta beyond the false aneurysm is heavily atheromatous.

CASE 4

History

▸ 62-year-old woman with systemic lupus erythematosus and renal insufficiency
▸ Presented with severe chest pains, lateral ST depression, and transient heart failure
▸ No past history of ischemic heart disease
▸ Had been observed for a saccular aneurysm arising off of the arch of the aorta, which had remained stable

Physical Examination

▸ BP initially 130/80 mm Hg, HR 90 bpm, RR normal
▸ No murmurs or rubs

Evolution and Outcome

▸ She underwent coronary angiography, which demonstrated an occluded large left circumflex artery as well as disease of the left anterior descending and right coronary arteries.

▸ Discussions were under way concerning myocardial revascularization options, including combined surgical procedure with aortic arch repair.
▸ She abruptly experienced salvos of asystolic episodes, then sustained asystole, from which she could not be resuscitated.

Comments

▸ Aortic saccular aneurysm associated with systemic lupus erythematosus
▸ Problematically concurrent pathologic processes—acute coronary syndrome (indicating antiplatelet and anticoagulant treatment) and aortic aneurysm (contraindicating antiplatelet and anticoagulant treatment)
▸ The basis of the aystolic arrest was unclear—myocardial ischemia, rupture of the heart, and rupture of the aneurysm were all possible.

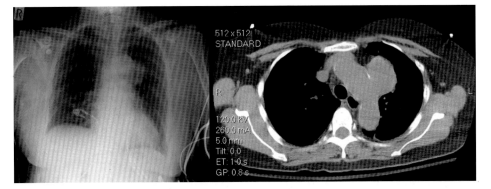

Figure 11-23. The chest radiograph (LEFT) reveals a prominent rounded lesion to the left of the aortic arch. No left pleural effusion. The non–contrast-enhanced axial CT scan (RIGHT) demonstrates a saccular cavity extending off the right wall of the arch—saccular aneurysm versus false aneurysm.

CASE 5

History

▸ 85-year-old man with chest pains
▸ Aortocoronary bypass 20 years before; CCS class II angina
▸ Mild symptoms of biventricular heart failure
▸ AAA repair 4 years before
▸ Recent melena—concern of aortoenteric (jejunal) fistula not substantiated by endoscopy
▸ CT at referring hospital demonstrated a large thoracoabdominal aneurysm.
▸ Renal insufficiency

Physical Examination

▸ BP initially 130/80 mm Hg, HR 80 bpm, RR normal
▸ Elevated venous pressures, right ventricular heave (right ventricular systolic pressure on echocardiography was 75 mm Hg)
▸ No murmurs or rubs

Evolution and Outcome

▸ Owing to concerns about general debility and frailty, the patient was not operated on.
▸ He survived more than a year.

Comments

▸ Thoracoabdominal aneurysm
▸ The initial AAA was not in isolation; the thoracic aorta was also enlarged at the time of the AAA repair. Within a few years, the thoracic aneurysm had enlarged to a major extent.
▸ An enormous amount of mural thrombus was associated with the thoracic aneurysm, as often happens with AAAs as well but not with ascending aortic aneurysms.
▸ Many comorbidities, as often occur in cases of thoracoabdominal aneurysm

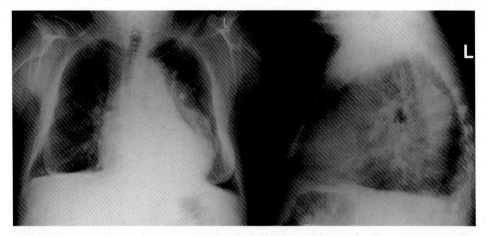

Figure 11-24. Chest radiograph shows cardiomegaly, some signs of left-sided heart failure, barrel chest, prior sternotomy, mildly enlarged aortic arch, and heavy intimal calcification of the aortic arch. Enlargement of the descending thoracic aorta is questionable. There is no left pleural effusion.

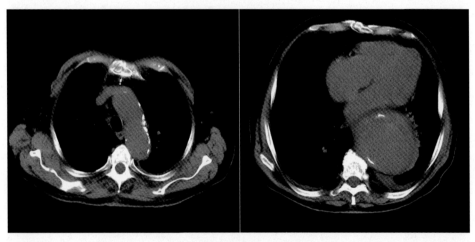

Figure 11-25. Non–contrast-enhanced axial CT scans. LEFT, There is heavy intimal calcification of the aortic arch. RIGHT, There is an enormous aneurysm of the descending retrocardiac aorta (12 cm). The location of the intimal calcification on the anterior wall of the descending aorta demonstrates that the layer inward of it is crescentic mural thrombus, which is faintly delineated.

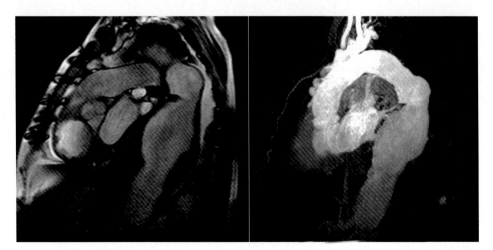

Figure 11-26. LEFT, Spin echo sequence MRI depicts the flowing blood within the lumen and clearly establishes the large amount of mural thrombus. RIGHT, Gadolinium-enhanced MRA. The saccular nature of the lumen of the thoracic aneurysm is apparent. Branch vessel depiction is good where there is no overlap. The mural thrombus and actual outside diameters of the aneurysm, though, are not apparent.

CASE 6

History

▸ 72-year-old man who had previously undergone endovascular repair of a proximal descending thoracic aneurysm
▸ The left subclavian artery had been excluded by the covered stent, resulting in a type II leak of moderate size.

Management and Outcome

▸ The leak was successfully addressed by coil embolization of the left subclavian artery.

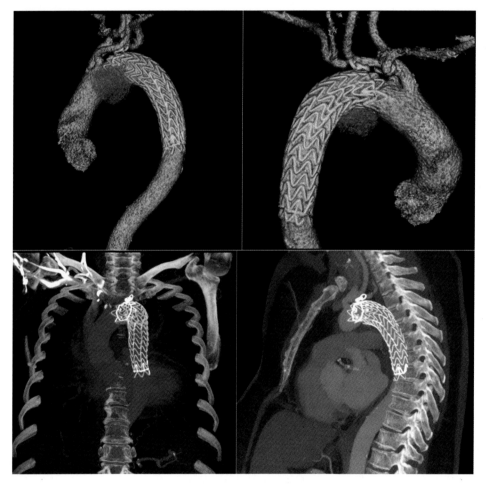

Figure 11-27. TOP, 3D reconstructions of contrast-enhanced CT scan. The type II leak is seen as blue hazy material under the arch to the left side. The leak was successfully addressed by coil embolization of the left subclavian artery. BOTTOM, The coil can be seen in the very proximal left subclavian artery in the CT reconstructions. (Courtesy of Mark Peterson, MD, Toronto, Canada.)

CASE 7

History and Physical Examination

▸ A 77-year-old man with a prior AAA surgical repair underwent evaluation for a known thoracic aneurysm, which, although large, was asymptomatic.

▸ He had previously experienced a myocardial infarction but was without angina or heart failure.

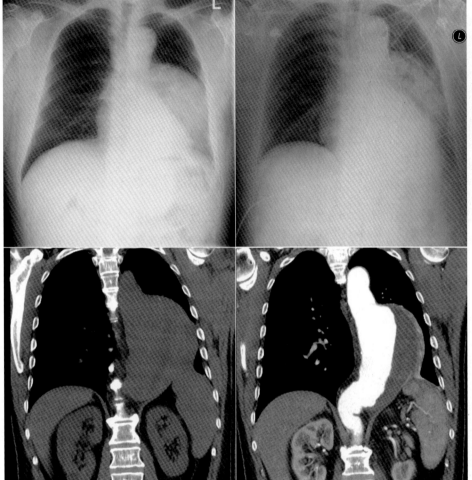

Figure 11-28. Corresponding posteroanterior chest radiographs and CT scans. TOP LEFT, Pre-EVAR posteroanterior chest radiograph reveals the very large aneurysm of the descending thoracic aorta. There does not appear to be a pleural effusion. TOP RIGHT, Post-EVAR image reveals the stents extending from the proximal descending aorta down to the diaphragm. BOTTOM, Non–contrast-enhanced and contrast-enhanced coronal CT scans depict the aneurysm and the very large amount of mural thrombus.

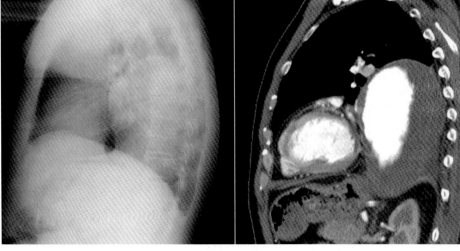

Figure 11-29. Corresponding lateral chest radiograph and CT scan. The enormity of the descending thoracic aneurysm is apparent as it exceeds the size of the heart.

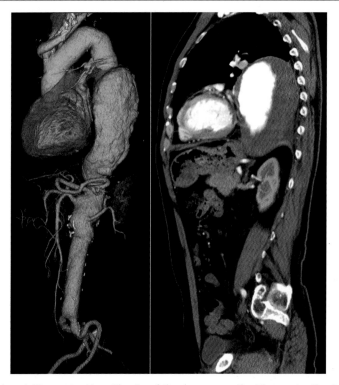

Figure 11-30. 3D (LEFT) and sagittal (RIGHT) CT reconstructions. The size of the aneurysm on the 3D reconstruction is underrepresented as the reconstruction is performed with use of only contrast-enhanced voxels; therefore, the mural thrombus and wall are not included. The sagittal reconstruction readily expresses the true size of the aneurysm and the amount and location of thrombus. The 3D reconstruction and this sagittal plane reconstruction depict the surgically repaired abdominal aorta, which has an unnatural tubular shape and regularity imparted by the graft.

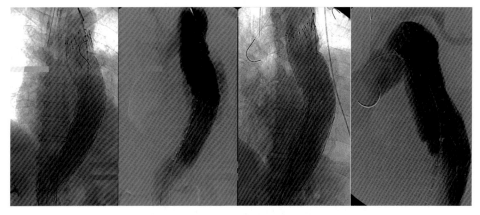

Figure 11-31. Angiography during EVAR. LEFT TWO IMAGES, After initial deployment. There is a type I leak arising from the proximal margin and seen on both the left and right sides of the aorta. RIGHT TWO IMAGES, The leak has been successfully sealed by redeployment of the proximal portion.

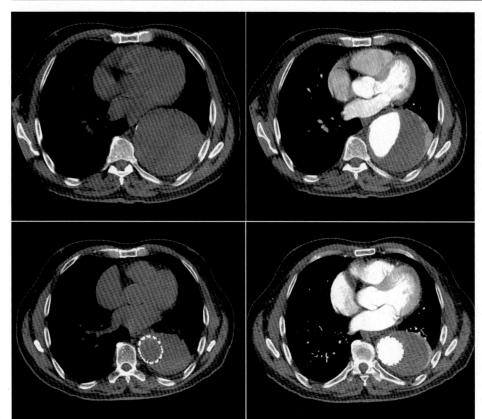

Figure 11-32. Axial CT scans without contrast enhancement (LEFT IMAGES) and with contrast enhancement (RIGHT IMAGES), before EVAR (TOP ROW) and after EVAR (BOTTOM ROW). The size of the aneurysm has diminished after EVAR. There is no endoleak.

CASE 8

History and Physical Examination

▸ A 67-year-old woman was evaluated for chronic cough.
▸ A chest radiograph detected an enlarged aorta.
▸ She was a former 40-pack/year smoker and hypertensive for a decade.
▸ Investigations revealed only mild emphysema.
▸ There was no murmur of aortic insufficiency.

Surgical Procedure

▸ It was recommended that the patient undergo a two-stage procedure on the aorta, as the aneurysmal length was too great to be approached by a single procedure.
▸ First stage: surgical tube graft replacement of the ascending aorta and arch, sewing the distal anastomosis to the distal arch, leaving an elephant trunk in the distal arch and proximal descending aorta
▸ Second stage: endovascular repair of the descending aorta, anchored to the elephant trunk

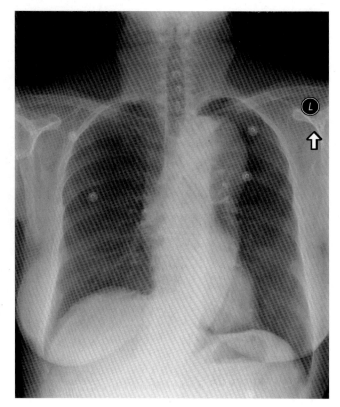

Figure 11-33. The chest radiograph shows enlarged ascending aorta (hilar overlay), arch, and descending aorta. There is no intimal calcium. The cardiopericardial silhouette is normal. There are no pleural effusions.

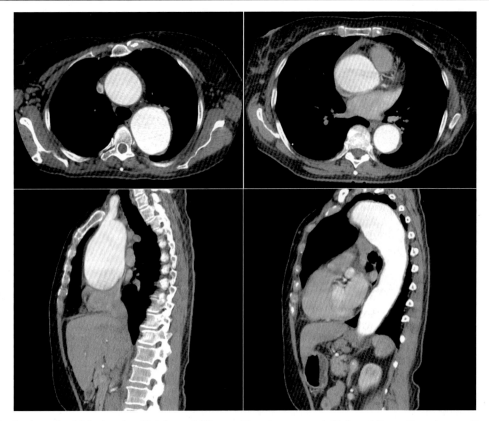

Figure 11-34. Contrast-enhanced axial (TOP) and sagittal (BOTTOM) CT scans. There is aneurysmal dilation of the aortic root, ascending aorta, arch, and most of the descending thoracic aorta. The aorta resumes a more normal caliber behind the left atrium. There are no intimal flaps, and there is only a small amount of mural thrombus in the descending aorta.

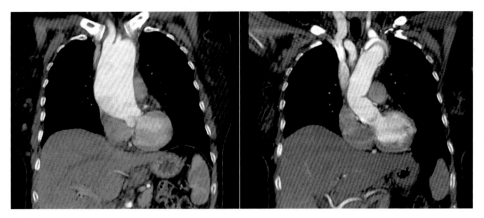

Figure 11-35. Contrast-enhanced CT scans, coronal views before (LEFT) and after (RIGHT) surgical tube graft replacement. The diameter of the tube graft is far less than that of the aneurysm. There is a degree of folding of the tube graft because of the high degree of curvature of the aorta in this case and the length of the tube graft. The distal anastomosis is in the distal arch, and the tube graft continues beyond as an elephant trunk.

11

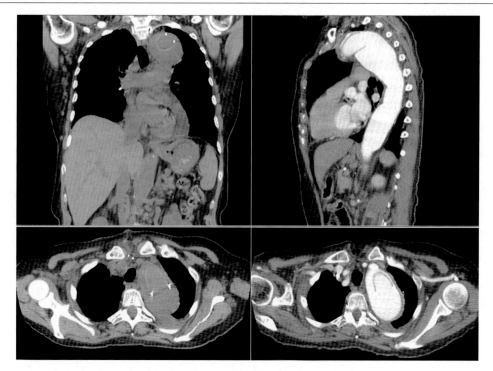

Figure 11-36. Non–contrast-enhanced and contrast-enhanced CT scans after elephant trunk procedure. The free end of the graft distal to the anastomosis is obvious, especially as there are radiopaque markers at the distal margin of the tube graft.

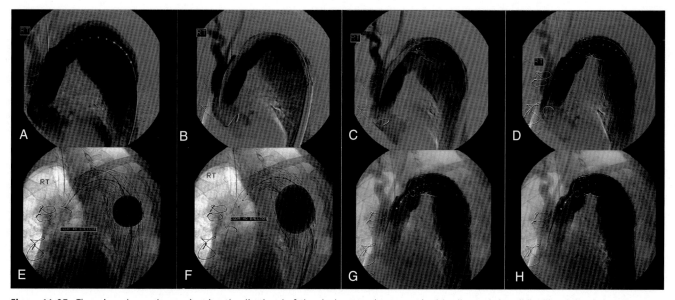

Figure 11-37. Thoracic endovascular repair using the distal end of the elephant trunk as a proximal landing and the mildly dilated distal thoracic aorta as a distal landing zone. **A,** Aortography reveals the normalized diameter of the ascending aorta by the tube graft replacement and the still aneurysmal distal arch and descending aorta. **B,** First stent graft being positioned to land in the elephant trunk. **C** and **D,** Deployment of the first stent graft and the second stent graft into the first. **E** and **F,** Dilation of the overlapping segment of stent grafts. **G** and **H,** After the procedure. There is a small type II endoleak, probably due to the left subclavian artery. The left subclavian artery has been excluded by the TEVAR procedure.

References

1. Elefteriades JA: Thoracic aortic aneurysm: current approach to surgical timing. ACC Curr J Rev 2002;11:82-88.

2. Masuda Y, Takanashi K, Takasu J, et al: Expansion rate of thoracic aortic aneurysms and influencing factors. Chest 1992;102:461-466.

3. Coady MA, Rizzo JA, Hammond GL, et al: What is the appropriate size criterion for resection of thoracic aortic aneurysms? J Thorac Cardiovasc Surg 1997;113:476-491.

4. Pape LA, Tsai TT, Isselbacher EM, et al: Aortic diameter > or = 5.5 cm is not a good predictor of type A aortic dissection: observations from the International Registry of Acute Aortic Dissection (IRAD). Circulation 2007;116:1120-1127.

5. Agmon Y, Khandheria BK, Meissner I, et al: Is aortic dilatation an atherosclerosis-related process? Clinical, laboratory, and transesophageal echocardiographic correlates of thoracic aortic dimensions in the population with implications for thoracic aortic aneurysm formation. J Am Coll Cardiol 2003;42:1076-1083.

6. Faxon DP, Creager MA, Smith SC Jr, et al: Atherosclerotic Vascular Disease Conference: Executive summary: Atherosclerotic Vascular Disease Conference proceeding for healthcare professionals from a special writing group of the American Heart Association. Circulation 2004;109:2595-2604.

7. Ricco JB, Cau J, Marchand C, et al: Stent-graft repair for thoracic aortic disease: results of an independent nationwide study in France from 1999 to 2001. J Thorac Cardiovasc Surg 2006;131:131-137.

8. Pelletier M, Mitchell S: Thoracic endovascular stent grafts. Can J Cardiol 2005;21:197.

9. Dagenais F, Normand JP, Turcotte R, Mathieu P: Changing trends in management of thoracic aortic disease: where do we stand with thoracic endovascular stent grafts? Can J Cardiol 2005;21:173-178.

10. Dake MD: Endovascular stent-graft management of thoracic aortic diseases. Eur J Radiol 2001;39:42-49.

11. Appoo JJ, Moser WG, Fairman RM, et al: Thoracic aortic stent grafting: improving results with newer generation investigational devices. J Thorac Cardiovasc Surg 2006;131:1087-1094.

12. Greenberg RK, West K, Pfaff K, et al: Beyond the aortic bifurcation: branched endovascular grafts for thoracoabdominal and aortoiliac aneurysms. J Vasc Surg 2006;43:879.

13. Safi HJ, Miller CC III, Estrera AL, et al: Staged repair of extensive aortic aneurysms: morbidity and mortality in the elephant trunk technique. Circulation 2001;104:2938-2942.

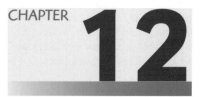

CHAPTER 12

Abdominal Aortic Aneurysms

KEY POINTS

▶ The etiology of AAA formation is unknown; inflammation is a participant, and biochemical (matrix metalloproteinase) processes may be involved.

▶ The natural history consists of progressive increase in size to approximately 55 mm, when risk of rupture rises exponentially. The 55-mm threshold should be interpreted with some concern for size of the patient.

▶ Survival is inversely proportional to AAA size.

▶ AAAs are less common but higher risk in women.

▶ Smoking is a strong risk factor for AAA development.

▶ Hypertension increases the rate of aneurysm formation and rupture.

▶ COPD increases both the rate of rupture and the operative risk of aortic repair.

▶ Whether AAAs are caused by atherosclerosis is unclear; however, what is undeniable is that many patients with AAA have concurrent clinically important coronary artery disease, which in elective cases should be well stratified before operative repair.

▶ Surgical repair, if patient factors are low risk, should be entertained for AAAs ≥5 cm.

▶ Endografts are increasingly used and subject to ongoing device development.

Abdominal aortic aneurysm (AAA) remains an underdetected lesion of enormous cost in morbidity, mortality, and finance. AAA is the tenth leading cause of death in adult men. About 15,000 deaths per year in the United States are recognized to be due to AAA; the true number is higher because prehospital, often sudden death is often not accounted for. Although elective surgical repair in low-risk cases carries an average 6% mortality, the mortality of operating on ruptured AAAs averages 50% (40% to 95%), although survivors can do well. In the United States, 40,000 abdominal aortic reconstructions are performed per year, leading to more than a billion dollars of in-hospital costs.

There is no universally accepted single definition of AAA. Most often, though, it refers to a localized dilation of the abdominal aorta (usually infrarenal) with an increase in diameter of 150% or more of expected (typical value used for defining an AAA is ≥3 cm, although some studies have used ≥3.5 cm and even ≥4.0 cm). All layers of the wall are present. The localized aspect of morphology is the most important feature. Some authors have indexed AAA diameter to body variables such as body surface area, weight, and height.

Women are only one third as likely to have AAAs as are men; however, rupture is four times more likely in women and more likely to be fatal.[1] AAA anatomy encroaching on the renal arteries is more common in women.[2] Almost all women who present with AAA are older than 70 years.

The actual incidence in asymptomatic individuals is still unknown, and the determined number is strongly influenced by both the study population and the definition of AAA. AAA incidence varies fourfold according to the definition and population studied.[3] In necropsy studies, it is found in 4.7% of men and 1.7% of women 56 to 74 years of age. Large (125,000-person) population screening studies report it as affecting 4.3% of men and 1.0% of women 50 to 79 years of age. Overall, about 5% of men older than 65 years have an AAA, although most are small. The more widespread use of ultrasonography and computed tomography (CT) for screening and nonscreening purposes increased the detection rate of AAAs sevenfold during the last 4 decades. This change in clinical detection, coupled with an aging population, is responsible for an increasing number of cases.

The majority of AAA patients (75% to 90%) have hypertension, and many are smokers (as many as 50% to 90% in some studies). Concurrent vasculopathies and comorbidities are common and are highly relevant with respect to surgical and percutaneous procedures, operative risk, and nonoperative risk. Vasculopathies include coronary artery disease, peripheral vascular (iliofemoral) disease, cerebrovascular disease, atherosclerotic renovascular disease, and other aneurysms (e.g., thoracic). Common comorbidities include COPD (which increases rupture risk as well as presents a problem with respect to surgery), hypertension and related complications, and renal insufficiency.

CLINICAL PRESENTATION OF ABDOMINAL AORTIC ANEURYSM

AAA is often an "incidental" finding. Most patients do not know that they have an AAA and are diagnosed in the course of unrelated investigations. Most AAAs are asymptomatic and remain asymptomatic until rupture. Pain resultant from AAA expansion indicates threatened rupture. Pain attributable to the AAA is usually of recent development, constant, and located in the mid abdomen, pelvis, or lumbar region.

Rupture generally presents with flank or abdominal pain, hypotension, or abdominal distention. Other presenting signs may be shock, cardiac arrest, aortic thrombosis and lower extremity thromboembolism, embolization of mural thrombus, in situ thrombosis, and infection (endovascular infection) that leads to rupture.

PHYSICAL DIAGNOSIS OF ABDOMINAL AORTIC ANEURYSM

In slender patients, an expansible epigastric mass fairly reliably indicates an AAA. A mass overlying the aorta may simulate the findings of an AAA. An AAA is usually located to the LEFT of the midline. However, in obese patients, few AAAs can be detected by palpation. As body weight continues to increase, the challenge to clinically detect AAAs will only increase further. Studies have demonstrated widely ranging accuracy of physical diagnosis for the detection of AAA, with sensitivity of 33% to 100%, specificity of 75% to 100%, and positive predictive value of 14% to 100%.[4]

As would be expected, the sensitivity of physical diagnosis for the detection of AAA depends on the size of the AAA and waist circumference of the patient (Table 12-1).[5] In a series of 198 patients with AAA presenting during a 3-year period, 48% were detected clinically, 37% were detected radiographically, and 15% were detected at laparotomy.[6] Average diameter of palpable AAAs

was 6.42 ± 1.24 cm; average diameter of nonpalpable AAAs was 4.86 ± 1.38 cm.[6]

Hence, physical examination has limitations in regard to AAA detection. The average diameter of a palpated AAA is already beyond the usual surgical size threshold. Tenderness to palpation is associated with risk of rupture. Abdominal bruits are common, whether they are due to tortuosity or associated atherosclerotic narrowings of iliac, renal, or other visceral arteries. Femoral pulses, if they are reduced, signify concurrent atherosclerotic disease.

PATHOLOGY AND MORPHOLOGY OF ABDOMINAL AORTIC ANEURYSM

Approximately 95% of AAAs are infrarenal and less than 5% are juxtarenal and suprarenal (Figs. 12-1 and 12-2). Such aneurysms are considerably more complicated to operate on. Most are fusiform and some are saccular. Most AAAs extend to the aortoiliac bifurcation, and some involve the iliac arteries. The wall of an AAA is usually thicker than that of normal aorta, but the wall is histologically disorganized. The majority of AAAs have histologic evidence of inflammation; 5% to 10% involve a prominent (gross) inflammatory response of the anterior and lateral aspects, akin to retroperitoneal fibrosis. This often renders surgery more difficult.

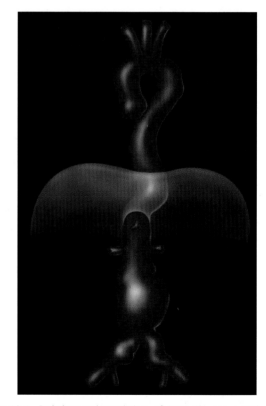

Figure 12-1. Pathology and morphology of AAAs. The aneurysmal dilation of the abdominal aorta is usually infrarenal and is commonly associated with elongation, tortuosity, and mild dilation of the thoracic aorta as well as with iliac aneurysms and tortuosity.

Table 12-1. Sensitivity of Physical Diagnosis for the Detection of Abdominal Aortic Aneurysm

Size	Sensitivity
AAA 3.0-3.9 cm	61%
AAA 4.0-4.9 cm	69%
AAA >5.0 cm	82%
Waist circumference <100 cm	91%
Waist circumference ≥100 cm	53%

AAA, abdominal aortic aneurysm.
From Fink HA, Lederle FA, Roth CS, et al: The accuracy of physical examination to detect abdominal aortic aneurysm. Arch Intern Med 2000;160:833-836.

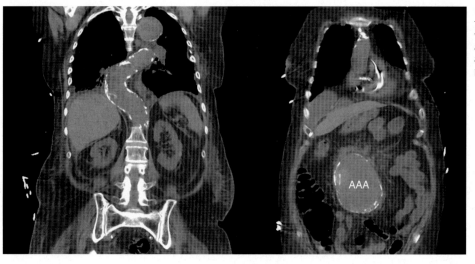

Figure 12-2. CT scans showing the marked tortuosity of the thoracic aorta in a patient with a very large (85-mm) AAA. The iliac arteries were just as tortuous. The thoracic aorta is typically elongated and tortuous in patients with AAAs.

PATHOGENESIS OF ABDOMINAL AORTIC ANEURYSM FORMATION

The pathogenesis of AAA formation remains unknown. No satisfactory solitary explanation exists. Atherosclerosis is a highly controversial cause despite is coexistence in most patients because it also could be an effect of injury to the aortic wall or it may be a comorbidity. Certainly, atherosclerosis is concurrent in a large number of cases. There are occasional post-traumatic, mycotic, and congenital AAAs. Formerly (in the early 20th century), most aortic aneurysms were syphilitic or tuberculous. Fifteen percent to 20% of cases have a family history.

Smoking is the strongest risk factor for AAA; 90% of patients in some studies have a history of smoking. The risk of AAA is six to seven times higher in heavy smokers, and smoking increases the expansion rate by at least 25%. Underlying biochemical abnormalities (e.g., matrix metalloproteinase, interleukin, C-reactive protein) are of current interest. Hypertension is a weak risk factor for AAA incidence, dilation, and rupture.[7]

NATURAL HISTORY OF ABDOMINAL AORTIC ANEURYSM

A sufficient knowledge of the natural history of AAAs is elusive. It is known that AAA diameter increases yearly. Population-based studies suggest an expansion rate of about 0.2 cm/year; CT and ultrasound imaging suggests a rate of 0.4 (0.3 to 0.6) cm/year. Therefore, most small (4- to 5.5-cm) AAAs reach surgical consideration size in 3 to 5 years. The larger the AAA, the faster the expansion (Fig. 12-3). Survival is inversely proportional to AAA size.[3,7] Once an AAA has formed, expansion until rupture and death is inevitable, unless it is preceded by death from other causes.

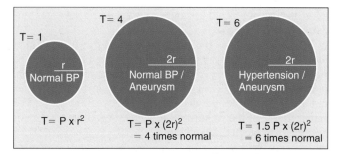

Figure 12-3. Expansion of aneurysms is driven by wall tension. According to the law of Laplace, tangential wall tension (T) is proportional to intraluminal pressure (P) and to the square of the radius.

Effect of Beta-Blockade on the Growth Rate of Abdominal Aortic Aneurysm

The effect of beta-blockade on AAAs will not be well understood until randomized prospective trials are performed. Small retrospective series of patients with AAAs larger than 3 cm suggest that the annual growth rate is reduced by beta-blocker use (0.17 cm/year versus 0.44 cm/year).[8] Population-based case-control studies have not observed lesser risk of AAA rupture among patients using beta-blockers.[9] Interestingly, angiotensin-converting enzyme inhibitors were associated with a lower incidence of rupture but angiotensin receptor blockers were not, nor were calcium channel blockers or alpha-blockers.[9]

ABDOMINAL AORTIC ANEURYSM RUPTURE

AAA rupture is held to be the third leading cause of sudden death.[10] There is an overall 90% mortality to rupture, with 75% prehospital mortality. There is a 50% salvage rate by surgery among patients who arrive to the hospital alive. The surgical survival is 25% if there is cardiac arrest, refractory shock, hematocrit below 25% (indicating extensive internal blood loss), or age 80 years or older.

Most patients whose AAAs rupture into the peritoneal cavity exsanguinate internally within minutes and expire suddenly. Most patients who survive to make it into the hospital have ruptures partially contained within the retroperitoneum.

The signs of an AAA (midline pulsatility) are often less prominent once the AAA has ruptured, shock has developed, and hematoma is clinically obscuring the aorta. For this reason, clinical decision to proceed to urgent operative repair is often made on the basis of no other apparent cause of shock (such as no indices of myocardial infarction or sepsis) with prior knowledge of an AAA or bedside suspicion of an AAA.

Symptoms are variable, but midline abdominal pain radiating posteriorly into the back is usual. Signs of hypovolemic shock are usual. Blood pressure is a notably poor index of cardiac output in a generally previously hypertensive population. Some patients are actually hypertensive after rupture if the magnitude of the hypertensive response to pain exceeds the degree of blood loss. Time-consuming misdiagnoses commonly include myocardial infarction (abnormal electrocardiogram but not acute), pancreatitis (history of ethanol use and severe epigastric pain and tenderness), and urosepsis.

AAA rupture is the initial presentation in a substantial number of cases. Factors associated with increasing likelihood of rupture include larger AAA diameter, presence of hypertension, presence of COPD or smoking, and aneurysm body diameter more than two times the diameter of the neck (Fig. 12-4). The actual trigger of the rupture event is unknown. Rupture cannot be accurately predicted in all cases.

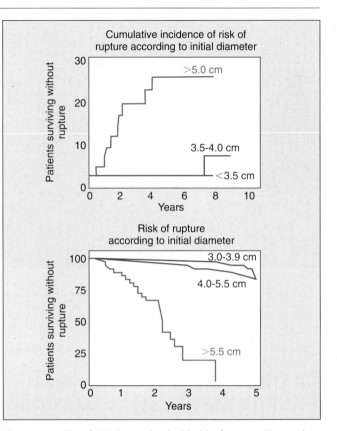

Figure 12-4. Size of AAA is associated with risk of rupture. (Top panel from Nevitt MP, Ballard DJ, Hallett JW Jr: Prognosis of abdominal aortic aneurysms: a population-based study. N Engl J Med 1989;321:1009-1014. Bottom panel from Powell JT, Greenhalgh RM: Clinical practice: small abdominal aortic aneurysms. N Engl J Med 2003;348:1895-1901.)

Sites of Abdominal Aortic Aneurysm Rupture

Retroperitoneal rupture is the most common; the rupture may be temporarily retarded, allowing diagnosis and intervention. Most hover for a matter of hours, but a few hover for days to weeks with obtuse signs such as fever (inflammation), abdominal pains, and anemia (occult blood loss from bleeding). However, rupture will resume, usually fatally. Retroperitoneal rupture is typically accompanied by pain (back, abdominal, or flank), abdominal or flank distention, and hypotension.

Intraperitoneal rupture is catastrophic because of rapid internal exsanguination. AAAs may rupture into other spaces, most notably the duodenum, producing an aortoenteric fistula (usually due to erosion of the tube graft from a prior repair into the overlying distal duodenum), or the inferior vena cava or another vein, producing a large arteriovenous fistula (rare).

The rate of AAA rupture relates to the initial diameter. AAAs smaller than 4 cm rupture at an average rate of 2% per year (10% per 5 years), those 4 to 5 cm rupture at an average rate of 3% per year (3% to 12% per 5 years), and those larger than 5 cm rupture at an average rate of 5% to 8% per year (25% to 40% per 5 years). Therefore, as risk of rupture rises sharply above 5.5 cm, there is general agreement that aneurysms larger than 5.5 cm should be operated on, assuming fitness of the patient.[11]

SCREENING FOR ABDOMINAL AORTIC ANEURYSM

The "rule of thumb" concerning the size of normal abdominal aorta is that it is the size of the person's thumb. Not indexing to body size, the normal abdominal aorta is 1.75 cm at 25 years of age and 2.25 cm at 55 years of age.

Unselective screening with ultrasound examination of asymptomatic individuals is feasible but low yield. Usually less than 5% have an AAA and less than 1% have an AAA larger than 4 cm. The cost-effectiveness of unselective screening is unclear.

Selective screening (age 55 to 80 years, hypertension, aneurysms of the femoral or popliteal arteries, family history of AAA) by ultrasound examination is also not well established but may be more cost-effective.

Aneurysms and Mural Thrombus

The lumen of an AAA nearly always contains mural thrombus, the formation of which is favored by the stasis within the capacious lumen. Thrombus has the potential to reduce the angiographic (luminal) depiction of the aneurysm size (a common occurrence) as well as the potential for embolization (acutely or chronically) to the distal limb or infection.

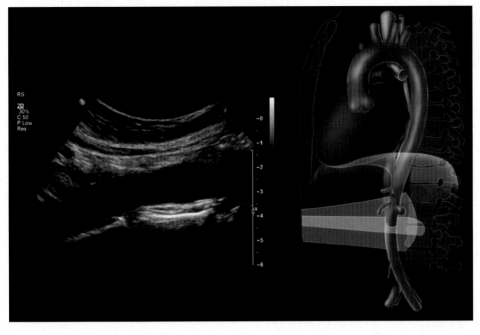

Figure 12-5. Vascular ultrasonography. In this single view, the aorta is seen in long axis through the majority of its abdominal course. The ability of ultrasonography to screen for abdominal aneurysms is evident.

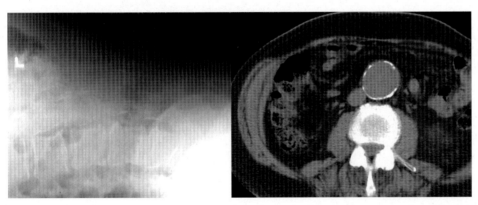

Figure 12-6. LEFT, Lateral shoot-through abdominal radiograph. RIGHT, Non–contrast-enhanced CT axial scan. The radiographic diameter of the AAA is 51 mm. The CT diameter is 50 mm.

ABDOMINAL AORTIC ANEURYSM IMAGING

Ultrasonography is the most appropriate test for screening and serial testing (Fig. 12-5). CT is a very useful test, especially when ultrasonography is inadequate and for EVAR planning. Axial views do not reliably depict renovascular or iliac disease (Figs. 12-6 to 12-12). As current multidetector CT (MDCT) technology affords most of what conventional aortography does, aortography is less used for diagnosis or planning purposes but is increasingly used as the platform to perform EVAR. Magnetic resonance (MR) imaging is a standard preoperative test at many centers because it avoids the contrast nephropathy risks of aortography and CT (Figs. 12-13 and 12-14). Table 12-2 offers an extensive comparison of these imaging modalities with regard to their suitability for imaging of AAAs.

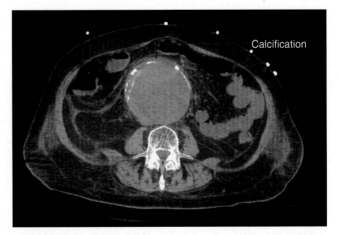

Calcification

Figure 12-7. Non–contrast-enhanced CT scan. The diameter of the AAA can be measured without use of contrast material; here it is 85 mm. Note the calcification.

Table 12-2. Modality Comparison for Abdominal Aortic Aneurysm Imaging

Modality	Advantages	Disadvantages	Comments
Ultrasonography (US)	The simplest test for imaging of AAAs Demonstrates location, size, thrombus, and fluid US can be performed in emergencies at bedside. US is accurate and reproducible ±0.6 cm.	US is poor at depicting branch (visceral) details. US may not determine the relation of the AAA to renal artery anatomy accurately. US does not reliably depict rupture. US is technologist expertise and time dependent.	US is a good screening test for AAAs. US may not be a sufficient test from which to plan an elective operation in complicated cases, although operations can be prompted by US and tailored to findings at the time of the operative repair.
Computed tomography (CT)	Demonstrates location, size, mural thrombus, adjacent fluid, and mural calcification CT can be performed in emergencies but not at bedside. MDCT acquisition is very fast. CT is fair at depicting branch details. CT may be more accurate than US. Current MDCT allows extensive off-line analysis that enables EVAR planning.	Cost, contrast nephropathy, allergy, ionizing radiation Lack of bedside portability CT may introduce confusion about the upper anatomic extent if only axial images are available and the AAA neck long axis is oblique. CT offers little beyond US for basic diagnosis. CT is very useful to assess symptomatic AAAs and invaluable for depiction of rupture.	CT is not recommended for screening. CT is very good for comparative serial studies. CT is useful to plan elective surgery in complicated cases.
Magnetic resonance (MR)	Demonstrates location, size, thrombus, fluid, ± calcium Displays coronal, sagittal, and transverse views MR can be performed in emergencies but not at bedside. MR is good but not excellent at depicting branch details. MR can be performed after endograft insertion.	Expensive, less available MR cannot be performed if the patient has a pacemaker, ICD, or ferromagnetic clips. MR does not depict occlusive disease well.	MR has no actual advantage over US or CT other than better imaging than US and minimal contrast nephropathy.
Aortography	Excellent depiction of branch vessels Demonstrates location. Size is variably underrepresented.	Does not depict thrombus; therefore underrepresents the true diameter Does not depict periaortic fluid (rupture) Cannot be performed at bedside Nephrotoxicity, contrast allergy, cost, access complications	Not essential (but useful) for management Particularly useful if suspected renovascular hypertension, juxtarenal AAA, or concurrent iliofemoral occlusive disease introduces the need to assess branch vessels A standard component of endovascular repair procedures

AAA, abdominal aortic aneurysm; EVAR, endovascular aortic repair; ICD, implantable cardioverter defibrillator; MDCT, multidetector computed tomography.

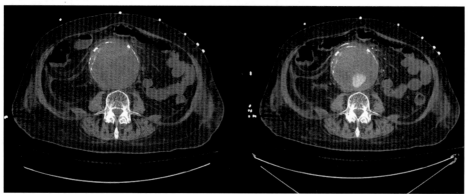

Figure 12-8. LEFT, Non–contrast-enhanced CT scan depicting AAA lumen and a large mural thrombus. RIGHT, Contrast-enhanced scan shows the same large AAA. Only the contrast-enhanced image details how much of the AAA is thrombus filled and the size of the lumen, which is remarkably small.

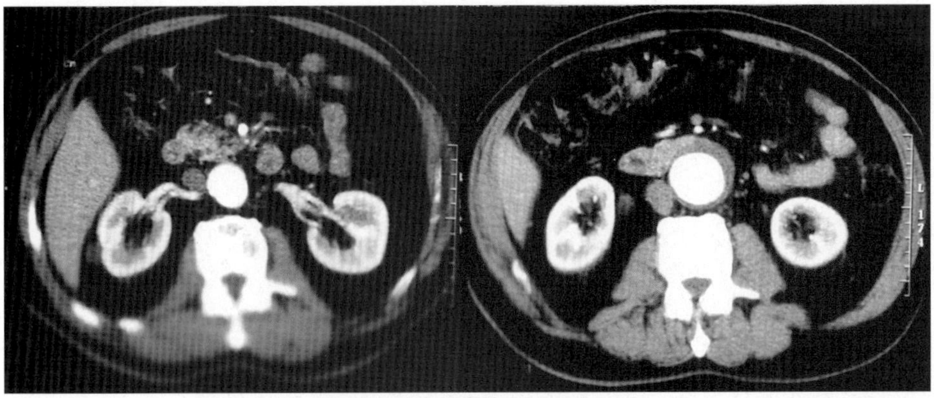

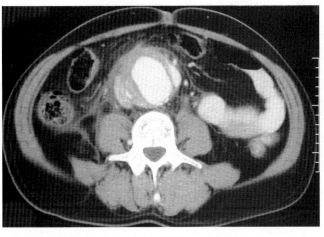

Figure 12-9. Contrast-enhanced CT axial scans at different levels. LEFT, At the level of the renal artery. The aortic diameter is normal. RIGHT, At the infrarenal level. The widening neck of the infrarenal AAA is apparent.

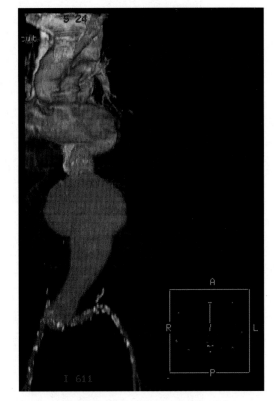

Figure 12-10. Contrast-enhanced axial CT scan showing an AAA rupture. Note haziness around the AAA with streaking between tissue planes, indicating leakage of blood out of the AAA.

Figure 12-11. Contrast-enhanced axial CT scan with 3D image reconstruction. The saccular nature of an infrarenal AAA (lumen) is apparent on this 3D reconstruction.

ABDOMINAL AORTIC ANEURYSM TREATMENT

Medical Management of Abdominal Aortic Aneurysms

The concern of AAA rupture often dominates the management of patients with AAA; however, among all AAA patients, more than half will die of other cardiovascular diseases (principally of myocardial infarction). This is more true for patients with smaller AAAs and less true for patients with larger AAAs. Medical management consists of efforts to reduce myocardial infarction and stroke risk factors through smoking cessation, cholesterol management, blood pressure control, and the like.

No specific form of medical therapy has been well shown to reduce risk of expansion. Beta-blockers, although validated to reduce the rate of root dilation in some patients with Marfan syndrome, have not been established to be effective in AAA patients.[3,9]

Recommended surveillance intervals depend on baseline size of an AAA. For those 3.0 to 4.5 cm, the recommended interval is 12 months; those 4.5 to 5.5 cm should be followed up every 6 months.[12]

If the criteria for surgery are 5.5 cm in men and 5 cm in women, then, by use of such criteria, approximately 5% of observed AAA patients would achieve consideration for surgery for each visit.[7]

Management algorithms for asymptomatic and symptomatic AAAs are shown in Figure 12-15.

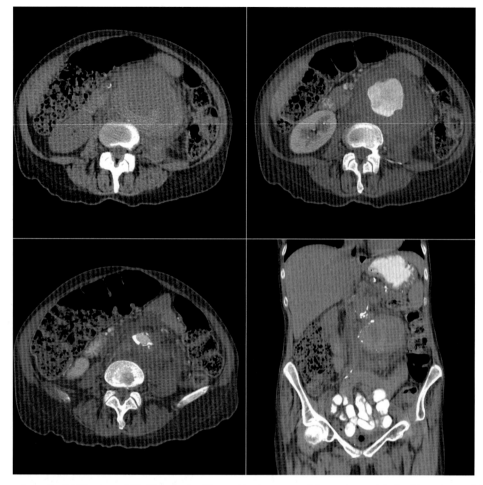

Figure 12-12. CT scan of a patient with a large AAA. There is streaking and haziness around the aorta consistent with rupture and leakage.

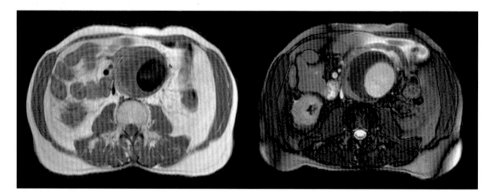

Figure 12-13. MR transaxial images taken in a patient with renal insufficiency to avoid CT contrast dye–related nephrotoxicity. An AAA is imaged in the two views known as black blood angiography (LEFT) and time-of-flight angiography (RIGHT). The T1:T2 imaging in both views displays a large AAA with substantial amount of crescentic thrombus.

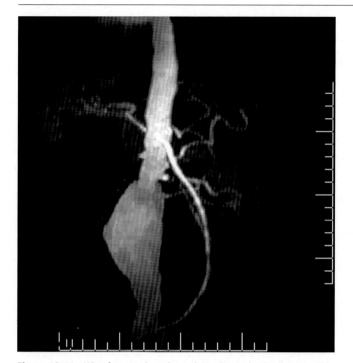

Figure 12-14. MR reformatted maximum intensity projection images. This gadolinium-enhanced view shows an infrarenal AAA. The lumen of the AAA is well depicted by the gadolinium enhancement, as are the branch vessels of the abdominal aorta. The mural thrombus is ambiguously depicted.

Surgical Management of Abdominal Aortic Aneurysms

The overall elective surgical mortality of nonruptured AAAs is 3% to 6%. Elective surgical mortality for patients older than 80 years is more than 10%. The overall surgical mortality of ruptured AAAs is 50%.[13]

Surgical approach consists of laparotomy and retroperitoneal dissection under general anesthesia, followed by cross-clamping of the aorta above the aneurysm and below the renal arteries. This is the time of greatest hemodynamic stress on the heart (rise in blood pressure and greatest demand for myocardial blood supply) as there is no flow to the lower extremities during the cross-clamp period. The aneurysm is incised. A tube graft is sewn to the normal aorta above the aneurysm and to the aortic bifurcation or to the iliac arteries below. The aneurysm is trimmed and sewn over the tube graft (Fig. 12-16).

Long-term outcome of immediate repair compared with surveillance of small AAAs has been studied by several groups. The United Kingdom Small Aneurysm Trial[1] included 1090 patients from 60 to 76 years of age and with AAA diameter of 4 to 5.5 cm (mean, 4.6 ± 0.4 cm). They were randomized to early elective surgery versus ultrasound surveillance and followed up for a mean of 8 years (6 to 10 years). Average survival was 6.7 years in the early elective surgery group and 6.5 years in the surveillance group ($P = .29$; NS). In terms of mortality, 30-day operative mortality in the early surgery group was 5.5%, giving an early survival disadvantage. At 3 years, the curves crossed; and by 8 years, the mortality of the early surgery group was 7.4% ($P = .03$) less, but more of the early surgical patients had stopped smoking. The majority of the surveillance group (75%) was operated on

within the time course of the study. The Veterans Affairs Cooperative Study[14] included 1136 patients from 50 to 79 years of age with AAA diameter of 4 to 5.4 cm who were without high surgical risk. They were randomized to early elective surgery versus ultrasound surveillance and followed up for a mean of 3.5 years (3.5 to 8 years). All-cause mortality and AAA mortality were not different between the two groups. The rupture rate in the surveillance group was 0.6% per year. Total operative mortality in the early surgery group was 2.7%, which is commendably low and eliminates the concern that excessive mortality from surgery confounded the results. The majority of the surveillance group (61%) was operated on within the time course of the study.

Indications for elective repair in asymptomatic patients are threefold. Diameter of more than 5.5 cm is the key indication, and there are abundant data supporting this. Aneurysm diameter remains the strongest predictor, albeit imperfect, of risk of rupture. Surgical repair versus surveillance for aneurysms 40 to 55 mm has not been shown to improve mortality.[14] Expansion in size of more than 0.5 or 1.0 cm during 12 months is also an indication for surgery, although there are fewer data to support this.[11] Tenderness or painfulness of an AAA is considered by many surgeons to be a sign of impending rupture, but it is a somewhat controversial notion.[15] Indications for urgent repair are development of symptoms that reliably predict rupture and rupture itself.

Operative risks depend on both aneurysm factors (Is the proximal anastomosis straightforward, that is, is there a sufficient infrarenal neck? Are the renal arteries involved by the aneurysm or by occlusive disease?) and the patient factors, particularly coronary artery disease, pulmonary disease, left ventricular function, renal function, and iliac and femoral disease (Figs. 12-17 and 12-18). Hence, the risk and the decision for elective repair are individualized.

Preoperative assessment of AAA patients is summarized in Table 12-3.

Endovascular Aortic Repair for Abdominal Aortic Aneurysms

Within a decade, endovascular aortic repair (EVAR) for AAA has emerged as a feasible and successful therapy in many patients (Figs. 12-19 to 12-23).[16,17] It has been performed for elective repair and for rupture,[18] has been rapidly adopted in some regions,[19] and currently accounts for 50% of AAA repair.[20] EVAR avoids laparotomy, retroperitoneal operation, and cross-clamping of the aorta, and its use is associated with lesser blood loss and need for blood product support and shorter ICU and hospital stay. Successful EVAR is associated with exclusion of the aneurysm, reduction of the aneurysm size, and no endoleak.

The EVAR 1 and DREAM randomized trials established improved early results compared with open surgical repair.[21,22] The EVAR 1 trial (endovascular aneurysm repair versus conventional open AAA repair) included 1082 patients (983 men, 99 women), with a mean aneurysm diameter of 6.5 cm, who were randomized to EVAR versus open surgical repair. The 30-day mortality was 1.7% in the EVAR group and 4.7% in the open surgery group ($P = .009$).[21] The DREAM (Dutch Randomized Endovascular Aneurysm Management) trial included 345 patients with a mean aneurysm diameter of 5 cm who were randomized to EVAR versus open surgical repair. In the EVAR group, operative mortality was 1.2%, and severe complications occurred in

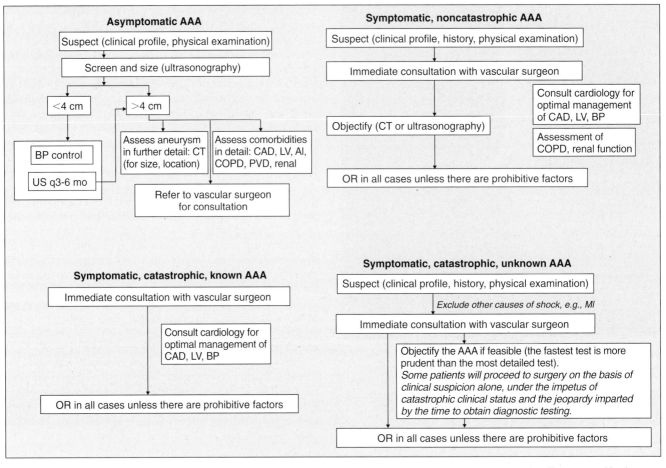

Figure 12-15. Algorithms for management of asymptomatic and symptomatic abdominal aortic aneurysm (AAA). AI, aortic insufficiency; BP, blood pressure; CAD, coronary artery disease; COPD, chronic obstructive pulmonary disease; CT, computed tomography; LV, LEFT ventricle; MI, myocardial infarction; OR, operative repair; PVD, peripheral vascular disease; US, ultrasonography.

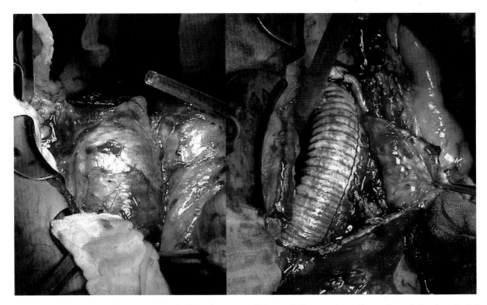

Figure 12-16. Surgical AAA repair. LEFT, A 7-cm AAA. RIGHT, Graft replacement. Tube graft is sewn into the neck and distal end of the AAA, from within the AAA. (Image courtesy of Alan Lossing, MD, Toronto, Canada.)

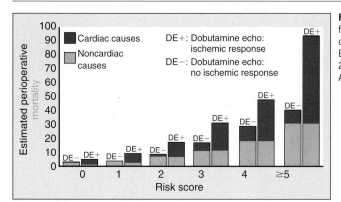

Figure 12-17. Perioperative risk prediction of surgical AAA repair. Risk factors include COPD, angina, myocardial infarction, diabetes mellitus, congestive heart failure, stroke, and renal failure. (From Kertai MD, Boersma E, Poldermans D: Small abdominal aortic aneurysms. N Engl J Med 2002;347:1112-1115. Copyright © [2001] Massachusetts Medical Society. All rights reserved.)

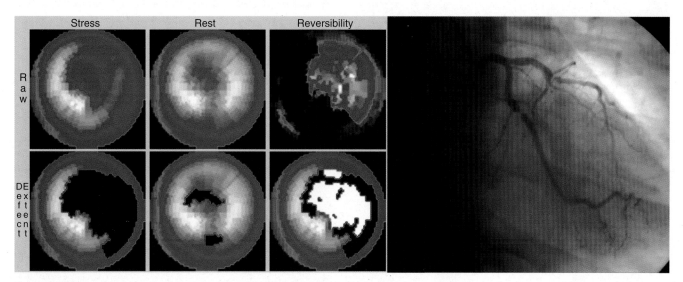

Figure 12-18. A 77-year-old man with a 7-cm AAA; 100 pack/year smoker, hypertensive. Severe COPD. Stable angina, CCS class III. LEFT, Large anterior perfusion defect is seen at stress. RIGHT, Coronary angiogram shows severe left anterior descending coronary artery and left circumflex lesions.

Table 12-3. Preoperative Assessment of Abdominal Aortic Aneurysm Patients

Establish the extent and severity of CAD. More than one third of perioperative deaths are due to complications of CAD, as more than one third of deaths in the 5 years after AAA repair are also due to CAD. One third of AAA patients have severe, surgically addressable CAD.

Revascularize if usual indications exist.

Assess left ventricular function.

Assess the presence and severity of aortic insufficiency (which will increase when the aorta is cross-clamped during surgery).

Control the blood pressure. Institute beta-blockade to attenuate blood pressure rise and myocardial ischemia when the aorta is cross-clamped.

Assess pulmonary function. Impaired pulmonary function (<50% predicted forced vital capacity, forced expiratory volume in 1 second) may preclude abdominal surgery under general anesthesia. Stopping smoking for 3 months reduces postoperative respiratory and ventilator problems.

Assess renal function as renal impairment is a surgical concern.

AAA, abdominal aortic aneurysm; CAD, coronary artery disease.

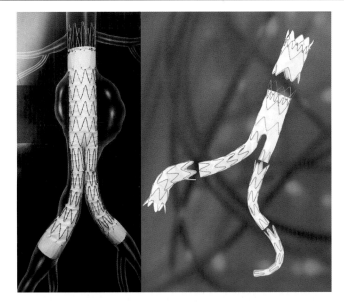

Figure 12-19. Percutaneous endografts. LEFT, Zenith percutaneous endograft. (Courtesy of Cooke Canada, Inc.) RIGHT, Talent percutaneous endograft. (Courtesy of Medtronic Canada, Inc.)

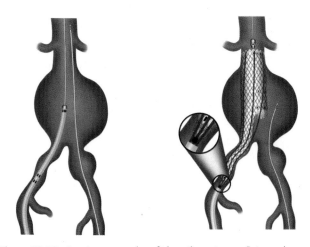

Figure 12-20. Percutaneous endograft insertion—1. LEFT, Retrograde bifemoral cannulation and insertion of main device. RIGHT, Deployment (release and expansion) of main device. (Courtesy of Cooke Canada, Inc.)

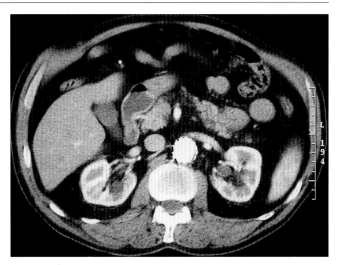

Figure 12-22. Contrast-enhanced axial CT scan after endograft insertion. Note the stent-like appearance of the wires in the abdominal aorta.

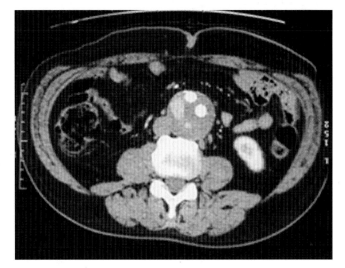

Figure 12-23. Contrast-enhanced axial CT scan. There is a persistent leak around the endograft. Note the partial contrast opacification of lumen (within copious thrombus) away from the lumen of the legs of the endograft.

Figure 12-21. Percutaneous endograft insertion—2. LEFT, Deployment of the other arm. (Courtesy of Cooke Canada, Inc.) RIGHT, Radiographic appearance.

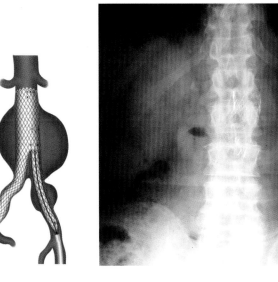

4.7%. In the open surgery group, operative mortality was 4.6%, and the rate of serious complications was 9.8%.[22] EVAR therapy for ruptured AAA appears to be associated with lower mortality (32% versus 51%; *P* = .001).[23]

However, early, intermediate, and late complications do occur. Long-term complications include endograft thrombosis, persisting primary (type I) endoleak, late secondary (type II) endoleak, device migration (>10 mm), increase in aneurysm diameter, graft infection, and rupture.[24] The true long-term course after EVAR devices is unknown. Numerous centers have experience, but only a few are highly experienced. Cost issues are relevant for many hospitals ($10,000 to $15,000 for the stent alone). Vascular access is an issue if there is iliac disease or if the vessel is not sufficiently large; in 90% of female patients, vascular anatomy precludes the procedure. A neck length greater than 1.5 to 2 cm (landing zone) is needed. Many ruptured AAAs have larger neck sizes. Endoleaks occur in many patients, and although the frequency decreases over time, new late endoleaks develop in some patients. Up to 5% of endografted AAA patients will still experience AAA growth, and 0.8% will still experience rupture. The annual secondary intervention rate is approximately 5% (EUROSTAR registry: 4.5%).[25] There is a commitment to ongoing, lifelong clinical and imaging follow-up. Therefore, EVAR is a developing technology and technique.[2]

Although endovascular repair in patients who are fit candidates for surgical repair is still controversial, there is prominent momentum toward endovascular repair for patients who are at high risk for surgery because of advanced comorbidities.[26]

CASE 1

History and Physical Examination

- 56-year-old hypertensive male smoker
- AAA followed up with ultrasound examination for 5 years; now AAA measures 55 mm
- Referred for elective surgery on the basis of size and acceptable operative risks
- Father died of a ruptured AAA
- No abdominal or back pains, no angina
- BP 160/87 mm Hg, HR 90 bpm
- Normal cardiac examination findings
- Palpable AAA
- Normal pulses, without bruits

Evolution and Management

- Clinical impression was that of an AAA without rupture, as confirmed by surgery.

- No significant comorbidities
- Preoperative BP control with beta-blocker
- Tube graft inserted
- Uneventful outcome

Comments

- AAA found incidentally by ultrasound examination (for gallstone pains) and followed up for 5 years until surgical threshold was reached
- Despite its palpability on examination, it was found only through testing for other reasons.
- Risk factors in this case were family history, smoking, and hypertension.
- Laminated mural thrombus within
- Usual morphology of infrarenal location

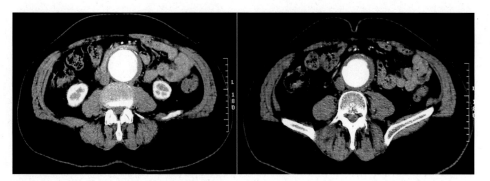

Figure 12-24. Contrast-enhanced axial CT scan images. A 5.5-cm AAA with a small amount of anterior calcification and a thin crescent of laminated thrombus on the left side.

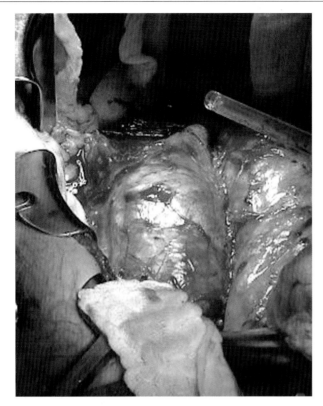

Figure 12-25. AAA surgery: surgical exposure.

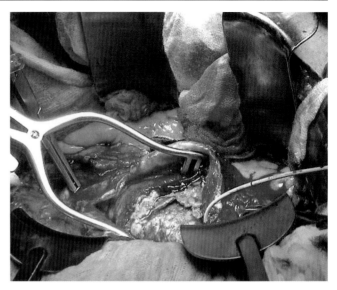

Figure 12-27. AAA surgery: the AAA is now incised, and the inside is exposed. The thrombus is seen between the spreader tips as a 2- to 3-mm-thick yellowish layer on the posterior wall that has partially separated off the AAA. There is a balloon catheter down the iliac arteries to prevent embolization of thrombus during the procedure.

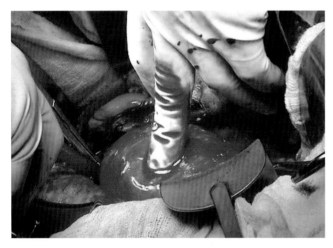

Figure 12-26. AAA surgery: containing surgical bleeding.

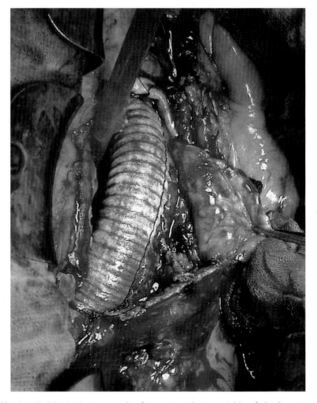

Figure 12-28. AAA surgery: the forceps on the RIGHT side of the image are holding up the wall of the AAA. Tube graft sewn into the neck (TOP) and lower end (BOTTOM) of the AAA from within the AAA.

CASE 2

History and Physical Examination

▸ 63-year-old hypertensive male smoker
▸ AAA found "incidentally" on an abdominal ultrasound examination
▸ No abdominal or back pains, no angina
▸ Taking a diuretic for hypertension
▸ BP 178/98 mm Hg, HR 75 bpm
▸ Normal cardiac examination findings
▸ On deep palpation of the abdomen, the AAA was palpable
▸ Normal pulses, without bruits elsewhere

Evolution and Management

▸ Clinical impression was that of an AAA without rupture, as confirmed by surgery.

▸ No significant comorbidities
▸ Poorly controlled hypertension
▸ Preoperative BP control with beta-blocker
▸ Aortoiliac tube graft inserted
▸ Uneventful outcome

Comments

▸ Another "incidental" AAA
▸ Despite its palpability on examination, it was found through testing for other reasons.
▸ Risk factors of hypertension and smoking present
▸ Large amount of mural thrombus
▸ Usual morphology of infrarenal location

12

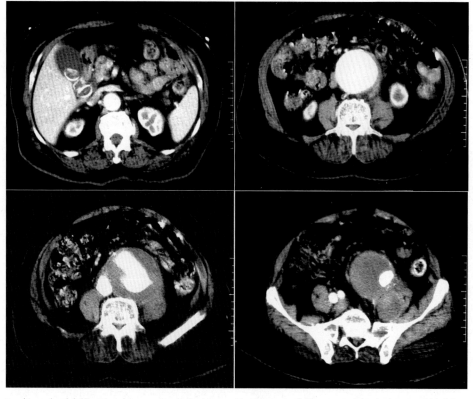

Figure 12-29. Contrast-enhanced axial CT scans show a normal diameter and appearance of the upper abdominal aorta. AAA (70 mm) with variable amount of mural thrombus.

CASE 3

History and Physical Examination

▸ 76-year-old obese man with a 65-mm infrarenal AAA "incidentally" found on an abdominal ultrasound examination
▸ Prior myocardial infarction, CCS class II angina
▸ Perfusion scan showed small, largely fixed inferior defect.
▸ No heart failure
▸ Advanced COPD, poor pulmonary function on testing; still smoking
▸ Hypertensive (170/100 mm Hg) on single agent
▸ AAA not palpable on examination because of obesity

Evolution and Management

▸ Clinical impression was that of an AAA without rupture.
▸ Very significant pulmonary morbidity and poorly controlled hypertension
▸ Endograft insertion was chosen in lieu of open surgery.
▸ Preoperative BP control with beta-blocker
▸ Uneventful outcome

Comments

▸ Another "incidental" and serendipitous finding of a large AAA, but in an older man with very relevant comorbidities and hidden by obesity
▸ Usual risk factor of hypertension present
▸ Usual morphology of infrarenal location
▸ Successful endograft deployment, no residual leak on follow-up CT scanning

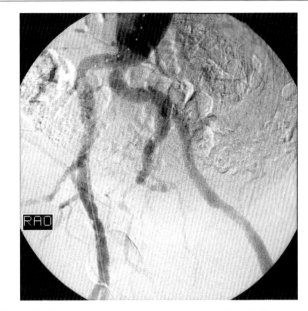

Figure 12-31. Aortogram shows an AAA ending at the aortoiliac bifurcation and tortuous iliac arteries.

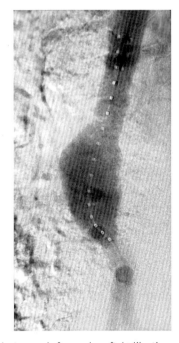

Figure 12-32. Aortogram before endograft (calibration markers). The AAA lumen is obvious, but mural thrombus does confound the determination of true AAA diameter by aortography. There is a suitable section of straight aorta above the AAA into which to land the upper part of the endograft-covered stent.

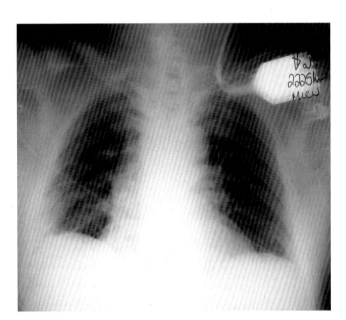

Figure 12-30. Chest radiograph shows an enlarged thoracic aorta, hilar overlay sign of ascending aortic dilation, intimal calcification at the knob of the aorta, and mediastinal widening due to the aorta or obesity.

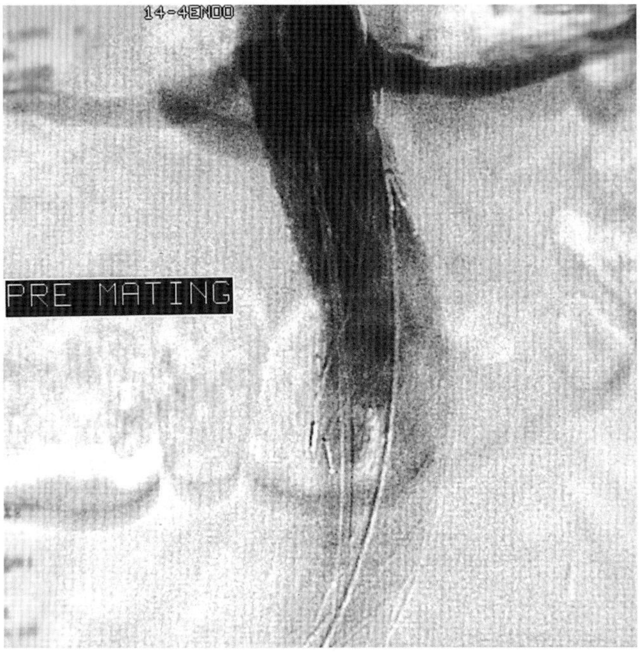

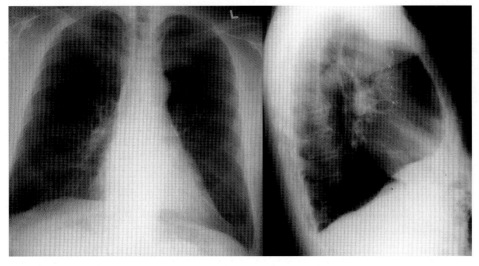

Figure 12-33. CT scan with contrast enhancement shows the main portion of the stent deployed in the infrarenal aorta.

CASE 4

History and Physical Examination

▸ A 67-year-old man with hypertension noticed a pulsation in his epigastrium after losing 20 pounds on a fad diet.
▸ Aortocoronary bypass 8 years previously, no symptoms of angina since; good exercise tolerance
▸ No symptoms of claudication or of cerebrovascular disease
▸ BP 145/90 mm Hg with antihypertensive monotherapy
▸ 8-cm AAA detected on ultrasound examination with a long infrarenal neck
▸ Given favorable anatomy for endograft, the patient was enrolled in a trial.
▸ After endograft insertion, he has been asymptomatic.

Comments

▸ AAA detected by the patient himself, despite being a well-known patient
▸ Infrarenal AAA with favorable anatomy and a good enduring outcome with endograft treatment
▸ Successful endograft insertion without procedural complications and without long-term complications (no persistent leak, no endograft migration, no progressive AAA dilation)
▸ With more antihypertensives, optimal BP control has been achieved.

Figure 12-34. Chest radiograph shows a normal cardiopericardial silhouette, clear lung fields, and surgical clips along the course of the left internal thoracic artery bypass graft. The appearance of the thoracic aorta is unremarkable.

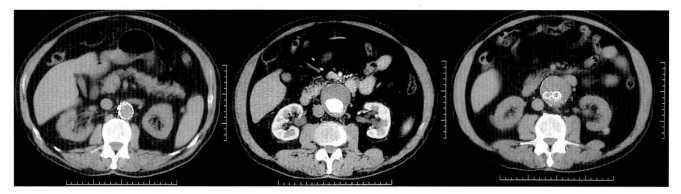

Figure 12-35. LEFT, Non–contrast-enhanced CT scan shows the stent wires apposed to the neck of the AAA as well as the radial artifacts from the stent wires. MIDDLE, Contrast-enhanced axial CT scan shows an AAA with eggshell calcification anteriorly. Thrombus surrounds the stent, with no dye outside the stent (no leak). RIGHT, The two legs of the stent can be seen within the lower body of the AAA. Eggshell calcification of the wall of the AAA can also be seen.

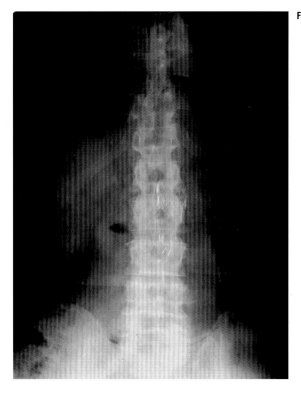

Figure 12-36. Abdominal radiograph shows a stent visible over the lumbar spine.

CASE 5

History

▸ A 68-year-old man with a history of hypertension, smoking, and COPD underwent EVAR of a 9.0-cm infrarenal aortic aneurysm.
▸ There was no history of peripheral arterial disease or imaging evidence of it.

Comments

▸ Infrarenal AAA
▸ Absence of peripheral arterial disease and large body habitus assist with EVAR delivery.
▸ Tortuosity of the aorta associated with aneurysmal disease
▸ Reduction of aneurysm size after successful exclusion by EVAR

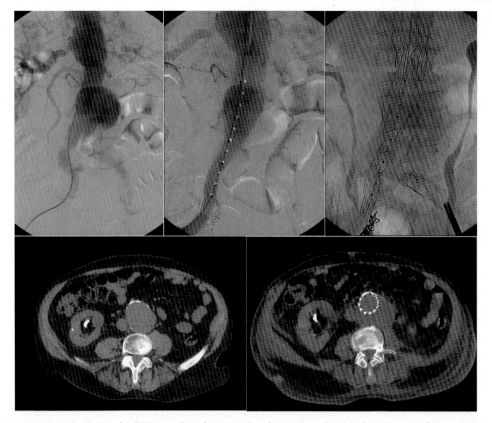

Figure 12-37. TOP IMAGES, Aortography during the EVAR procedure demonstrating the aneurysm (LEFT) and deployment of the main body of the graft (MIDDLE) and of the left iliac sleeve (RIGHT). The right internal iliac artery has been embolized; the coils are seen by the distal margin of the right iliac sleeve. BOTTOM IMAGES, Non–contrast-enhanced CT scans before (LEFT) and after (RIGHT) EVAR. There was no endoleak. The size of the AAA decreased after EVAR.

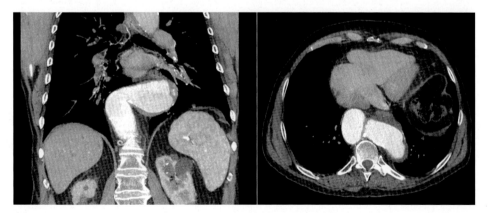

Figure 12-38. Contrast-enhanced CT images: coronal view (LEFT) and axial view (RIGHT). The elongation of the thoracic aorta associated with the AAA (and history of hypertension) is striking. There is a pseudocoarctation of the aorta above the diaphragm due to its elongation and restraint by the os of the diaphragm. The axial image is low and across the fold of the left inferior wall of the lower thoracic aorta.

CASE 6

History

▸ A 73-year-old male smoker with hypertension and COPD was found to have a large (8.8 cm) infrarenal AAA.
▸ He was asymptomatic.
▸ There was no history of coronary artery disease or peripheral arterial disease.

Comments

▸ Infrarenal AAA
▸ Absence of peripheral arterial disease and large body habitus assist with EVAR delivery.
▸ Successful EVAR placement, but type II endoleak and no reduction in aneurysm size

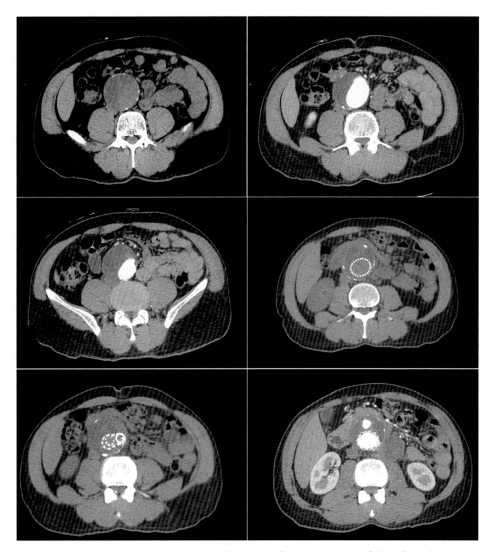

Figure 12-39. Axial CT scans. TOP LEFT, Pre-EVAR non–contrast-enhanced image revealing the large body of the infrarenal AAA and suggesting mural thrombus on the patient's right side. TOP RIGHT, Contrast-enhanced image establishing the large bulk of mural thrombus. MIDDLE, Pre-EVAR image (LEFT) and post-EVAR image (RIGHT) at the same level. BOTTOM LEFT, The iliac legs of the EVAR device are seen within the main body sleeve. BOTTOM RIGHT, Type II endoleak from what appeared to be lumbar arteries.

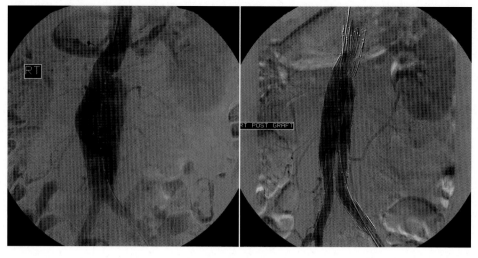

Figure 12-40. Aortography during EVAR. LEFT, Before deployment. RIGHT, After deployment. No leak was apparent at the time of operation.

12

References

1. Long-term outcomes of immediate repair compared with surveillance of small abdominal aortic aneurysms. N Engl J Med 2002;346:1445-1452.

2. Upchurch GR, Eagleton MJ: Endovascular abdominal aortic aneurysm repair. ACC Curr J Rev 2002;11:94-96.

3. Faxon DP, Creager MA, Smith SC Jr, et al: Atherosclerotic Vascular Disease Conference: Executive summary: Atherosclerotic Vascular Disease Conference proceeding for healthcare professionals from a special writing group of the American Heart Association. Circulation 2004;109:2595-2604.

4. Lynch RM: Accuracy of abdominal examination in the diagnosis of non-ruptured abdominal aortic aneurysm. Accid Emerg Nurs 2004;12:99-107.

5. Fink HA, Lederle FA, Roth CS, et al: The accuracy of physical examination to detect abdominal aortic aneurysm. Arch Intern Med 2000;160:833-836.

6. Karkos CD, Mukhopadhyay U, Papakostas I, et al: Abdominal aortic aneurysm: the role of clinical examination and opportunistic detection. Eur J Vasc Endovasc Surg 2000;19:299-303.

7. Powell JT, Greenhalgh RM: Clinical practice: small abdominal aortic aneurysms. N Engl J Med 2003;348:1895-1901.

8. Leach SD, Toole AL, Stern H, et al: Effect of beta-adrenergic blockade on the growth rate of abdominal aortic aneurysms. Arch Surg 1988;123:606-609.

9. Hackam DG, Thiruchelvam D, Redelmeier DA: Angiotensin-converting enzyme inhibitors and aortic rupture: a population-based case-control study. Lancet 2006;368:659-665.

10. Nevitt MP, Ballard DJ, Hallett JW Jr: Prognosis of abdominal aortic aneurysms: a population-based study. N Engl J Med 1989;321:1009-1014.

11. Scott RA, Kim LG, Ashton HA: Assessment of the criteria for elective surgery in screen-detected abdominal aortic aneurysms. J Med Screen 2005;12:150-154.

12. Brady AR, Thompson SG, Fowkes FG, et al: Abdominal aortic aneurysm expansion: risk factors and time intervals for surveillance. Circulation 2004;110:16-21.

13. Ernst CB: Abdominal aortic aneurysm. N Engl J Med 1993;328:1167-1172.

14. Lederle FA, Wilson SE, Johnson GR, et al: Immediate repair compared with surveillance of small abdominal aortic aneurysms. N Engl J Med 2002;346:1437-1444.

15. Cronenwett JL, Murphy TF, Zelenock GB, et al: Actuarial analysis of variables associated with rupture of small abdominal aortic aneurysms. Surgery 1985;98:472-483.

16. Howell MH, Strickman N, Mortazavi A, et al: Preliminary results of endovascular abdominal aortic aneurysm exclusion with the AneuRx stent-graft. J Am Coll Cardiol 2001;38:1040-1046.

17. Teufelsbauer H, Prusa AM, Wolff K, et al: Endovascular stent grafting versus open surgical operation in patients with infrarenal aortic aneurysms: a propensity score–adjusted analysis. Circulation 2002;106:782-787.

18. Hechelhammer L, Lachat ML, Wildermuth S, et al: Midterm outcome of endovascular repair of ruptured abdominal aortic aneurysms. J Vasc Surg 2005;41:752-757.

19. Leon LR Jr, Labropoulos N, Laredo J, et al: To what extent has endovascular aneurysm repair influenced abdominal aortic aneurysm management in the state of Illinois? J Vasc Surg 2005;41:568-574.

20. Nowygrod R, Egorova N, Greco G, et al: Trends, complications, and mortality in peripheral vascular surgery. J Vasc Surg 2006;43:205-216.

21. Greenhalgh RM, Brown LC, Kwong GP, et al: Comparison of endovascular aneurysm repair with open repair in patients with abdominal aortic aneurysm (EVAR trial 1), 30-day operative mortality results: randomised controlled trial. Lancet 2004;364:843-848.

22. Prinssen M, Buskens E, Blankensteijn JD: Quality of life after endovascular and open AAA repair. Results of a randomised trial. Eur J Vasc Endovasc Surg 2004;27:121-127.

23. Dillavou ED, Muluk SC, Makaroun MS: Improving aneurysm-related outcomes: nationwide benefits of endovascular repair. J Vasc Surg 2006;43:446-451.

24. Torsello G, Osada N, Florek HJ, et al: Long-term outcome after Talent endograft implantation for aneurysms of the abdominal aorta: a multicenter retrospective study. J Vasc Surg 2006;43:277-284.

25. Hobo R, Buth J: Secondary interventions following endovascular abdominal aortic aneurysm repair using current endografts: A EUROSTAR report. J Vasc Surg 2006;43:896-902.

26. Iannelli G, Monaco M, Di TL, et al: Endovascular vs. open surgery of abdominal aortic aneurysm in high-risk patients: a single-center experience. Thorac Cardiovasc Surg 2005;53:291-294.

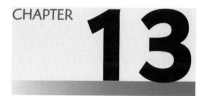

Endovascular Therapy for Thoracic Aortic Pathology

Mark D. Peterson and Edward B. Diethrich

KEY POINTS

▶ Deployment of a covered stent graft through the femoral artery avoids a thoracotomy incision, aortic cross-clamping, and the physiologic perturbations associated with open surgery.

▶ The only FDA-approved indication is treatment of degenerative aneurysms of the descending thoracic aorta. Many specialized centers currently treat a wide variety of thoracic pathologic processes with stent grafts.

▶ High-quality imaging is critical to ensure successful endovascular repair. Thin-cut, contrast-enhanced CT has emerged as the preoperative imaging study of choice because it provides most of the needed information for the planning of endovascular procedures and because of its widespread availability.

▶ The Gore TAG thoracic endoprosthesis is the only FDA-approved stent graft available for use in the United States. Several others are used clinically as part of

investigational protocols, including the Cook Zenith TX2 thoracic TAA endovascular graft and the Medtronic Talent thoracic stent graft.

▶ Stent graft repair introduces a set of complications distinct from those observed after open surgical repair.

  ▸ The requirement for frequent post-intervention imaging also exposes patients to both repeated high-doses of radiation and intravenous contrast material.

  ▸ The long-term durability of stent grafts has also not been firmly established.

▶ Hybrid endovascular-open procedures are being used to treat patients whose proximal or distal landing zones are close (<20 mm) to critical branch vessels.

▶ Highly specialized centers are gaining increasing experience with branched endografts to treat thoracoabdominal aneurysms.

Until a landmark paper demonstrating the safe and effective treatment of thoracic aortic aneurysms with endovascular stent grafts by Dake and colleagues[1] in 1994, conventional open surgery was the only effective treatment of thoracic aortic disease. During the last decade, the confluence of refined endovascular techniques and improved devices combined with widespread commercial availability of stent grafts has fueled an explosion of centers that offer endovascular stent grafting to treat a wide range of thoracic aortic disease. Although the Food and Drug Administration (FDA) has approved only one stent graft device for treatment of descending thoracic aortic aneurysms, the desire to avoid the morbidity associated with traditional open repair has broadened both the spectrum of thoracic aortic diseases treated and the segments of the proximal and distal aorta deemed suitable for stent grafting. Endovascular surgeons currently have the ability to stent the thoracic aorta from the distal aortic arch down to the aortic bifurcation. Specialized centers are also gaining experience with

stent grafting of the aortic arch and, in very select cases, the ascending aorta. In this chapter, we review the indications, the principles and techniques, and the pitfalls associated with endovascular stent grafting for thoracic aortic diseases. Finally, we review hybrid endovascular-open surgical procedures and future developments of stent graft therapy.

INDICATIONS FOR ENDOVASCULAR REPAIR

The FDA has approved endovascular stent graft therapy solely for the treatment of degenerative aneurysms of the descending thoracic aorta.[2] Stent graft therapy for the descending thoracic aorta has several distinct advantages over open surgery. Compared with

Table 13-1. Etiology of Thoracic Aortic Disease Treated at the Arizona Heart Institute Between 2000 and 2006 (n = 289)

Etiology	N (%)
Aneurysm	119 (41%)
Type B dissection	
Acute	45 (16%)
Chronic	43 (15%)
Penetrating ulcer	30 (10%)
Contained rupture	16 (5.5%)
Pseudoaneurysm	16 (5.5%)
Traumatic transection	10 (3.5%)
Aortobronchial fistula	7 (2.4 %)
Atheroembolic aorta	2 (0.7%)
Coarctation repair	1 (0.3%)

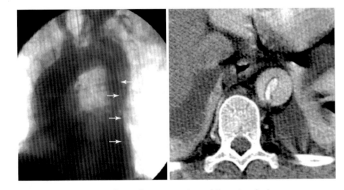

Figure 13-2. Type B dissection presenting with malperfusion. Intraoperative aortogram (LEFT) demonstrates contrast material in both the true and false lumens with arrows depicting the intimal flap. Axial CT scan (RIGHT) shows almost complete separation of the intima from the outer aortic layers with contrast material within the smaller true lumen.

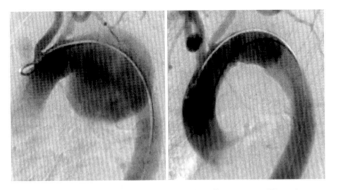

Figure 13-1. Endovascular repair of a distal arch aneurysm. Thoracic aortogram before stent graft deployment (LEFT) and after endovascular exclusion (RIGHT).

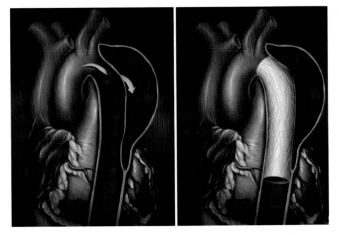

Figure 13-3. Principles of endovascular repair for type B dissection. Illustration depicting endovascular exclusion of the primary intimal tear (LEFT) with a covered stent graft (RIGHT). (Courtesy of the Arizona Heart Institute.)

open surgery, deployment of a covered stent graft through the femoral artery avoids a thoracotomy incision, aortic cross-clamping, and the physiologic perturbations associated with open surgery. Many specialized centers currently treat a wide variety of thoracic pathologic processes with stent grafts (Table 13-1).[3-7]

Because randomized clinical trial data comparing open surgery and endovascular repair do not exist, the decision to treat a patient with a thoracic stent graft must balance patient factors with the anticipated risks and benefits. For example, a young patient with a large aneurysm may tolerate open repair, and placement of a stent graft with undetermined long-term durability may not be prudent. In contrast, elderly patients with chronic obstructive pulmonary disease may potentially benefit greatly by avoiding a thoracotomy. In general, indications for endovascular repair parallel the indications for open repair. Asymptomatic patients with fusiform aneurysms of the thoracic aorta of greater than 5.5 cm can be considered for endovascular repair (Fig. 13-1).[8]

The ability to intervene quickly and less invasively with stent grafts compared with open surgery may be particularly applicable to the treatment of disease that requires urgent attention, such as in some cases of type B dissections, traumatic aortic transections, and contained aortic rupture. Indications for endovascular repair of type B dissections are similar to the indications for open repair and include rupture (or impending rupture),

intractable pain, hypertension refractory to medical management, and evidence of end-organ malperfusion (Fig. 13-2). The primary goals of endovascular repair for type B dissections are to restore perfusion to the true lumen and to cover the site of the primary intimal tear; it is not necessary to treat all segments of the dissected aorta (Figs. 13-3 and 13-4). Complete obliteration of the false lumen occurs more often in treatment of acute type B dissections than of chronic type B dissections, which may contain varying amounts of thrombus in the false lumen. Figure 13-5 demonstrates persistent compromise of the true lumen despite placement of a proximal descending thoracic aortic stent graft. Uncovered stainless steel Z stents may be required to provide additional radial force at the distal end of the covered stent graft to improve true lumen perfusion.

Endovascular stent grafts may be particularly well suited for trauma patients presenting with a traumatic aortic transection (Fig. 13-6).[7,9-11] Intra-abdominal organ, closed head, and orthopedic injuries often accompany traumatic aortic transections; therefore, avoiding the morbidity of open surgery, including the requirement for systemic anticoagulation, is desirable. The goal of stenting aortic transections, which usually occur at the level of the aortic isthmus, is to cover the intimal flap and the associated

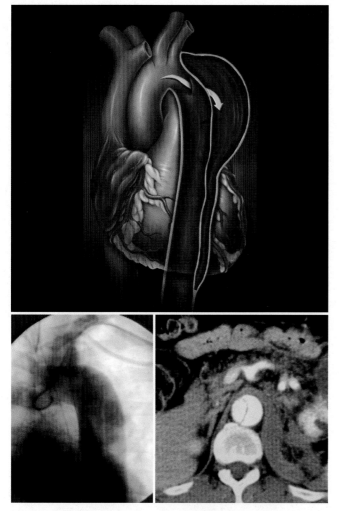

Figure 13-4. Type B dissection depicted by graphic aortogram (TOP), with pigtail catheter inserted through the left subclavian (BOTTOM LEFT), and axial CT scan demonstrating true (smaller) and false lumens in the distal thoracic aorta (BOTTOM RIGHT).

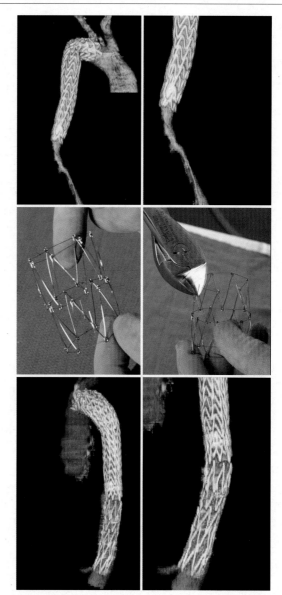

Figure 13-5. Reconstructed CT scans after stent graft deployment showing persistent compromise of the distal false lumen (TOP ROW). Stainless steel Gianturco Z stents (MIDDLE LEFT) with barbs manually removed (MIDDLE RIGHT). Reconstructed CT scans after reintervention to deploy Z stents at the distal seal zone, with a corresponding improvement in true lumen patency (BOTTOM ROW).

pseudoaneurysm (Fig. 13-7). The left subclavian artery is covered by the proximal end of the stent graft in many cases to allow a suitable proximal seal zone (Fig. 13-8). These cases extend the limits of stent graft therapy because many of the patients are young with small aortic diameters, small access vessels, and a narrow inner radius of the aortic arch.

PRINCIPLES AND TECHNIQUES OF ENDOVASCULAR REPAIR

Successful endovascular repair of aortic disease requires a convergence of open surgical and interventional skills. At the Arizona Heart Institute, cardiac or vascular surgeons with extensive training in catheter-based procedures perform all of the aortic endovascular procedures; however, in many centers, these cases are performed by a multidisciplinary team consisting of either a cardiac or vascular surgeon and an interventional radiologist or cardiologist. Not only must the surgical team be comfortable with

exposure of the femoral arteries, but the team should be comfortable with retroperitoneal exposure of the iliac arteries and distal aorta when the common femoral or external iliac arteries are of insufficient size to permit passage of a large-bore sheath. The surgical team should also be comfortable with open repair of the thoracic aorta in the event of a procedural catastrophe, such as aortic rupture or retrograde type A dissection. A Task Force on Endovascular Surgery convened by the Society of Thoracic Surgeons has also recommended minimum training requirements for the acquisition of catheter-based skills necessary to perform endovascular surgery.[12] The position statement of the Society of Thoracic Surgeons recommends a minimum of 25 wire-catheter placements, comfort with large-bore femoral cannulation, and participation in either 10 abdominal or 5 thoracic stent graft procedures.

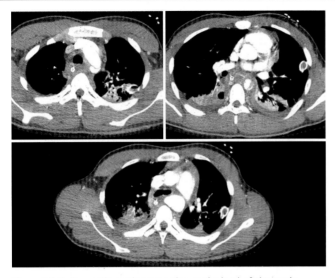

Figure 13-6. Traumatic aortic transection at the level of the aortic isthmus. Axial contrast-enhanced CT scan demonstrating an intimal flap (TOP LEFT), intraluminal thrombus (TOP RIGHT), and pseudoaneurysm with periaortic hematoma (BOTTOM).

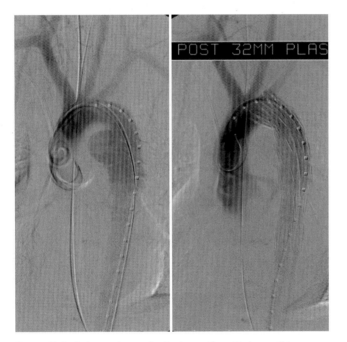

Figure 13-7. Endovascular repair of a traumatic aortic transection. LEFT, Aortogram showing a large pseudoaneurysm at the level of the aortic isthmus. RIGHT, Stent graft repair of traumatic disruption with partial coverage of the left subclavian artery origin.

IMAGING

High-quality preoperative and intraoperative imaging is critical to ensure successful endovascular repair. A high-quality preoperative imaging study permits careful planning of all aspects of the endovascular procedure, including device diameter and length selection, anticipated number of devices required, preferred access site, proximity to important branch vessels, and potential need for extra-anatomic bypass when coverage of one or more critical aortic branches (such as the origin of the left common

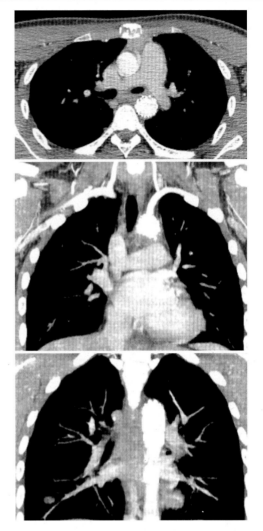

Figure 13-8. Postoperative CT scan 1 month after endovascular repair of a traumatic aortic transection. TOP, Axial contrast-enhanced CT scan confirming complete exclusion of pseudoaneurysm and intimal flap. MIDDLE, Coronal reconstruction demonstrating patent left subclavian artery despite partial coverage of the origin. BOTTOM, Additional coronal slice showing resolution of periaortic hematoma and no endoleaks.

carotid artery) is anticipated. Thus, the preoperative imaging study must accurately define the pathologic process; the diameter and quality of the aorta at the prospective proximal and distal seal zones; the length of aorta requiring stent graft coverage; and the quality, size, and tortuosity of the aorta and access vessels. Thin-cut, contrast-enhanced computed tomography (CT) has emerged as the preoperative imaging study of choice because it provides most of this information and is widely available. CT scans performed for endovascular case planning should image the chest, abdomen, and pelvis, including the common femoral arteries to determine the adequacy of the access vessels. In addition, digital reconstructions of CT scans allow more accurate estimation of aortic diameter and the length of the aortic pathologic process because the thoracic aorta is often tortuous and analysis of axial cuts alone would lead to overestimation of the aortic diameter. Figure 13-9 illustrates the principle of center line of flow analysis whereby computerized software algorithms select the center of the aortic lumen as determined from axial, coronal, and sagittal images and then reconstruct the images perpendicular to the

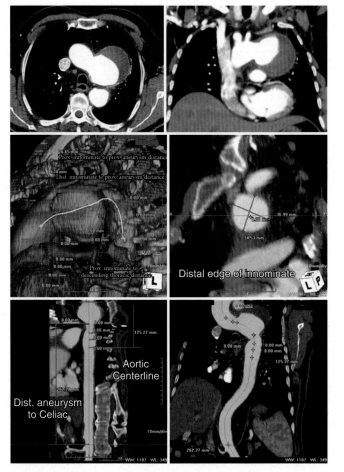

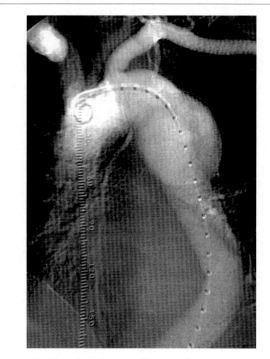

Figure 13-10. Thoracic aortogram with proximal aneurysm.

Figure 13-9. Axial (TOP LEFT) and coronal (TOP RIGHT) contrast-enhanced CT scans demonstrating a large arch aneurysm. Center line of flow analysis (MIDDLE LEFT) and corresponding two-dimensional reconstructions (MIDDLE RIGHT AND BOTTOM).

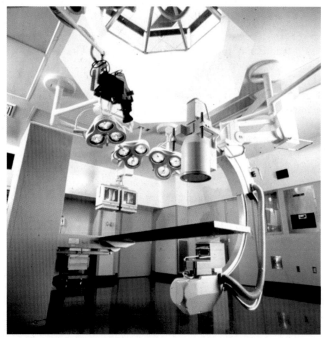

Figure 13-11. Hybrid operating room–endovascular suite at the Arizona Heart Institute, with a fixed, ceiling-mounted imaging system. (Courtesy of the Arizona Heart Institute.)

center line for accurate determination of the aortic diameter. This type of analysis and three-dimensional reconstructions were critical for evaluating the length of the proximal landing zone. Initial study of the axial and coronal slices suggested a potentially suitable proximal landing zone distal to the innominate artery, which would have allowed a hybrid approach composed of a carotid-carotid bypass followed by stent grafting of the mid arch distal to the innominate artery. However, careful analysis of the center line of flow images revealed a proximal landing zone of less than 15 mm; therefore, we planned on a strategy of total arch debranching, followed by stent grafting of the entire arch, with the proximal landing zone in the ascending aorta.

Recent improvements in CT image quality have largely rendered preoperative angiography unnecessary. Nevertheless, fluoroscopy and aortography remain the principal intraoperative imaging tools (Fig. 13-10). Whereas many straightforward endovascular procedures can be performed adequately in an interventional radiology suite or in an operating room with a portable C-arm, we strongly encourage the development of a fully functional hybrid endovascular-surgical operating suite, such as the one illustrated in Figure 13-11. A hybrid suite combines a high-quality, ceiling-mounted fixed image intensifier and x-ray tube (C-arm) with a room equipped to perform a full range of both interventional and conventional surgical procedures. These types of dedicated facilities are ideally suited for performance of hybrid surgical and endovascular procedures, in some extreme cases including the use of cardiopulmonary bypass, which is becoming increasingly more common. Clearly, the superior imaging and higher heat tube capacity obtained with a fixed, ceiling-mounted system compared with a portable C-arm facilitates procedural success in complex and lengthy endovascular procedures.

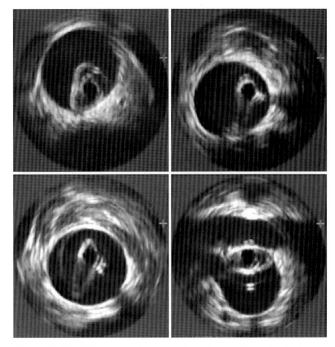

Figure 13-12. IVUS images obtained before stent graft repair of a type B dissection showing nearly complete separation of intimal and outer aortic layers (TOP AND BOTTOM LEFT). Representative section taken at the level of the renal arteries and renal vein (BOTTOM RIGHT).

Additional intraoperative imaging tools include transesophageal echocardiography and intravascular ultrasonography (IVUS). IVUS is particularly important during endovascular repair for urgent disease, such as contained aortic rupture or traumatic aortic transection, when preoperative case planning may be limited. IVUS allows the operator to measure several important parameters for stent graft sizing and placement, including the aortic diameter, the length of the proximal and distal landing zones, the distance between the landing zone and critical branch vessels, and the quality of the aorta at the site of the prospective landing zones (i.e., amount of mural thrombus, atherosclerotic plaque, and calcification). In addition, IVUS is very useful in defining the true and false lumens in type B dissections and may help identify the site of the primary intimal tear (Fig. 13-12).

DEVICES

The Gore TAG thoracic endoprosthesis (W. L. Gore & Associates, Flagstaff, AZ) is the only FDA-approved stent graft available for use in the United States. This device is constructed from an expanded polytetrafluoroethylene tube graft supported by a self-expanding stent constructed from nitinol that runs along its external surface (Fig. 13-13). The stent graft also contains radiopaque gold marker bands at the base of the device flares to facilitate device positioning at the proximal and distal landing zones. The device deploys in situ from the center toward both the proximal and distal ends simultaneously to minimize the potential for graft migration (Fig. 13-14).

Several other thoracic stent grafts are used clinically in the United States as part of investigational protocols, including the

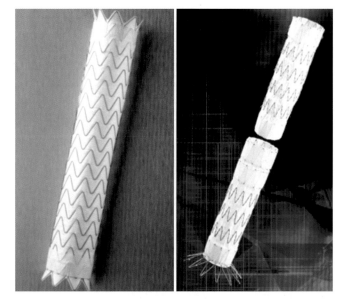

Figure 13-13. Thoracic endovascular stent grafts. Gore TAG device approved for clinical use in the United States (LEFT) and modular two-piece Cook TX2 thoracic stent graft (RIGHT).

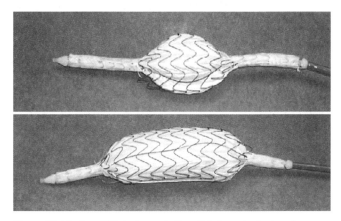

Figure 13-14. Gore TAG deployment. Gore TAG thoracic stent graft deploys from the center (TOP) toward both proximal and distal ends (BOTTOM) to minimize risk of graft migration during deployment.

Cook Zenith TX2 thoracic TAA endovascular graft (Cook Medical Inc., Bloomington, IN) and the Medtronic Talent thoracic stent graft (Medtronic Inc., Minneapolis, MN). These devices are used in Canada under special access granted by Health Canada on a per case basis. The Cook Zenith TX2 graft is available as a single or two-piece device and is fabricated from a woven polyester tube graft reinforced with independent stainless steel Z stents that allows the graft to conform to the tortuosity of the aorta (see Fig. 13-13). The inherent radial strength of the Z stents secures the graft to the aorta within the seal zones; staggered barbs at the proximal end and an uncovered bare stent at the distal end provide additional fixation.

DEVICE SIZING

Patients with thoracic aortic disease are selected for potential endovascular repair on the basis of several important anatomic features gleaned from the CT scans. The femoral and iliac arteries must be sufficiently large to permit passage of a large-bore introducer sheath. Sheath sizes vary, depending on the size of the endoprostheses, but they are generally in the range of 20 to 24 Fr (outer diameter of 7.6 to 9.2 mm). Predicting the ability of an introducer sheath to pass through the femoral and external iliac arteries by the size of the vessels alone may be difficult; relatively normal vessels will stretch, whereas calcified or tortuous vessels may not. If the sizes of the common femoral or external iliac arteries are considered marginal, we recommend suturing a 10-mm Dacron graft directly to the common iliac artery or distal abdominal aorta to provide access, rather than risk rupture of the external iliac artery.[13] At the termination of the procedure, the Dacron graft is either divided and oversewn or anastomosed to the common femoral artery. Iliac artery rupture is a devastating complication and usually is manifested when the sheath is withdrawn. The operator should always be prepared for this potential complication with a series of angioplasty balloons to temporarily tamponade the bleeding. Additional covered stent grafts should be available for potential endovascular repair of a ruptured iliac artery; otherwise, definitive repair would require open exploration.

The next step in case planning involves determination of graft size. The graft size is determined by the diameter of the aorta in the proximal and distal landing (seal) zones. The efficacy of endovascular stent grafts for successful exclusion of thoracic aortic disease is largely determined by the adequacy of fixation at the proximal and distal landing zones (Fig. 13-15). Effective seal is primarily generated by the inherent radial force of the stent graft against the native aorta and thus requires 10% to 20% oversizing of the stent graft to the native aortic diameter. Because the Gore TAG device is available in diameters ranging from 26 to 40 mm and the Cook Zenith TX2 is available in diameters of 22 to 42 mm, the range of aortic diameters suitable to act as a landing zone for a stent graft ranges from 23 to 37 mm and 20 to 38 mm, respectively. Thus, patients with small native aortas, such as a young patient with a traumatic aortic transection, or patients with

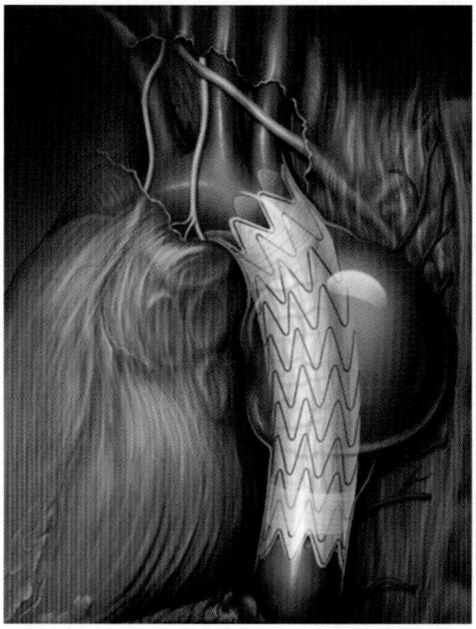

dilated aortas at the site of the prospective landing zone may not be appropriate candidates for stent grafting. The length of the seal zone at the proximal and distal landing zone must be at least 20 mm to ensure adequate fixation. Greater lengths of normal aorta are advisable to achieve effective seal when the landing zone involves a curved segment of aorta, such as the distal arch, or a tapered segment. Most endovascular specialists require a minimum of 20 mm from the origin of the left subclavian and the celiac arteries to avoid unplanned coverage. If extension of the proximal or distal landing zone is necessary to obtain an adequate seal, coverage of one or more branch vessels is possible if the appropriate extra-anatomic bypass has been performed (see later).[14,15]

The number of stent grafts required in a given patient depends on the length of the aortic pathologic process. The Cook Zenith TX2 graft is available in lengths ranging from 115 to 208 mm; the Gore TAG device is available in 100-, 115-, and 200-mm lengths, depending on the graft diameter. When more than one stent graft is required, the companies advise at least 50 mm of graft-to-graft overlap for similarly sized devices and 30 mm for grafts of unequal size. The latter scenario occurs when the diameters of the proximal and distal landing zones differ by more than 20%.

PROCEDURAL TECHNIQUES

Endovascular repair of thoracic aortic disease can be performed under local, spinal, or general anesthesia. Unless the patient is considered at very high risk for postoperative pulmonary complications, we prefer a general anesthetic. Standard intraoperative monitoring is employed, including multiple arterial monitoring lines. We place cerebrospinal fluid drains selectively in patients at high risk for paraplegia, such as patients with a history of abdominal aortic aneurysm repair, patients in whom coverage of the entire thoracic and abdominal aorta is planned, and patients presenting with contained aortic rupture. If paraplegia or paraparesis develops postoperatively in patients who did not receive a cerebrospinal fluid drain, we will insert a spinal drain and start a high-dose dexamethasone protocol. We also maintain a systolic blood pressure above 140 mm Hg for the first 24 hours after stent deployment.

Arterial access is obtained by exposing the common femoral artery through either a small oblique incision 2 to 3 cm above the groin crease or a longitudinal incision directly over the artery. A 5 or 6 Fr sheath is inserted percutaneously through the contralateral common femoral artery to allow insertion of a pigtail catheter. Once access is obtained on both sides, regular stiffness 0.035-inch, 260-cm guide wires are inserted bilaterally to allow a full IVUS examination and positioning of the pigtail catheter for aortography. The C-arm should be perpendicular to the aortic arch; a left anterior oblique angle of 45 degrees is generally sufficient. After standard aortography and IVUS examinations are completed, the proximal and distal landing zones are marked, the systolic blood pressure is lowered to less than 100 mm Hg, and the endoprosthesis is deployed over a double-curved, stiff Lunderquist wire (LES3, Cook Medical Inc.). A post-deployment aortogram confirms adequacy of seal between the stent graft and the aortic wall at the proximal and distal landing zones. If a proximal or distal type I endoleak is detected, a semi-compliant profiling balloon is used to ensure full apposition of

Figure 13-15. Principles of thoracic endografting. Endovascular exclusion of aortic disease requires a segment of nonaneurysmal proximal and distal aorta of at least 20 mm.

the stent graft with the aortic wall. The distal seal zone is ballooned first, followed by the proximal seal zone and then the graft-to-graft overlap, if more than one device was deployed. Once the final aortogram demonstrates no significant endoleaks, the sheaths and wires are removed, the common femoral artery is repaired, and the patient is awakened to allow a cursory neurologic examination.

A non–contrast-enhanced and contrast-enhanced CT scan is performed before hospital discharge and then at 1, 6, and 12 months and annually thereafter. If an endoleak or aneurysm sac expansion is identified at 1 month, a repeated CT scan is performed at 3 months.

PITFALLS OF ENDOVASCULAR REPAIR

Despite rapidly increasing enthusiasm of patients and physicians to embrace endovascular stent graft therapy, there are no prospective, randomized clinical trials comparing open surgical and endovascular repair for thoracic aortic diseases. Most of the published results of endovascular repair are derived from small to medium-sized case series or registries.[8] The results from these studies are often compared with the results from open surgical therapy, which are also invariably derived from single centers. Meaningful comparisons between endovascular and open surgical repair are further confounded either by comparison of modern endovascular results with older surgical literature or by comparison of endovascular results with "contemporary" open surgical management published by large-volume, specialized referral centers with highly trained surgeons. Nevertheless, endovascular repair for thoracic aortic disease is generally associated with acceptable rates of death and major morbidity: operative mortality, 0% to 10.2%; stroke, 0% to 6.8%; and paraplegia, 0% to 6%.[8]

Stent graft repair also introduces a set of complications distinct from those observed after open surgical repair (Table 13-2). The requirement for frequent postintervention imaging also exposes patients to both repeated high doses of radiation and intravenous contrast material. The long-term durability of stent grafts has also not been firmly established.

An endoleak is defined by the presence of blood outside the lumen of the stent graft but contained within the aneurysm sac, as evidenced by an intraoperative or postoperative imaging study. An endoleak implies a connection between the lumen of the endoprosthesis and the aneurysm sac. Endoleaks are classified according to standard nomenclature.[16] A type I endoleak results from failure to achieve adequate seal at either the proximal or distal seal zone and is thus classified as either a proximal (type Ia) or distal (type Ib) endoleak. A type II endoleak is the result of retrograde blood flow into the aneurysm sac from a patent branch vessel, such as intercostal, left subclavian, inferior mesenteric, hypogastric, lumbar, or accessory renal arteries. Figure 13-16 illustrates an example of a type II endoleak from a patent left subclavian artery. This endoleak was successfully treated by retrograde coil embolization of the origin of the left subclavian, performed percutaneously through the left brachial artery (Fig. 13-17). Two additional types of endoleak are also reported: disruption of the graft material, resulting in blood flow into the aneurysm sac, or lack of seal between two contiguous endografts is termed a type III endoleak; blood flow through the graft pores, without an obvious tear in the graft, is termed a type IV endoleak. Type I and II endoleaks, the most commonly observed endoleaks, have been reported in up to one quarter of patients after endovascular repair.[8] Large type I endoleaks generally require reintervention to establish effective seal. As a first step, we attempt repeated profile ballooning to improve apposition of the graft with the aortic wall. If this fails, we extend the proximal or distal landing zone with an additional covered stent graft. In contrast,

Table 13-2. Complications Associated with Endovascular Repair for Thoracic Aortic Disease

Endoleak (types I-IV)

Graft collapse

Graft migration

Retrograde aortic dissection

Aortic rupture (stent strut)

Access complications

  Iliac rupture

  Iliac dissection

Contrast-induced renal failure

Reintervention

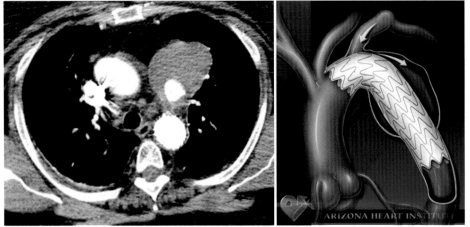

Figure 13-16. LEFT, Contrast-enhanced CT scan demonstrating contrast material within the excluded aneurysm sac from a patent left subclavian artery (type II endoleak). RIGHT, Graphic illustrating a type II endoleak from a patent left subclavian artery. (Right image courtesy of the Arizona Heart Institute.)

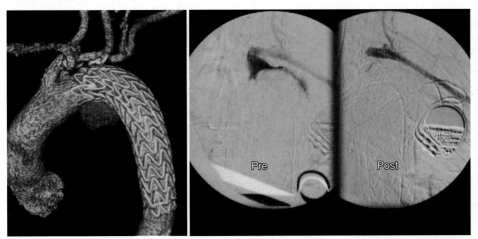

Figure 13-17. Endovascular repair of a type II endoleak emanating from the left subclavian artery. LEFT, Reformatted CT scan shows embolization coils deposited adjacent to the endograft at the origin of the left subclavian artery. RIGHT, Retrograde arteriogram performed through the left brachial artery confirms seal of type II endoleak.

type II endoleaks may be treated conservatively and observed with repeated imaging; however, evidence of aneurysm sac expansion or large type II endoleaks mandate reintervention, such as collateral vessel embolization. Type III endoleaks are usually treated with placement of an additional covered stent graft.

HYBRID ENDOVASCULAR AND OPEN REPAIR

In recent years, many groups have extended the limits of endovascular therapy by developing hybrid procedures to treat patients whose proximal or distal landing zones are close (<20 mm) to critical branch vessels.[14-18] Many of these patients would be very high risk patients for conventional arch or thoracoabdominal surgery. Hybrid procedures combine open surgery, usually some form of extra-anatomic rerouting or debranching procedure, and stent graft therapy to treat patients with complex aortic disease.

Various different extra-anatomic rerouting procedures have been developed to permit deployment of a conventional stent graft either across the entire aortic arch or at varying points distal to one of the brachiocephalic vessels. Figure 13-18 illustrates representative 64-slice CT scans from a patient with a large calcified aneurysm discovered at the base of the innominate artery. The options for the patient included a conventional arch replacement (Fig. 13-19, left), involving cardiopulmonary bypass and circulatory arrest, and a total great vessel debranching with aortic arch stenting (Fig. 13-19, right). The latter procedure, performed off-pump through a sternotomy, involved suturing of a bifurcated Dacron graft from the ascending aorta to the innominate and left common carotid arteries, followed by antegrade delivery of a single stent graft through a side branch sutured onto the primary Dacron graft. Figure 13-20 illustrates another form of extra-anatomic rerouting because the aneurysm begins in the mid distal arch. The preoperative imaging confirmed that adequate seal could be obtained by landing the stent graft distal to the origin of the innominate artery. Blood flow was established to the left common carotid through a carotid-carotid bypass, and then the aneurysm was excluded by landing a single stent graft just beyond the innominate artery origin (see Fig. 13-20). Postoperative imaging studies confirm carotid patency as well as absence of endoleaks (Fig. 13-21).

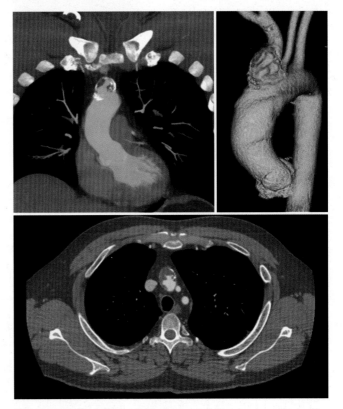

Figure 13-18. Preoperative contrast-enhanced CT scan of a patient with a large, calcified aneurysm at the base of the innominate artery shown in coronal plane (TOP LEFT), 3D reconstruction (TOP RIGHT), and axial plane (BOTTOM).

Stent grafts are also used to complete staged repairs of extensive ascending, arch, and descending thoracic aortic aneurysms. Figure 13-22 demonstrates intraoperative photographs of a patient with a massive 10-cm ascending, 7-cm arch, and 6-cm descending aneurysm. The ascending and arch aneurysms were repaired simultaneously (stage I) with a composite valve-graft conduit and a total arch replacement with elephant trunk. The distal end of the elephant trunk was marked with three large metallic clips (Fig. 13-23). CT images obtained after the patient was discharged home revealed thrombus adjacent to the elephant trunk in the proximal descending aorta and contrast material

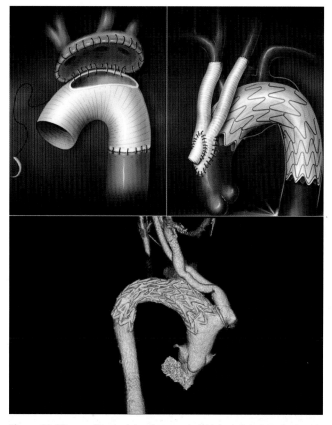

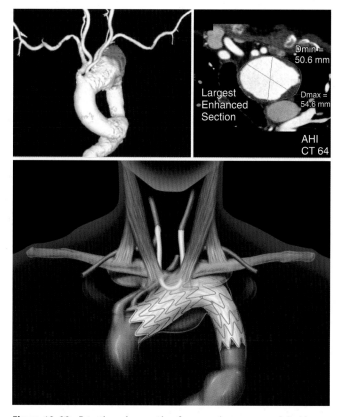

Figure 13-19. TOP, Standard (LEFT) versus hybrid (RIGHT) arch replacement. BOTTOM, Volume-rendered 3D contrast-enhanced CT scan revealing the stent graft (wire), its exclusion of the arch aneurysm, and the reconstructed arch vessels.

Figure 13-20. Extrathoracic rerouting for an arch aneurysm originating distal to the innominate artery. TOP, Preoperative reformatted CT image of a large arch aneurysm starting in the mid transverse arch. BOTTOM, Illustration demonstrating endovascular exclusion of the arch aneurysm with a proximal landing zone distal to the origin of the innominate artery and a carotid-to-carotid bypass. (Bottom image courtesy of the Arizona Heart Institute.)

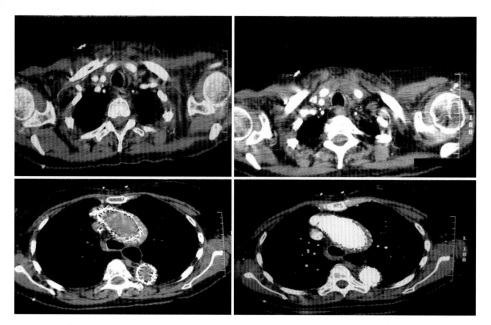

Figure 13-21. Contrast-enhanced CT scan after hybrid repair of mid arch aneurysm. Axial slices depict patent carotid-carotid bypass (TOP LEFT), native carotid arteries (TOP RIGHT), and endograft in arch and proximal descending thoracic aorta without contrast enhancement (BOTTOM LEFT) and with contrast enhancement (BOTTOM RIGHT).

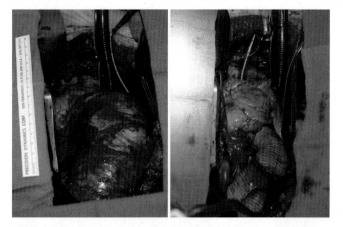

Figure 13-22. Stage I repair of a large ascending, arch, and descending thoracic aortic aneurysm. LEFT, Intraoperative photograph demonstrates a 10-cm ascending aortic aneurysm. RIGHT, Photograph after completion of an elephant trunk, arch replacement, and Bentall procedure.

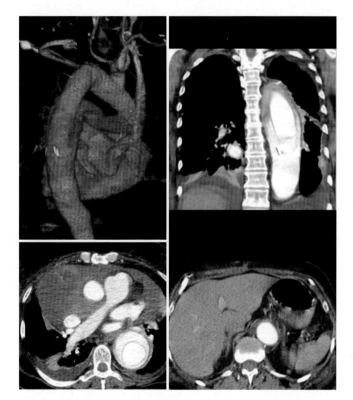

Figure 13-23. Postoperative contrast-enhanced CT scan demonstrates metallic clips marking the distal end of the Dacron elephant trunk graft (TOP LEFT). Coronal (TOP RIGHT) and axial (BOTTOM LEFT) cuts through proximal descending thoracic aorta show contrast material within and surrounding the elephant trunk. Axial cut in the distal descending thoracic aorta shows a suitable distal landing zone for a stent graft (BOTTOM RIGHT).

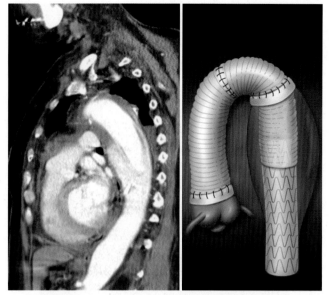

Figure 13-24. Parasagittal reconstruction demonstrating elephant trunk with surrounding thrombus proximally and contrast material distally (LEFT). Illustration shows endovascular exclusion of descending aneurysm with stent graft deployed into the elephant trunk proximally (RIGHT). The stent graft is deployed distally in a nonaneurysmal segment of aorta. (Right image courtesy of the Arizona Heart Institute.)

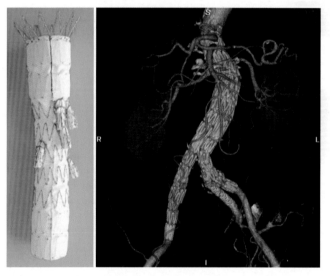

Figure 13-25. Branched endograft for thoracoabdominal aneurysm repair (LEFT) and reconstructed CT scan after repair (RIGHT).

both within the lumen and surrounding the graft in the mid descending aorta. The second stage of the procedure was completed 8 weeks after the initial procedure by insertion of a stent graft into the elephant trunk graft with access obtained through the femoral artery (Fig. 13-24). The distal landing zone was several centimeters above the celiac, where the aorta measured 34 to 35 mm.

FUTURE DEVELOPMENTS

Endovascular stent graft therapy for the treatment of complex aortic disease promises continued growth with improved devices and delivery systems. Highly specialized centers are gaining increasing experience with branched endografts to treat thoracoabdominal aneurysms (Fig. 13-25).[19] These grafts permit stent graft coverage of segments of the aorta that contain critical side branches, such as the celiac, superior mesenteric, and renal arteries. Stent grafts are custom designed to a particular patient's anatomy on the basis of detailed preoperative imaging, with a main body for covering the diseased aorta and side branches to

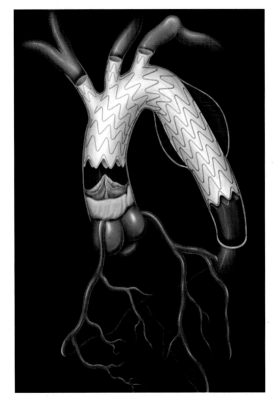

Figure 13-26. Illustration depicting future branched grafts to treat aortic arch aneurysms. (Courtesy of the Arizona Heart Institute.)

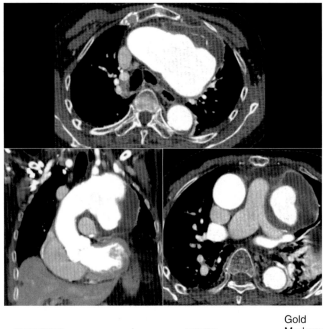

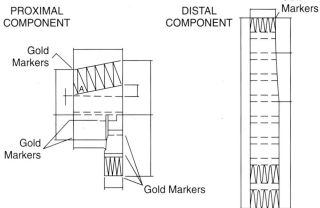

PROXIMAL COMPONENT

DISTAL COMPONENT

Gold Markers

Gold Markers

Gold Markers

Gold Markers

Figure 13-27. Contrast-enhanced CT scans of a patient with an arch and proximal descending aortic aneurysm. TOP, Axial scan demonstrating aneurysm at the arch level with a small amount of mural thrombus. MIDDLE, Coronal plane (MIDDLE LEFT) and axial plane (MIDDLE RIGHT) demonstrating preserved diameter of the ascending aorta and significant aneurysm of the mural thrombus within the proximal descending aorta. Custom design of proximal (BOTTOM LEFT) and distal (BOTTOM RIGHT) components of a composite stent graft for endovascular repair of the aneurysm.

ensure continued perfusion of vital organs. Stent grafts with side branches have also been implanted in the aortic arch (Fig. 13-26). Figure 13-27 illustrates preoperative CT scans from a patient awaiting coverage of the entire aortic arch, from the ascending to the descending aorta. The custom-designed graft is composed of two devices. The first piece is bifurcated, and the proximal portion will achieve seal in the ascending aorta with one branch routed into the innominate and the second into the aortic arch. A second stent graft will be deployed from the femoral artery with sufficient graft-graft overlap in the arch to achieve seal. The proximal descending aorta will be the distal seal zone for the second device.

At present, disease involving the ascending aorta meeting standard criteria for repair almost always requires conventional open surgery. Highly specialized centers have successfully treated patients with very selective pathologic processes confined to the ascending aorta. Figure 13-28 illustrates the case of a patient who had an expanding pseudoaneurysm from previous aortocoronary bypass grafting. The patient had undergone multiple previous cardiac surgical procedures and was deemed very high risk for open repair. A custom-made stent graft was deployed in the ascending aorta above the sinotubular junction to cover the base

of the pseudoaneurysm. Follow-up CT scans demonstrated a resolving pseudoaneurysm.

In summary, increasingly improved endovascular stent grafts and delivery systems will continue to expand the number and complexity of cases amenable to stent graft therapy for the treatment of a wide spectrum of aortic disease. Until more clinical research validates current stent grafting practices, physicians treating patients with stent grafts must judiciously balance the potential risk and benefits.

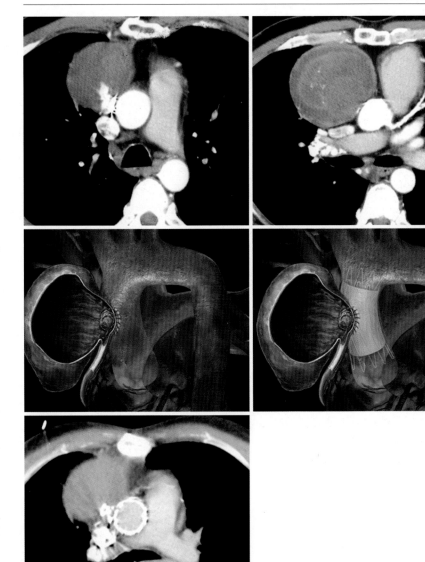

Figure 13-28. Initial experience with endovascular repair of the ascending aorta. Axial contrast-enhanced CT scan after attempted coil embolization of pseudoaneurysm neck (TOP LEFT). Repeated CT scan performed 4 months later demonstrating rapid enlargement of pseudoaneurysm (TOP RIGHT). Illustration of a large pseudoaneurysm emanating from the proximal anastomosis of an occluded saphenous vein graft to the right coronary artery (MIDDLE LEFT) and exclusion of pseudoaneurysm with a custom-made stent graft (MIDDLE RIGHT). Postoperative 1-year CT scan showing the stent graft in the ascending aorta with a marked reduction in the size of the pseudoaneurysm (BOTTOM LEFT). (Middle images courtesy of the Arizona Heart Institute.)

References

1. Dake MD, Miller DC, Semba CP, et al: Transluminal placement of endovascular stent-grafts for the treatment of descending thoracic aortic aneurysms. N Engl J Med 1994;331:1729-1734.

2. Makaroun MS, Dillavou ED, Kee ST, et al: Endovascular treatment of thoracic aortic aneurysms: results of the phase II multicenter trial of the GORE TAG thoracic endoprosthesis. J Vasc Surg 2005;41:1-9.

3. Cambria RP, Brewster DC, Lauterbach SR, et al: Evolving experience with thoracic aortic stent graft repair. J Vasc Surg 2002;35:1129-1136.

4. Song TK, Donayre CE, Walot I, et al: Endograft exclusion of acute and chronic descending thoracic aortic dissections. J Vasc Surg 2006;43:247-258.

5. Wheatley GH III, Gurbuz AT, Rodriguez-Lopez JA, et al: Midterm outcome in 158 consecutive Gore TAG thoracic endoprostheses: single center experience. Ann Thorac Surg 2006;81:1570-1577.

6. Fattori R, Nienaber CA, Rousseau H, et al: Results of endovascular repair of the thoracic aorta with the Talent Thoracic stent graft: the Talent Thoracic Retrospective Registry. J Thorac Cardiovasc Surg 2006;132:332-339.

7. Schumacher H, Bockler D, Tengg-Kobligk H, Allenberg JR: Acute traumatic aortic tear: open versus stent-graft repair. Semin Vasc Surg 2006;19:48-59.

8. Svensson LG, Kouchoukos NT, Miller DC, et al: Expert consensus document on the treatment of descending thoracic aortic disease using endovascular stent-grafts. Ann Thorac Surg 2008;85(Suppl):S1-S41.

9. Orford VP, Atkinson NR, Thomson K, et al: Blunt traumatic aortic transection: the endovascular experience. Ann Thorac Surg 2003;75:106-111.

10. Reed AB, Thompson JK, Crafton CJ, et al: Timing of endovascular repair of blunt traumatic thoracic aortic transections. J Vasc Surg 2006;43:684-688.

11. Neschis DG, Moaine S, Gutta R, et al: Twenty consecutive cases of endograft repair of traumatic aortic disruption: lessons learned. J Vasc Surg 2007;45:487-492.

12. Kouchoukos NT, Bavaria JE, Coselli JS, et al: Guidelines for credentialing of practitioners to perform endovascular stent-grafting of the thoracic aorta. Ann Thorac Surg 2006;81:1174-1176.

13. Diethrich EB: Technical tips for thoracic aortic endografting. Semin Vasc Surg 2008;21:8-12.

14. Czerny M, Gottardi R, Zimpfer D, et al: Transposition of the supraaortic branches for extended endovascular arch repair. Eur J Cardiothorac Surg 2006;29:709-713.

15. Melissano G, Civilini E, Bertoglio L, et al: Results of endografting of the aortic arch in different landing zones. Eur J Vasc Endovasc Surg 2007;33: 561-566.

16. Chaikof EL, Blankensteijn JD, Harris PL, et al: Reporting standards for endovascular aortic aneurysm repair. J Vasc Surg 2002;35:1048-1060.

17. Kpodonu J, Diethrich EB: Hybrid interventions for the treatment of the complex aortic arch. Perspect Vasc Surg Endovasc Ther 2007;19:174-184.

18. Diethrich EB, Ghazoul M, Wheatley GH, et al: Surgical correction of ascending type A thoracic aortic dissection: simultaneous endoluminal exclusion of the arch and distal aorta. J Endovasc Ther 2005;12:660-666.

19. Greenberg RK, Lytle B: Endovascular repair of thoracoabdominal aneurysms. Circulation 2008;117:2288-2296.

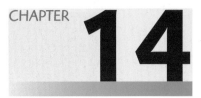

CHAPTER **14**

Diseases of the Aortic Root

KEY POINTS

- The aortic root is one of the most often diseased segments of the aorta and has the highest risk for development of secondary cardiac complications.
- Aortic diseases, if they involve the root, may incite cardiac complications such as aortic insufficiency, fistulas, coronary compromise with myocardial ischemia, pericardial effusions, and tamponade.
- Infection of the aortic valve may extend distally into the aortic root.

The aortic root is notable for being one of the most commonly—and variably—diseased segments of the aorta (Table 14-1). Furthermore, root disease has a profound effect on aortic valve function, commonly necessitating concurrent surgical repair or replacement of the aortic valve. The aortic root has several very important anatomic relations that include supporting the aortic valve, giving rise to the coronary arteries, and residing entirely within the pericardial space. Hence, aortic valve insufficiency, coronary compromise with myocardial ischemia, and leakage or rupture resulting in tamponade are all regular occurrences. Aortic valvular and annular infection may extend into the aortic root, causing abscesses, fistula, dehiscence, and rupture. The aortic root is one of the principal sites of intimal tears initiating aortic dissection and the most common site of thoracic aortic aneurysms.

SINUS OF VALSALVA ANEURYSMS AND FISTULAS

Aneurysms of the sinuses of Valsalva may be single or multiple. Aneurysms of the right sinus are the most common. If it is large and bulbous, a sinus of Valsalva aneurysm may compress adjacent structures or obstruct adjacent cavities into which they prolapse. Fistulization of an aortic root sinus into an adjacent chamber may occur, again usually into the right atrium or ventricle but occasionally into the left atrium, producing a continuous murmur (Fig. 14-1).

ABSCESSES OF THE AORTIC ROOT

Endocarditis of the aortic valve or of an aortic valve replacement may extend into the aortic annulus and aortic root as an abscess. Abscesses are usually detected by echocardiography. Transesophageal echocardiography is considerably more sensitive than transthoracic echocardiography (Figs. 14-2 and 14-3). If an abscess has emptied into the bloodstream, then it appears blood filled and echolucent, and color Doppler flow mapping demonstrates flow within. If the abscess remains full of necrotic infected material, it usually is bright and complex appearing. Abscesses are notorious for breaking down and are therefore considered an indication for surgical débridement and repair.

AORTIC ROOT SURGERY

Surgery for aneurysms of the aortic root can be performed with an in-hospital and 30-day mortality of 4% (composite root replacement, 4%; valve-sparing root replacement, 3.7%), a stroke rate of 1%, and a reoperation rate for bleeding of 4%. At 5, 10, 15, and 20 years, survival rates are 93% (88%-97%), 79% (71%-87%), 67% (57%-79%), and 52% (36%-69%), respectively.[1] Freedom from other cardiovascular events is as follows: reoperation, 72% (54%-86%); endocarditis, 99% (92%-100%); and thromboembolism, 91% (77%-98%).[1] Reoperation is most commonly required because of failure of valve-sparing root reconstruction, Marfan syndrome, older age, and need for concomitant surgery for mitral insufficiency.

251

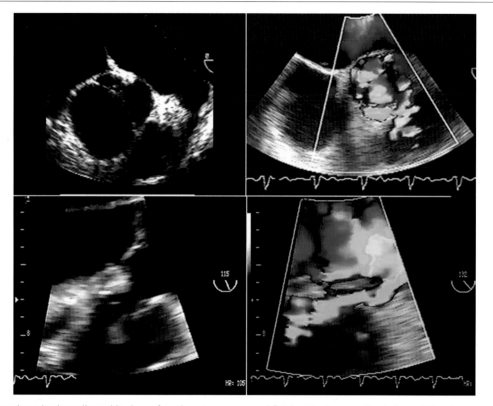

Figure 14-1. Transesophageal echocardiographic views of aortic root aneurysm and fistula. TOP, Cross-sectional views of the sinuses. BOTTOM, Oblique view of the fistula. There is asymmetric dilation of the sinuses of Valsalva, with a fistulous track into the right ventricular outflow tract. The fistulous track from the right sinus of Valsalva into the right ventricular outflow tract can be seen with 2D imaging but is far more obvious with color Doppler flow mapping.

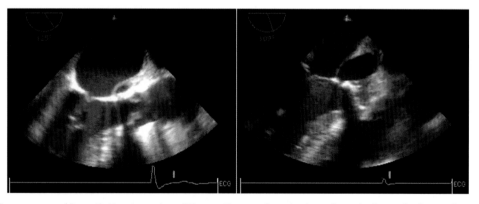

Figure 14-2. *Staphylococcus aureus* bioprosthetic valve endocarditis. LEFT, Transesophageal echocardiography long-axis view at the aortic valve level shows a small abscess cavity along the posterior wall of the aortic root, which pulses in systole. Native aortic valve viridans endocarditis. RIGHT, Transesophageal echocardiography long-axis view at the aortic valve level shows the same finding.

Table 14-1. Diseases of the Aortic Root

Aortic atherosclerotic plaques

Root and ascending aortic aneurysms

   Annuloaortic ectasia

   Post-stenotic dilation

   Bicuspid aortic valve–associated dilation

Sinus of Valsalva

   Aneurysms

   Fistula

Aortic root dissection

Traumatic disruption of the root and ascending aorta

Specific diseases

   Giant cell aortitis

   Takayasu's aortitis

   Arthropathies

   Systemic lupus erythematosus–associated aortitis

   Rheumatoid arthritis–associated aortitis

   Syphilis-associated aortitis

   Luetic aortitis

Complications of infective endocarditis

   Abscesses

   Fistula

Complications of aortic valve replacement

   Pseudoaneurysms

   Fistula

   Dissection

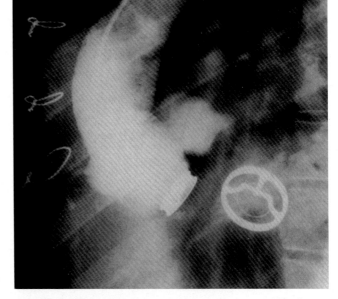

Figure 14-3. This aortogram demonstrates a large abscess within the aortic root wall, caused by *Staphylococcus aureus* endocarditis of the Bjork-Shiley aortic valve replacement. (Image courtesy of Robert J. Chisholm, MD, Toronto, Canada.)

CASE 1

History and Physical Examination

▸ A 37-year-old man with Down syndrome presented with progressive leg and scrotal swelling for 2 months.
▸ No shortness of breath or orthopnea
▸ No chest pain
▸ Normal BP, HR, RR, afebrile
▸ Obese
▸ Markedly elevated jugular venous pressure; massive leg and scrotal edema
▸ Heart sounds distant; no abnormal sounds or murmurs

Evolution and Outcome

▸ Sinus of Valsalva aneurysm, without fistula, obstructive to the right side of the heart at the tricuspid annulus level
▸ Surgical excision was discussed but declined.
▸ The patient died of gram-positive sepsis and a mixed septic and obstructive shock picture.

Comments

▸ Unusually narrow-necked and large sinus of Valsalva aneurysm, obstructing the tricuspid orifice, causing right-sided heart failure

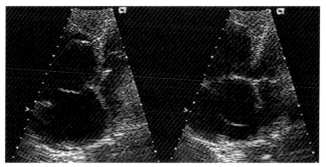

Figure 14-4. Transthoracic echocardiography, apical views in diastole (LEFT) and systole (RIGHT). A thin-walled, fluid-filled mass is seen in the right side of the heart and exhibits motion. The left panel shows the mass more apically, and the right panel shows the mass more basally.

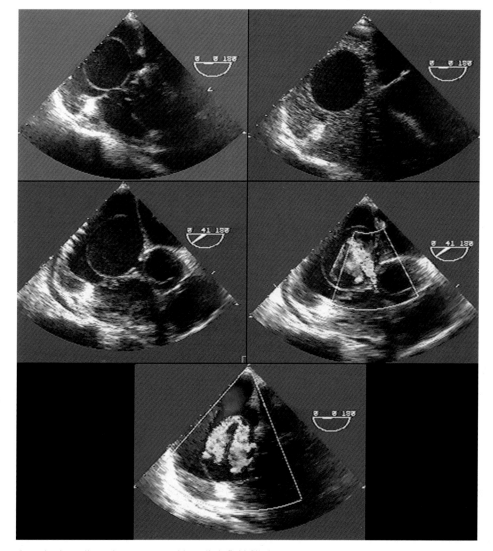

Figure 14-5. Transesophageal echocardiography. TOP LEFT, A thin-walled, fluid-filled mass is seen in the enlarged right atrium. TOP RIGHT, Injection of agitated saline contrast demonstrates that the mass does not communicate with the right side of the heart. MIDDLE LEFT, There is a communication with the aortic root. MIDDLE RIGHT, A systolic jet enters the rounded mass from the aortic root. BOTTOM, The systolic jet entering from the aortic root does not exit the cystic mass into the right atrium.

CASE 2

History and Physical Examination

▸ 31-year-old man, asymptomatic
▸ 4/6 continuous murmur at the base of the heart

Evolution and Outcome

▸ Clinical diagnosis was a bicuspid aortic valve and an aortic root to right atrium fistula.
▸ Echocardiography and catheterization confirmed the diagnosis.

▸ Surgery confirmed a bicuspid aortic valve and an aortic root to right atrium–right ventricle fistula.
▸ The fistula straddled the tricuspid valve.
▸ A small Dacron patch was used to close the defect.
▸ Uneventful postoperative course

Comments

▸ Asymptomatic but large left-to-right shunt from a sinus of Valsalva fistula
▸ Associated bicuspid aortic valve

14

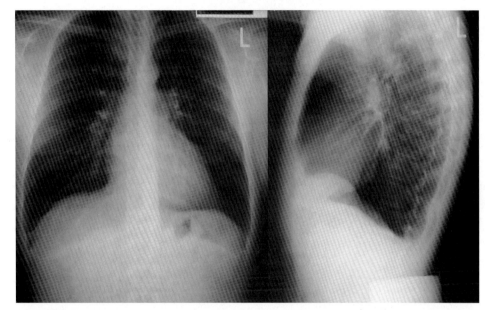

Figure 14-6. Chest radiograph shows no abnormality to the aortic contour.

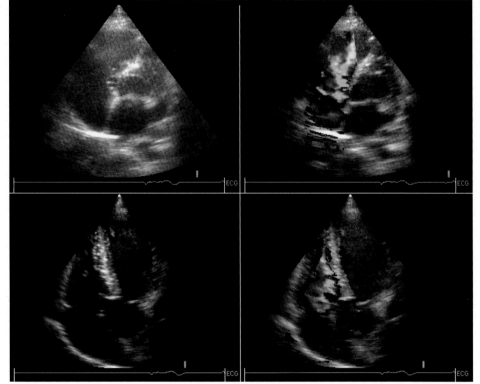

Figure 14-7. Transthoracic echocardiography. TOP, Parasternal short-axis views. BOTTOM, Apical 4-chamber views. A jet of blood flow enters the right ventricle just anterior to the tricuspid valve.

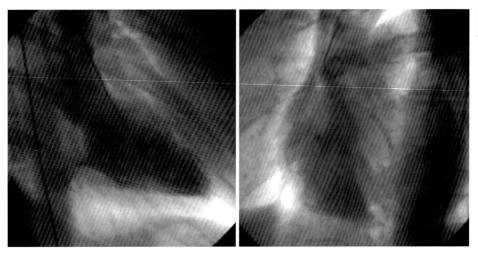

Figure 14-8. LEFT, Contrast ventriculogram. RIGHT, Aortogram. There is opacification of the right atrium from either injection.

CASE 3

History and Physical Examination

▸ 42-year-old man with a recently noted murmur
▸ No cardiovascular complaints
▸ Normal BP, HR
▸ Normal jugular pressure
▸ Continuous murmur at the base of the heart

Evolution and Management

▸ Clinical impression was that of a right sinus of Valsalva fistula into the right atrium and a trileaflet aortic valve, as confirmed by surgery.

▸ Patch closure was performed.
▸ Uneventful outcome

Comments

▸ Sinus of Valsalva fistula with mild left-sided heart volume

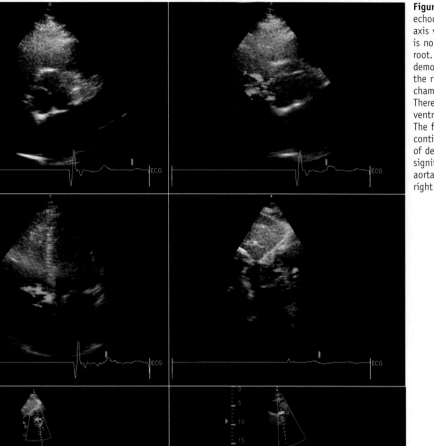

Figure 14-9. Transthoracic echocardiography. TOP, Parasternal short-axis views at the base of the heart. There is no definite abnormality of the aortic root. Color Doppler flow mapping, though, demonstrates flow from the aortic root into the right ventricle. MIDDLE LEFT, Apical 4-chamber view. MIDDLE RIGHT, Subcostal view. There is a systolic jet into the right ventricle from the aortic root. BOTTOM LEFT, The flow into the right ventricle is continuous. BOTTOM RIGHT, Suprasternal view of descending thoracic aortic flow. There is significant flow reversal in the thoracic aorta due to the fistulous flow into the right side of the heart.

14

CASE 4

History and Physical Examination

▶ A 45-year-old man with a Bjork-Shiley aortic valve prosthesis presented with fevers and weight loss.
▶ Blood cultures yielded *Enterococcus*.
▶ There was no clinical evidence of heart failure.
▶ Initial echocardiography confirmed normal functioning of the aortic prosthesis and the lack of aortic insufficiency.

Management

▶ It was decided to treat the valve conservatively (nonsurgically).
▶ An 8-week course of IV antibiotics was initiated.
▶ The patient presented 6 weeks later with presyncope.

▶ The blood pressure was 60/– mm Hg, and there was evidence of shock.

Evolution and Outcome

▶ Emergent surgery was performed.
▶ The aortic root was circumferentially an abscess.
▶ There was little viable tissue to provide anchor to surgical repair.
▶ The patient did not survive surgery.

Comments

▶ The perfidious nature of medical treatment of mechanical valve replacement endocarditis is evident.
▶ The entire aortic root was destroyed and rendered nonviable by the endocarditis.

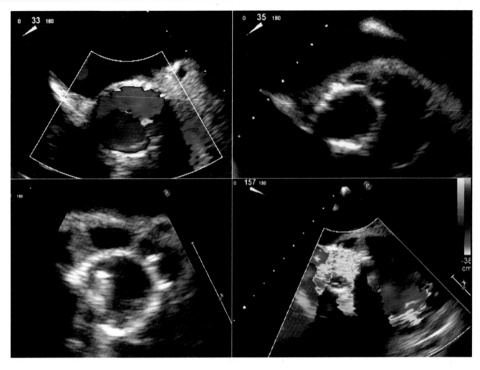

Figure 14-10. TOP LEFT, Transesophageal echocardiographic image during the initial hospitalization. The aortic root is normal in appearance. TOP RIGHT, On representation, there is a large lucent crescent surrounding the aortic valve, consistent with an aortic root abscess. BOTTOM LEFT, Further depiction of the complex root abscess. BOTTOM RIGHT, Severe aortic insufficiency and flow around the aortic valve.

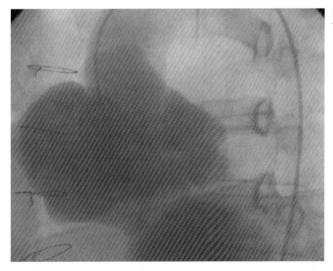

Figure 14-11. The aortogram shows an enormous and complex cavity around the aortic root and severe aortic insufficiency into the left ventricle.

Reference

1. Zehr KJ, Orszulak TA, Mullany CJ, et al: Surgery for aneurysms of the aortic root: a 30-year experience. Circulation 2004;110:1364-1371.

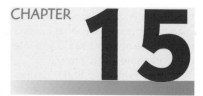

Congenital Bicuspid Aortic Valve–Associated Aortopathy

The prevalence of congenital bicuspid aortic valves is 0.5% to 2% of the adult population (2% of men, <0.5% of women).[1] This makes bicuspid valves one of the two most common forms of congenital heart disease recognized in adulthood, the other being atrial septal defects (Fig. 15-1). Bicuspid and unicuspid valves are probably the most common lesion responsible for aortic valve replacement in men.[2]

The clinical significance of bicuspid valves is manifold. They may become symptomatic from dysfunction (usually stenosis) or infection. They may be associated with significant cardiac or aortic and other vascular anomalies. Associated aortic anomalies and complications may be more clinically significant than the bicuspid valve lesion itself is; hence, the presence of a bicuspid valve should be recognized and aortic associations excluded.

The incidence of aortic dissection is 10 times greater in patients with bicuspid aortic valves.[3,4] A bicuspid aortic valve appears to compound the aortic risks of Marfan syndrome and pregnancy.[5] The presence of a bicuspid aortic valve and advanced age are more important risk factors for the development of aortic wall complications than are hemodynamic severity and prior surgical or angioplasty repair.[6]

The concept of an aortopathy associated with bicuspid aortic valves and due to a common error to explain the dilation, coarctation, and medial degeneration from which aneurysms and dissection arise has been proposed for decades and is increasingly

supported.[7] The concept of aortopathy proposes to explain the incidence of type or distal aortic dissection in patients with bicuspid aortic valves and the abnormal elasticity of the aorta in patients with nonstenotic bicuspid aortic valves.[8] Furthermore, approximately half of young people with functional disturbance associated with their bicuspid aortic valve have dilation of the ascending portion of the aorta.[9]

Bicuspid aortic valves and Marfan syndrome are the most common congenital and hereditary causes of aortic dissection. The incidence of bicuspid valves greatly exceeds that of Marfan syndrome (1% to 2% versus 0.01%).

In children and adolescents, specific cardiac, noncardiac, and coarctation associations appear to depend on the pattern of commissural fusion: right-left, right-noncoronary, or left-noncoronary (Table 15-1).[10]

CLINICAL PRESENTATIONS OF BICUSPID AORTIC VALVES

Aortic abnormalities associated with bicuspid aortic valves include dilation or aneurysm of the ascending aorta, the ascending aorta and the aortic root, or just the aortic root; aortic dissection; aortic rupture; coarctation of the aorta (50% to 80% of coarctation cases have an associated bicuspid aortic valve); and interruption of the aorta (35% of interruption cases have an associated bicuspid aortic valve).[1]

The most important cardiac presentations of bicuspid aortic valves include aortic stenosis and aortic insufficiency. Aortic stenosis is far more common than aortic insufficiency. Mixed aortic valve disease occurs. Pure aortic insufficiency begets the question of infectious endocarditis.

Other presentations of bicuspid aortic valves include infectious endocarditis, isolated ventricular septal defect, patent ductus arteriosus, and stroke. Bicuspid valves may also be discovered as an incidental finding and have normal function.

The site of dilation of the aorta associated with bicuspid aortic valves is usually the ascending aorta above the sinotubular

junction (44%), but it may include the sinotubular junction (15%), sinuses (20%), or annulus (7.5%).[9]

A bicuspid valve is suggested on physical examination by the presence of an ejection click or a systolic ejection murmur. However, a well-functioning bicuspid valve may be inaudible.

Echocardiography is the usual diagnostic test. Transthoracic echocardiography is usually adequate; transesophageal echocardiography offers an incremental yield. Steady-state free precession magnetic resonance imaging and gated cardiac computed tomography are also able to image the aortic valve. Some cases will remain ambiguous despite imaging. On the parasternal long-axis view, thickening may be present, an eccentric closure point (>1.5 : 1) is seen in some cases, and doming is often seen. Parasternal short-axis imaging reveals the elliptical orifice (football or fish mouth shaped) in *systole* (Fig. 15-2).

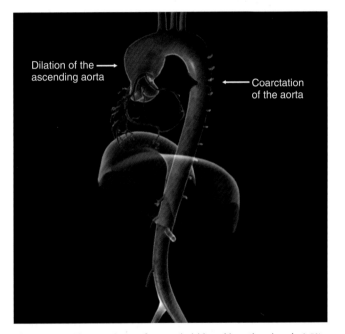

Figure 15-1. The prevalence of congenital bicuspid aortic valves is 0.5% to 2% of the adult population, making it one of the two most common forms of congenital heart disease recognized in adulthood.

Table 15-1. Cardiac, Noncardiac, and Coarctation Associations in Children and Adolescents with Bicuspid Valves

	Total	Valve Morphology		
		R-L	R-N	L-N
Isolated bicuspid valve	569	59%	40%	2%
Aortic coarctation	295	89%	11%	1%
Left-sided heart defects	155	79%	18%	3%
Non–left-sided heart defects	116	68%	31%	1%
All patients	1135	70%	28%	1%

R-L, right-left; R-N, right-noncoronary; L-N, left-noncoronary.
From Fernandes SM, Sanders SP, Khairy P, et al: Morphology of bicuspid aortic valve in children and adolescents. J Am Coll Cardiol 2004;44:1648-1651. Copyright Elsevier, 2004.

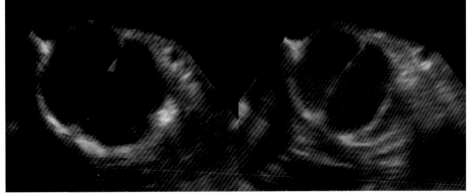

Figure 15-2. Bicuspid aortic valve. Left image (diastole) demonstrates two cusps and two sinuses. Right image (systole) reveals the elliptical orifice.

PROGRESSIVE DILATION OF THE AORTA

Progressive dilation of the proximal aorta occurs in patients with bicuspid aortic valves.[11] Sinus of Valsalva and sinotubular junction dilate at the rate of +0.5 mm/year; the ascending aorta dilates +0.9 mm/year. If the aortic root is dilated in the setting of a bicus-

pid aortic valve, it appears that the proximal aorta may continue to dilate, whether or not aortic stenosis or aortic insufficiency is surgically corrected.[12] In those cases, the ascending aorta may continue to dilate at a rate of +0.08 mm/year. Hypertension increases the rate of aortic dilation in the setting of bicuspid valves.[13] In normotensive individuals, the rate of dilation is +1.25 mm/year, which increases to +2.85 mm/year in hypertensive persons.

15

CASE 1

History

▸ 48-year-old man referred for evaluation of coronary artery disease (CAD)
▸ Previous anteroseptal myocardial infarction, class II angina since; NYHA class I shortness of breath
▸ CAD risk factors present: smoking, dyslipidemia; no hypertension
▸ No cardiovascular disease or peripheral vascular disease

Physical Examination

▸ BP 150/80 mm Hg, HR 60 bpm
▸ Normal carotid contour and volume
▸ Apex enlarged and displaced
▸ Mesoapical impulse present
▸ 3/6 SEM early peaking at left upper sternal border; no murmur of aortic insufficiency
▸ S_4
▸ Normal femoral pulses

Management and Evolution

▸ Optimal management was angiography to define coronary anatomy with a view to combined aortic root surgery (possibly valve sparing) and myocardial revascularization.
▸ The patient declined further work-up and treatment other than medical management.
▸ Prescribed antianginal, lipid-lowering, ACE inhibitor, and endocarditis prophylaxis therapy

Comments

▸ Bicuspid aortic valve–associated aortopathy with an aeurysmal ascending aorta
▸ Not associated with or complicated by significant functional disturbance; therefore, the dilation is not post-stenotic
▸ No coarctation or dissection of the aneurysmal segment

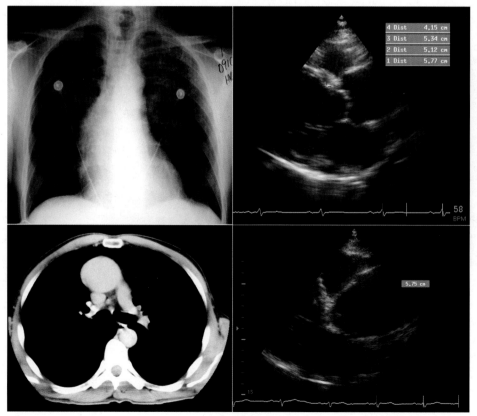

Figure 15-3. TOP LEFT, Chest radiograph shows mild cardiomegaly. Hilar overlay sign is present—the right hilum is obscured by an enlarged ascending aorta. Normal contour of the descending aorta. No rib notching. TOP RIGHT, Parasternal long-axis view of the ascending aorta, which is dilated, as is the root. The aortic valve is thickened. BOTTOM LEFT, Contrast-enhanced CT scan shows dilation of the ascending aorta but not of the descending aorta. No intimal flap. BOTTOM RIGHT, Right parasternal view of the ascending aorta, which again shows the ascending aortic dilation and no flap.

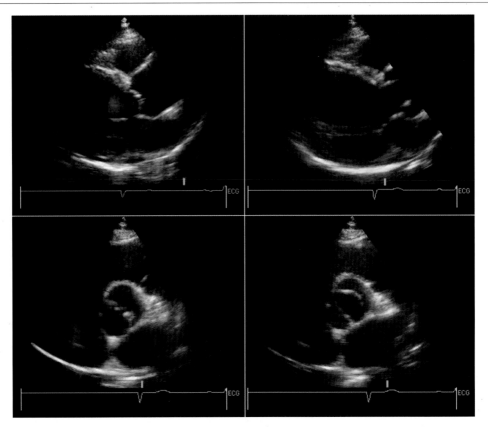

Figure 15-4. Transthoracic echocardiography. Parasternal long-axis views (TOP) and short-axis views (BOTTOM) demonstrate that the aortic valve is bicuspid, with a clearly elliptical orifice, but no doming.

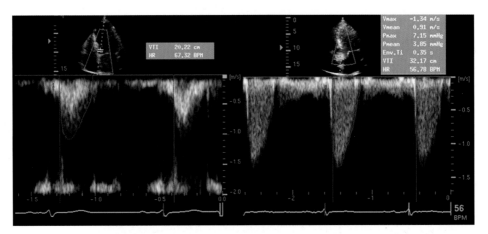

Figure 15-5. The aortic valve, although thickened, is not stenotic.

CASE 2

History

▸ 55-year-old woman, being evaluated for a murmur
▸ Smoker, hypertensive, receiving ACE inhibitor therapy
▸ No history of chest pains
▸ No shortness of breath, paroxysmal nocturnal dyspnea, edema
▸ Left calf claudication at 300 meters
▸ No family history of Marfan syndrome

Physical Examination

▸ Slim
▸ BP 165/90 mm Hg, HR 75 bpm
▸ Normal carotid pulses, left carotid bruit
▸ 2/6 SEM, 1/4 murmur of aortic insufficiency
▸ Normal apex
▸ Right femoral bruit and reduced pulse
▸ Absent right pedal and post-tibial pulses

▸ Good capillary filling
▸ No acute or chronic ischemic changes

Management and Outcome

▸ The aortic root was electively and uneventfully repaired with a tube (noncomposite) graft.
▸ The aortic valve was left in situ because it functioned well, other than mild insufficiency; thus, anticoagulation could be avoided.
▸ Endocarditis prophylaxis for the bicuspid aortic valve

Comments

▸ Bicuspid aortic valve–related aortopathy with aneurysmal dilation of the ascending aorta, complicated by localized chronic dissection within the aneurysm
▸ No associated coarctation responsible for her hypertension
▸ The timing of the occurrence of the dissection within the aneurysm remained unknown.

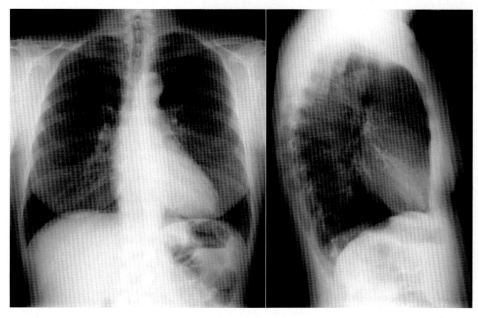

Figure 15-6. Chest radiographs show the hilar overlay sign of ascending aortic dilation, normal aortic knob (distal arch), mild cardiomegaly, and no coarctation signs.

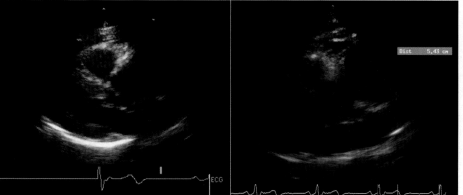

Figure 15-7. Transthoracic echocardiography, parasternal long-axis view (LEFT) and high left view (RIGHT). There is aneurysmal dilation of the ascending aorta (5.4 cm). No definite abnormalities within the aorta. The aortic valve is thickened.

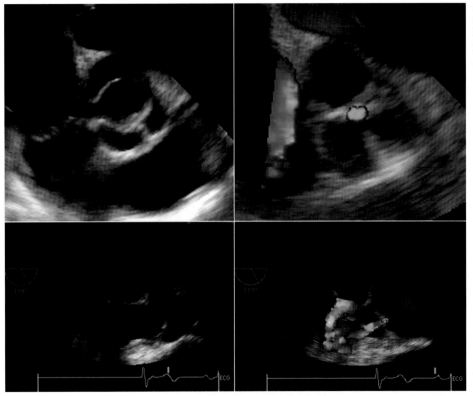

Figure 15-8. Transesophageal echocardiographic views. There is a bicuspid aortic valve with a raphe. The systolic orifice configuration is elliptical. There is a small central jet of aortic insufficiency. The valve domes in systole.

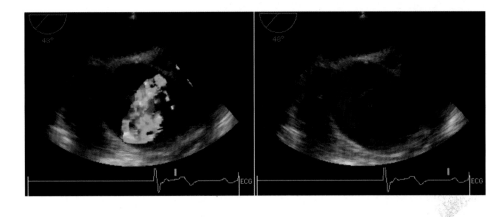

Figure 15-9. Transesophageal echocardiographic views of the ascending aorta. Dilated ascending aorta with a posterior dissection flap that partitions flow. The intimal flap is located only in the ascending portion and does not extend farther than the pulmonary artery level.

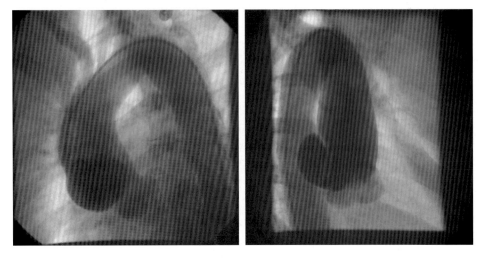

Figure 15-10. Aortography shows a dilated ascending aorta with retention of dye in the ascending aorta. An intimal flap is seen on the oblique view. Normal sinuses of Valsalva. No aortic insufficiency.

CASE 3

History

▸ A 62-year-old woman underwent remote repair of coarctation at 14 years; no specific details available.
▸ Normotensive until 55 years of age, then developed mild hypertension, controlled with an ACE inhibitor and assumed to be essential
▸ Known bicuspid aortic valve with mild insufficiency

Management

▸ Medical blood pressure control
▸ Endocarditis prophylaxis (for both the coarctation and the aortic valve)

Comments

▸ Small residual coarctation in the proximal descending aorta

15

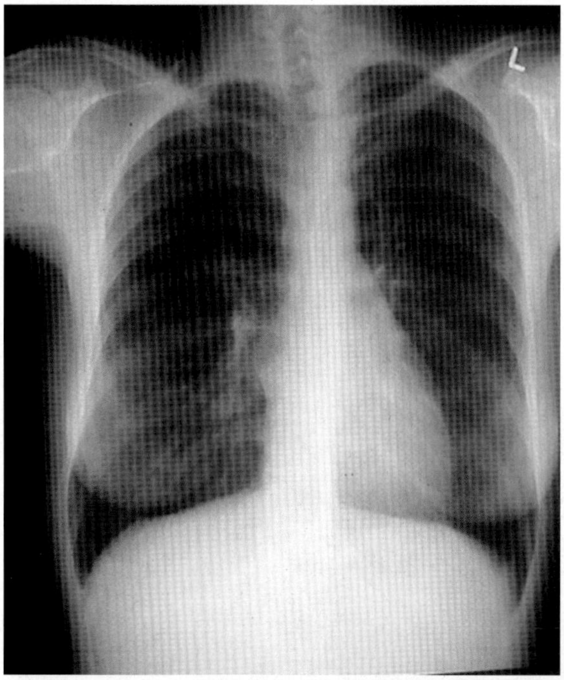

Figure 15-11. Chest radiograph shows normal heart size, normal aortic contour, and no rib notching.

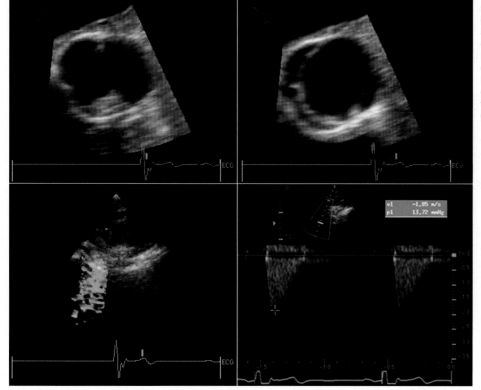

Figure 15-12. TOP, Diastolic (LEFT) and systolic (RIGHT) transesophageal echocardiographic zoom views of the aortic valve show an elliptical systolic orifice diagnostic of a bicuspid valve. BOTTOM LEFT, Suprasternal transthoracic echocardiographic color Doppler mapping reveals turbulence in the proximal descending aorta. BOTTOM RIGHT, Continuous wave Doppler detects very little residual gradient.

CASE 4

History

▸ A 62-year-old man presented to his family physician with atypical chest pains.
▸ Echocardiography revealed a dilated aortic root.
▸ Smoker, hypertensive
▸ No peripheral vascular disease, cardiovascular disease, angina, symptoms of congestive heart failure

Physical Examination

▸ BP 145/88 mm Hg (enalapril 20 mg bid)
▸ Normal carotid upstroke, contour, volume
▸ Normal peripheral pulses
▸ 1/6 SEM; no murmur of aortic insufficiency

Management and Outcome

▸ Surgical repair was elected because of the aneurysm of the ascending aorta.

▸ As the aortic valve was dysfunctional, valve replacement was performed.
▸ Histology showed focal medial necrosis of the aortic wall.
▸ Coronary angiography was normal.
▸ Underwent uneventful Bentall composite graft procedure (mechanical aortic valve and Dacron tube graft)
▸ Discharged in 5 days on anticoagulation
▸ Endocarditis prophylaxis for the aortic valve replacement

Comments

▸ The aortopathy was more significant than the functional disturbance of the aortic valve malformation, underscoring the point that bicuspid aortic valves should be recognized and their associations evaluated.

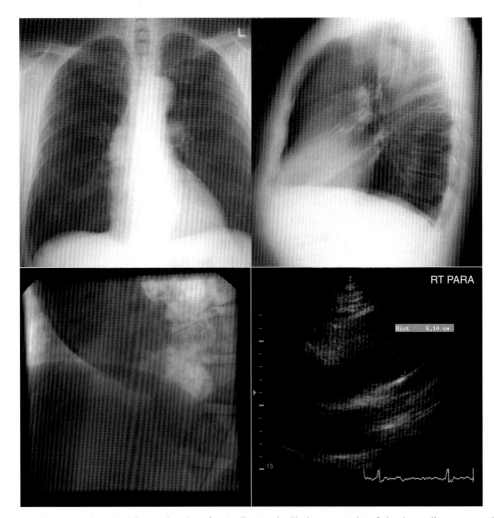

Figure 15-13. TOP, Chest radiographs show the hilar overlay sign of ascending aortic dilation, tortuosity of the descending aorta, and no rib notching. BOTTOM LEFT, Aortography shows a dilated ascending aorta and root with effacement of the sinotubular junction. Mild aortic insufficiency as well as a rightward displacement of the lateral wall of the aortic root, responsible for the overlay sign, is apparent. BOTTOM RIGHT, Right parasternal view of the ascending aorta, again underscoring the rightward displacement of enlargement of the ascending aorta.

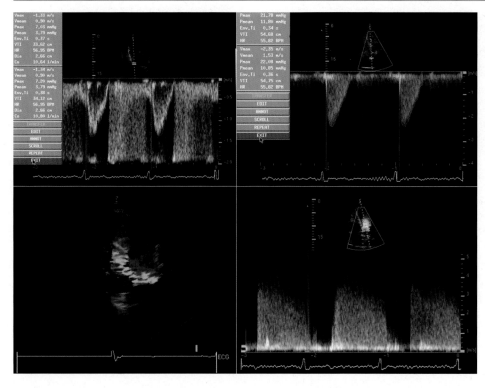

Figure 15-14. Bicuspid aortic valve hemodynamics: moderately increased total forward stroke volume (due to aortic insufficiency), no significant aortic valve gradient, and moderate aortic insufficiency by Doppler signs. The ascending aortic dilation is not associated with severe aortic stenosis (post-stenotic) and is localized rather than generalized, as is usual with severe aortic insufficiency. Therefore, the aortic enlargement has no clear relation to the aortic valve disease.

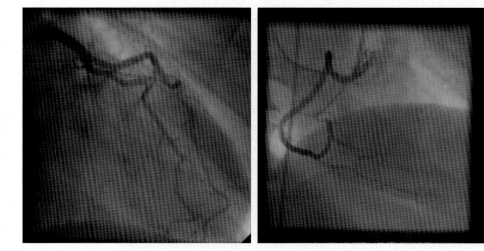

Figure 15-15. Normal left and right coronary angiography.

CASE 5

History

▸ 62-year-old man with CCS class III angina, taking medications
▸ CAD risk factors: hypertension, lifelong smoking
▸ No peripheral vascular disease or cardiovascular disease
▸ First attempt at coronary angiography foiled by inability to pass the wires from the femoral artery to the arch

Physical Examination

▸ BP 165/80 mm Hg in both arms
▸ Normal carotid upstroke and contour, increased volume
▸ 2/6 SEM, early peaking; no murmur of aortic insufficiency
▸ Normal apex
▸ Normal femoral pulses, no bruits

Comments

▸ Mild coarctation (10 mm Hg gradient) of the aorta associated with a bicuspid aortic valve, accounting for little of the hypertension

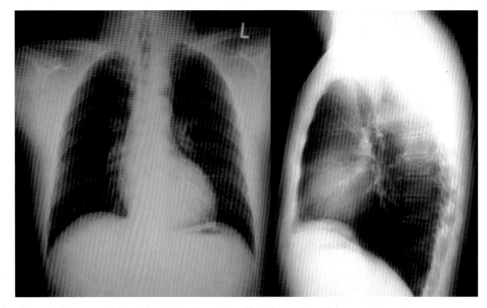

Figure 15-16. Chest radiograph shows normal heart size and aortic contour. There is no rib notching.

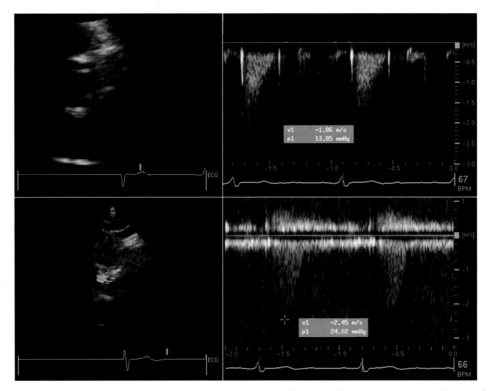

Figure 15-17. Transthoracic echocardiography. TOP, Bicuspid aortic valve without a significant gradient. BOTTOM, Suprasternal views of the proximal descending aorta. Turbulence is present, with a 24 mm Hg peak instantaneous gradient. Turbulent flow down the proximal descending aorta, which is itself poorly seen because of artifact.

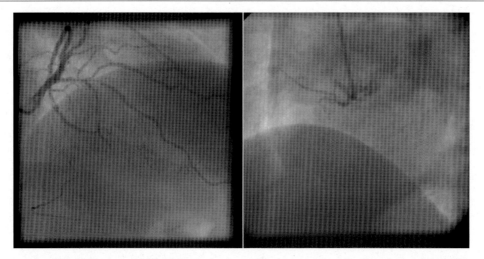

Figure 15-18. Coronary angiography shows severe proximal left anterior descending coronary artery disease and an occluded right coronary artery.

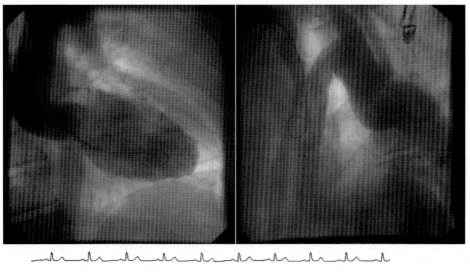

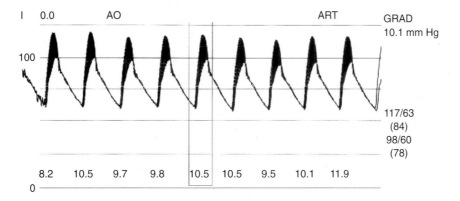

Figure 15-19. Contrast ventriculography and aortography show an abnormal elongation and angulation of the ascending aorta and a slight narrowing of the proximal descending aorta seen on the right upper image. The catheterization peak to peak gradient is 19 mm Hg, and the mean gradient is 10 mm Hg, consistent with the aortographic appearance and Doppler findings.

References

1. Cripe L, Andelfinger G, Martin LJ, et al: Bicuspid aortic valve is heritable. J Am Coll Cardiol 2004;44:138-143.

2. Roberts WC, Ko JM: Frequency by decades of unicuspid, bicuspid, and tricuspid aortic valves in adults having isolated aortic valve replacement for aortic stenosis, with or without associated aortic regurgitation. Circulation 2005;111:920-925.

3. Lindsay J Jr: Coarctation of the aorta, bicuspid aortic valve and abnormal ascending aortic wall. Am J Cardiol 1988;61:182-184.

4. Hagan PG, Nienaber CA, Isselbacher EM, et al: The International Registry of Acute Aortic Dissection (IRAD): new insights into an old disease. JAMA 2000;283:897-903.

5. Immer FF, Bansi AG, Immer-Bansi AS, et al: Aortic dissection in pregnancy: analysis of risk factors and outcome. Ann Thorac Surg 2003;76:309-314.

6. Oliver JM, Gallego P, Gonzalez A, et al: Risk factors for aortic complications in adults with coarctation of the aorta. J Am Coll Cardiol 2004;44:1641-1647.

7. McKusick VA: Association of congenital bicuspid aortic valve and Erdheim's cystic medial necrosis. Lancet 1972;1:1026-1027.

8. Grotenhuis HB, Ottenkamp J, Westenberg JJ, et al: Reduced aortic elasticity and dilatation are associated with aortic regurgitation and left ventricular hypertrophy in nonstenotic bicuspid aortic valve patients. J Am Coll Cardiol 2007;49:1660-1665.

9. Nistri S, Sorbo MD, Marin M, et al: Aortic root dilatation in young men with normally functioning bicuspid aortic valves. Heart 1999;82:19-22.

10. Fernandes SM, Sanders SP, Khairy P, et al: Morphology of bicuspid aortic valve in children and adolescents. J Am Coll Cardiol 2004;44:1648-1651.

11. Ferencik M, Pape LA: Changes in size of ascending aorta and aortic valve function with time in patients with congenitally bicuspid aortic valves. Am J Cardiol 2003;92:43-46.

12. Yasuda H, Nakatani S, Stugaard M, et al: Failure to prevent progressive dilation of ascending aorta by aortic valve replacement in patients with bicuspid aortic valve: comparison with tricuspid aortic valve. Circulation 2003;108(Suppl 1):II291-II294.

13. Kuralay E, Demirkilic U, Ozal E, et al: Surgical approach to ascending aorta in bicuspid aortic valve. J Card Surg 2003;18:173-180.

CHAPTER 16

Coarctation and Atresia of the Aorta

KEY POINTS

▸ Coarctation is a congenital narrowing of the aorta accounting for approximately 5% of congenital heart disease cases.

▸ Coarctation is often accompanied by other congenital cardiovascular malformations.

▸ There are infantile and adult types.

▸ It is often complicated by hypertension, stroke, congestive heart failure, and aortic dissection.

▸ The morphologic features of coarctation are readily recognized by TEE, CT, MRI, and aortography; the physiologic changes are diagnosed by echocardiography, MRI, and cardiac catheterization.

▸ Standard treatment of severe coarctation is surgery.

▸ The role of interventional techniques varies, depending on the center.

▸ Roles of angioplasty and stenting are evolving.

Coarctation is a congenital narrowing of the aorta, with variable location, length severity (gradient), and associated cardiovascular lesions. Coarctation accounts for approximately 5% of congenital heart disease cases. One half of coarctation cases occur without cardiac association (simple coarctation), and the other half have associated cardiac defects (complex coarctation).

Atresia is an interruption of the aorta characterized by complete luminal and anatomic discontinuity of the aorta. Interruption of the aorta may occur in several patterns. Interruption of the proximal descending aorta is the most common, although the arch and the abdominal and ascending aorta may also be interrupted. Interruption at each site has its specific clinical characteristics, if not classification and associations. For example, interruption of the aortic arch may occur distal to the left subclavian artery (type A), between the left subclavian artery and the left carotid artery (type B), or between the innominate artery and the left carotid artery (type C). Interruption of the aortic arch is usually associated with cardiac (bicuspid aortic valves are usual) and other vascular defects.[1]

Pseudocoarctation is a term used for folding, kinking, or buckling of the aorta resulting in a shelf that arises on the inside curvature, which mimics a coarctation narrowing but does not cause a gradient and is due only to excess elongation of the aorta (Figs. 16-1 and 16-2).

ETIOLOGY OF COARCTATION OF THE AORTA

The etiology of coarctation is unknown. The ductal theory proposes that contractile ductal tissue extended onto the periductal aorta, and when the ductus arteriosus contracted, the ductal tissue on the aorta contracted as well, narrowing it. Abnormal migration of ductal cells underlies this theory, which is supported by the temporal association of development of coarctation as the patent ductus arteriosus closes. This theory, however, cannot account for abdominal coarctation. The flow theory proposes that severe left-sided heart obstructive lesions reduce the flow into the aorta, leading to hypoplasia and narrowing.

TYPES OF COARCTATION OF THE AORTA AND ASSOCIATED ANOMALIES

The classic form of coarctation of the aorta is a discrete narrowing, which is visible as an indentation and located by (before, at,

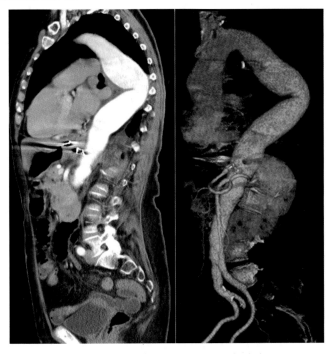

Figure 16-1. Contrast-enhanced CT images. LEFT, Sagittal view. RIGHT, Three-dimensional (3D) reconstruction. The aorta is aneurysmal in the ascending segment and is elongated and thereby unfolded, resulting in a kinked segment that by two-dimensional (2D) imaging suggests a coarctation; but there is no gradient, and the origin of the lesion is aneurysmal disease, not congenital coarctation.

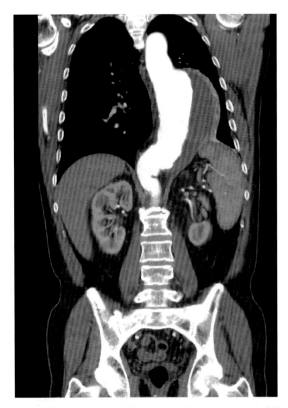

Figure 16-2. Contrast-enhanced CT scan revealing an aneurysm of the thoracic aorta (with a large volume of mural thrombus) and elongation and folding of the aorta at the diaphragmatic level with a shelf on the inside curvature due to the elongation of the aorta (pseudocoarctation).

or beyond) the aortic end of the ductus arteriosus. The infantile form of coarctation is preductal or juxtaductal. The adult form of coarctation is postductal. Typically, there is post-stenotic dilation that appears as a shelf that extends posteriorly and laterally into the aortic lumen. Atypical forms occur with longer lengths of narrowing and unusual location (arch, ascending aorta–arch, abdominal aorta).

Associated intracardiac lesions include bicuspid aortic valves, ventricular septal defects (VSDs), mitral valve defects, left-sided heart obstructive lesions, and many other lesions. Extracardiac (vascular) lesions include patent ductus arteriosus, "berry" aneurysms of intracranial arteries, and brachiocephalic vessel anomalies.

Bicuspid aortic valves are the most common association and are seen in 50% to 80% of infants with coarctation of the aorta. The presence of a bicuspid aortic valve and advanced age are more important risk factors for the development of aortic wall complications than are hemodynamic severity and prior surgical or angioplasty repair.[2] VSDs are typically perimembranous and large, with posterior infundibular malalignment and tendency to cause left ventricular outflow tract obstruction. Mitral valve defects include stenosis, parachute valve, and supravalvular stenosis. Patent ductus arteriosus is the most common associated vascular malformation, and its status is very important. Berry aneurysms of intracranial arteries are common.

The most important determinants of the pathophysiologic process are the severity of the coarctation, the relation of the coarctation to the ductus arteriosus, the acuity or chronicity of the lesion, and the associated cardiac malformations.

In the infantile form of coarctation (preductal, juxtaductal) of the aorta, the ductus arteriosus is supplying desaturated blood to the lower extremities and conferring differential cyanosis but maintaining blood flow to the lower half of the body. Spontaneous closure of the ductus arteriosus leads to ischemia of the kidneys and lower body and ductal shock. Prostaglandin E_1 infusion to reopen the ductus is lifesaving. Supplemental oxygen may cause the ductus to close and is therefore contraindicated. Associated cardiac dysfunction and malformations may complicate the hemodynamics; afterload mismatch from the hypertension may result in pulmonary edema and heart failure, and diastolic dysfunction of the left ventricle from left ventricular hypertrophy (LVH) or secondary endocardial fibroelastosis may occur.

In the adult form (postductal type), blood flow to the lower extremities is reduced, depending on the severity of the coarctation lesion and the degree of collaterals that have formed. As with the infantile form, associated cardiac dysfunction and malformations may complicate the hemodynamics (afterload mismatch from hypertension and diastolic dysfunction from LVH). Alleviation of the coarctation gradient does not necessarily alleviate hypertension, as intrinsic vascular abnormalities persist.

Clinical presentations of coarctation of the aorta depend on the age and type (infantile versus adult), the severity, and the associated cardiac malformations. In the infantile form, most cases are symptomatic because of heart failure. Some will present critically in ductal shock with acute heart failure and acidosis.

Many older children, adolescents, and young adults are asymptomatic and present with hypertension or murmurs or occasionally because of incidental detection of findings on chest radiography or echocardiography.

Prognosis of Coarctation of the Aorta

About 80% of untreated patients die by 50 years of age. Deaths occur from stroke (often hemorrhagic; death may occur from associated berry aneurysms), aortic dissection (from hypertension ± dilation of the ascending aorta), congestive heart failure (from hypertension ± bicuspid aortic valve lesions such as aortic stenosis and aortic insufficiency), and coronary artery disease (accelerated because of the hypertension).

PHYSICAL DIAGNOSIS FINDINGS OF COARCTATION OF THE AORTA

- Shock in some infant cases
- Differential cyanosis in infantile cases, and differential cyanosis and clubbing in long-term survivors with the infantile form
- Reduced or absent and delayed femoral and pedal pulses with strong upper extremity pulses
- Right arm cyanosis suggests an associated arch vessel anomaly, such as a right subclavian artery origin distal to the site of coarctation.
- Systolic ejection murmur from the coarctation may be heard anteriorly and also posteriorly, by the tip of the left scapula.
- Holosystolic murmurs are usually from an associated VSD.
- A continuous murmur may result from a tight coarctation or from large collaterals (which also may produce a sustained hum).
- Abnormalities imparted by associated cardiac malformations and complications

Collateral Vessel Formation

Collateral vessels form in the long term. Their absence in infants contributes to the intolerance of the hemodynamic disturbances imparted by the coarctation. Collaterals form to deliver blood to the descending aorta and its vascular distribution. The principal collateral beds are subclavian collaterals (internal thoracic arteries and transverse subscapular arteries), intercostal collaterals, vertebral arteries, and anterior spinal arteries. Collateral vessels can become very large and tortuous, even aneurysmal, and may generate an audible hum. Intercostal collaterals commonly produce notching because of their tortuosity, eroding adjacent bone, and reactive sclerosis. Intercostal collaterals are seen posteriorly along the inferior margin of the fifth to eighth ribs.

IMAGING OF COARCTATION OF THE AORTA

Physical examination findings and clinical context are indicators of the presence of coarctation, but ultimately the anatomic lesion and its hemodynamic severity need to be documented and the complications and associations determined. No single test reliably offers all of this information; therefore, proficiency with different

Table 16-1. Electrocardiographic and Chest Radiographic Findings in Coarctation of the Aorta

Electrocardiographic Findings	Chest Radiographic Findings
Arrhythmias are uncommon	Cardiac findings
In infants	In infants, there is almost always cardiomegaly.
RVH and RAD are usual.	In adults, heart size may be normal or increased.
LVH with strain is uncommonly seen in simple coarctation and suggests concurrent aortic stenosis.	Aortic findings
In older children and adults	Not seen in infants but are seen in older children and adults
LVH is common.	The figure-of-3 sign on the frontal chest radiograph is suggestive of coarctation and is due to pre-coarctation dilation of the aorta (and left subclavian artery), the site of narrowing, and post-stenotic dilation of the aorta.
RVH suggests a VSD or pulmonary hypertension.	Other vascular findings
	Rib notching of the fifth to eighth ribs is seen in one third of older children and adults with postductal coarctation.
	Pulmonary findings
	Findings of heart failure may be present.

LVH, left ventricular hypertrophy; RAD, right axis deviation; RVH, right ventricular hypertrophy; VSD, ventricular septal defect.

modalities is important. Electrocardiographic and chest radiographic findings in coarctation of the aorta are summarized in Table 16-1. Although the chest radiograph may suggest coarctation, it is not a sufficient or reliable test for this diagnosis or its associations (Figs. 16-3 to 16-9).

Echocardiography for Coarctation of the Aorta

Transthoracic echocardiography (TTE) is often able to detect, localize, and hemodynamically characterize coarctation of the aorta and its associated cardiac abnormalities. The smaller body size of infants and children and the regularity of the diagnosis among that population make echocardiography in the pediatric population very polished. In older children and adults, owing to larger body size, obesity, lung disease, and lesser incidence of coarctation and therefore proficiency with the diagnosis, the success of echocardiography is less. The most useful view is the suprasternal view. One aspect of the suprasternal 2D view that is vexing in regard to imaging an interruption of the proximal descending aorta is that the view, normally oblique, emerges out the side of the aorta in the proximal or mid descending portions; thus, a normal aorta and a complete coarctation or interrupted aorta look similar, and neither would have a conspicuous jet of blood flow acceleration to be imaged or recorded. Only some cases of interruption have a clearly abnormal proximal segment that is obvious by TTE.[1]

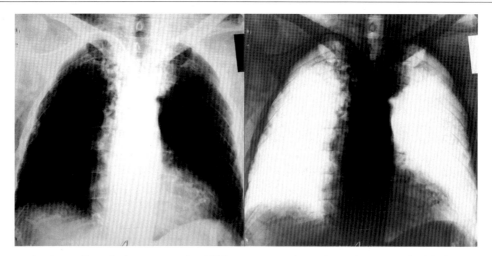

Figure 16-3. Anteroposterior chest radiographs (overpenetrated and high contrast to enhance the aortic contour; the right image is black-white inverted). The indentation of the coarctation is evident, as is the dilated pre-coarctation segment and left subclavian artery.

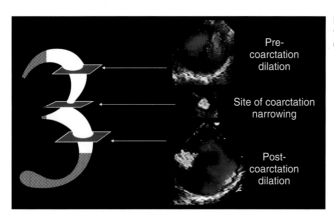

Pre-coarctation dilation

Site of coarctation narrowing

Post-coarctation dilation

Figure 16-4. The basis of the figure-of-3 sign is demonstrated by the TEE images of the aorta. Also note the narrow and high-velocity jet from the coarctation radiating into the descending aorta.

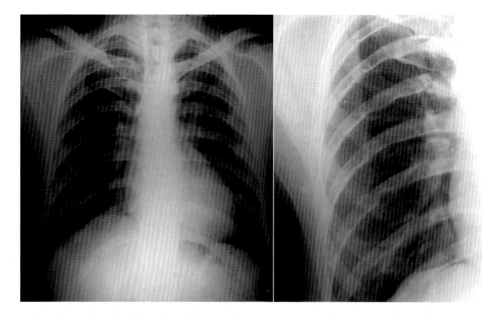

Figure 16-5. Anteroposterior chest radiographs of a patient with coarctation. LEFT, Conventional image. RIGHT, Black-white inverted. Rib notching is extensively present. The tortuosity of the enlarged collateralized subcostal arteries has resulted in rounded areas of erosion, with typical reactive sclerosis at their edges.

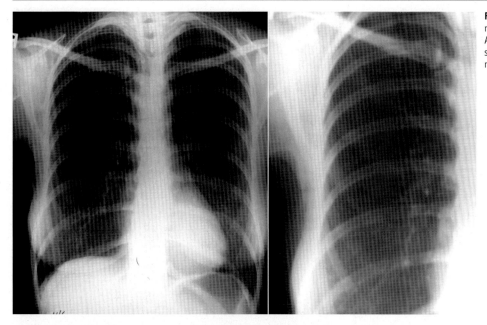

Figure 16-6. Anteroposterior chest radiographs of a patient with coarctation. Although the coarctation was tight and severe, there is very little if any rib notching.

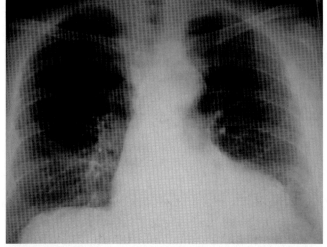

Figure 16-7. Anteroposterior chest radiograph. There is mild cardiomegaly and mild prominence of the distal arch. There is no clear figure-of-3 sign, and the rib notching is faint and partially obscured by lung markings despite the presence of severe coarctation.

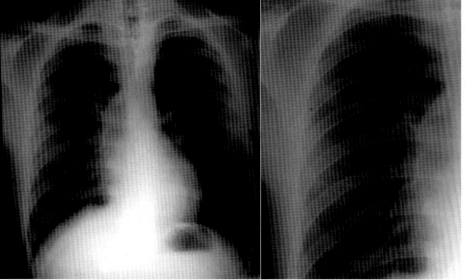

Figure 16-8. Hilar overlay sign (the dilated ascending aorta overlies the right hilum). The dilated and aneurysmal ascending aorta was associated with a bicuspid aortic valve. There is little rib notching despite the presence of significant coarctation.

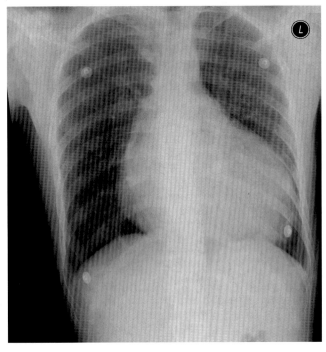

Figure 16-9. Rib notching is present bilaterally. There is significant cardiomegaly and pulmonary venous redistribution.

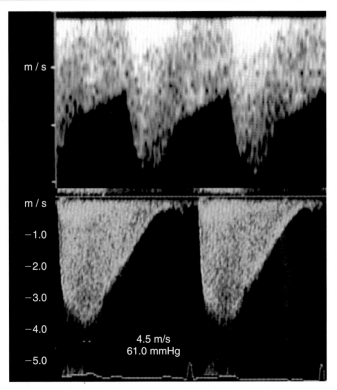

Figure 16-10. TTE suprasternal recording of flow velocity across coarctation. TOP, Note the elevated systolic velocity and widened spectral profile, continuous through diastole. BOTTOM, Note the widened spectral profile, continuing into diastole.

Two-dimensional images may reveal the narrowing in infants but are of limited usefulness in adults. Color Doppler mapping shows acceleration that correlates with the beginning of the coarcted segment.

Continuous wave Doppler interrogation sampled from the suprasternal position yields determination of gradients that correlate with catheterization measurements of gradients; but in the presence of complete coarctation, interruption, or atresia, the absence of a gradient is misleading as to the presence of the lesion.

In critically ill infants, echocardiography alone (without angiography) is preferable because it may obviate the need for and therefore the risks of catheterization. When echocardiography is not complete, catheterization is needed to complete the assessment.

Severe coarctation is characterized by a marked elevation of the systolic velocity across the site of coarctation, a spectral broadening of the systolic profile or increased diastolic antero-grade velocity (a diastolic tail), and a delayed upstroke of abdominal aortic flow compared with ascending aortic flow (Figs. 16-10 and 16-11).

Transesophageal echocardiography (TEE) offers little additional information in pediatric cases of coarctation, generally because TTE in experienced hands is comprehensive. In adults, TEE is better able than TTE to assess the anatomic substrate of coarctation. TEE estimates of gradient are less accurate than transthoracic estimates, as alignment for Doppler sampling occurs from limited sites. In severe coarctation, TEE often reveals portions of the bewilderingly complex collateral networks around the aorta, but never as completely as magnetic resonance imaging does (Fig. 16-12).

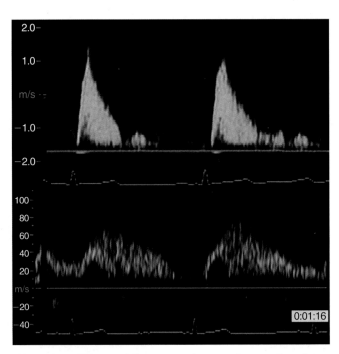

Figure 16-11. TTE spectral flow patterns in coarctation. TOP, Ascending aorta—rapid acceleration (velocity upstroke). BOTTOM, Abdominal aorta—reduced acceleration (velocity upstroke) akin to pulsus tardus.

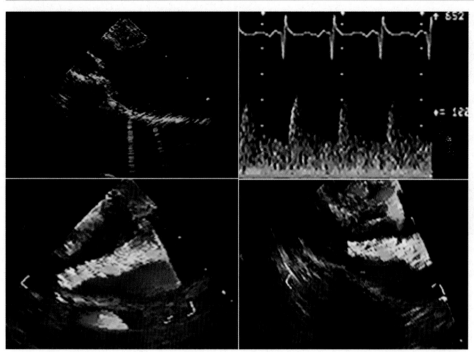

Figure 16-12. TEE views of coarctation. TOP LEFT, Longitudinal view of the proximal descending aorta revealing the narrowing of the coarctation site, with an oblique orientation and the sausage-like post-coarctation dilation. TOP RIGHT, Spectral display of continuous wave Doppler interrogation. There is continuous flow with a prominent diastolic component. Despite poor alignment for sampling, the peak velocity is more than 3 m/s, but more important, the profile is continuous with anterograde diastolic flow. BOTTOM, Color Doppler flow mapping demonstrates the jet emerging from the coarctation. The jet emerging from the coarctation is prominent but eccentric because of the oblique orientation of the coarctation segment. Between the aorta and the TEE probe are collaterals revealed by flow mapping.

Magnetic Resonance Imaging for Coarctation of the Aorta

Magnetic resonance imaging (MRI), particularly the gadolinium contrast–enhanced MR angiography (MRA) technique, is able to successfully image the anatomic details of the coarcted segment, the size of the arch and isthmus of the aorta, the status of the ductus, the extent of collaterals, and the associated vascular and cardiac abnormalities. The velocity-encoded phase-contrast technique is able to determine the flow and gradient across the coarctation. Given the generally vertical course of the descending aorta, sagittal and parasagittal 2D T1-weighted black blood views are also suitable for depiction of the coarctation anatomy (Figs. 16-13 to 16-16).

Contrast Angiography for Coarctation of the Aorta

Angiography and catheterization for solely diagnostic purposes are avoided, especially in infants, if echocardiography allows a complete assessment of the coarctation and the associated cardiac lesions. However, angiography and catheterization should still be performed for diagnostic purposes in the following circumstances: (1) in infants, if echocardiography is incomplete or inconclusive; (2) in older children; (3) in adults, especially when MRI is not available; and (4) as a platform for interventions (Fig. 16-17). Angiography offers excellent imaging of the location and extent of coarctation, the state of development of the isthmus and of the ductus and collaterals, and the associated great vessel anomalies (Figs. 16-18 and 16-19). Catheterization may be performed by radial (anterograde catheterization) or femoral (retrograde catheterization) access, but femoral access may be more difficult because of absent pulses. Other potential

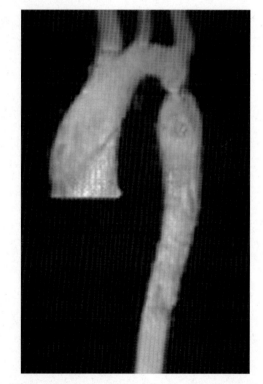

Figure 16-13. Gadolinium contrast–enhanced aortography and 3D reconstruction of the aorta. Note the coarctation, the mildly dilated ascending aorta, and the collateral vessel.

problems with retrograde catheterization include inability to pass a wire through the lesion and the catheter's increasing the gradient within the stenosis. When they are performed, catheterization and angiography form the basis of interventional techniques.

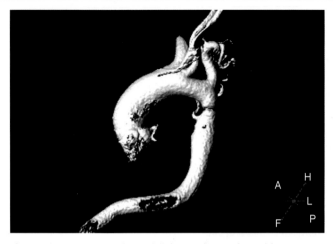

Figure 16-14. MRA. Rotating gadolinium contrast–enhanced image, allowing visualization of the aorta (aortic lumen) from different perspectives. The site of coarctation is discrete; collaterals are near it.

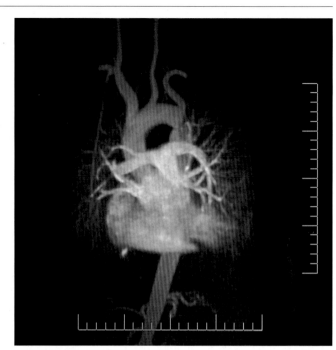

Figure 16-16. Rotating gadolinium contrast–enhanced MR aortography. The site and length of coarctation are depicted.

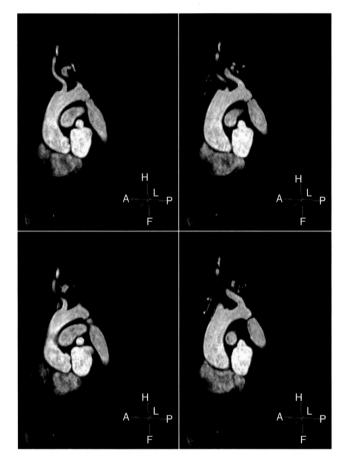

Figure 16-15. MRA. Gadolinium contrast–enhanced sequential sagittal images of the aorta. The level and length of coarctation are evident, but not the severity.

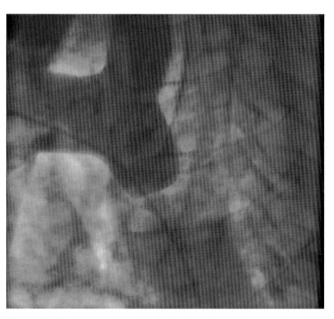

Figure 16-17. Aortography at the beginning of a stenting procedure. The catheter is through the coarctation, which is so tight that it is actually difficult to see a lumen through it. The aorta is dilated after the coarctation.

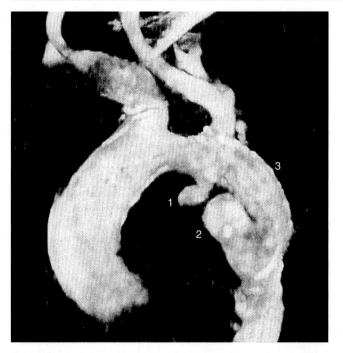

Figure 16-18. Aortography and 3D reconstruction. The excellent spatial resolution of aortography scanning is evident in this image. This 54-year-old woman with chest pain and a prior coarctation repair whose MRI and standard aortogram yielded ambiguous images underwent a 3D image reconstruction of an aortogram. The stumps of the prior repair (1 and 2) are clearly seen, as is the Dacron conduit (3). (From Boccalandro F, De La Guardia B, Smalling RW: Rotational aortogram with three-dimensional reconstruction in a case of repaired aortic coarctation. Circulation 2001;104:620-621.)

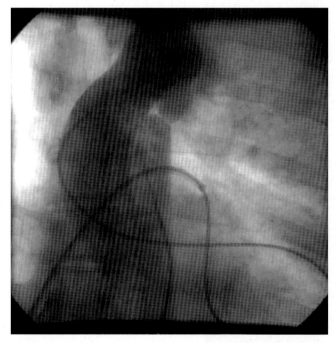

Figure 16-19. Conventional aortography. Contrast dye is being injected by transseptal catheterization. The site and length of coarctation are depicted (LEFT), as are the enlarged internal thoracic artery collaterals (RIGHT).

MANAGEMENT OF COARCTATION OF THE AORTA

16

Most infants (80%) with congestive heart failure due to coarctation will die, if they are untreated, within 12 months. Medical management is intended to improve hemodynamics and perfusion of the lower body in the short term only and potentially to allow time for the infant to grow. In cases of ductal shock, prostaglandin E_1 is infused to avoid and to treat lower extremity ischemia, renal failure, and acidosis. Many side effects do occur, although fewer with the lipid-coated form of prostaglandin E_1.

Restoration of patency of the aorta by surgery or balloon angioplasty is the priority. In infants, surgery is generally preferred to angioplasty, whose role as primary treatment is in evolution and controversial.

Balloon Angioplasty for Coarctation of the Aorta

There has been considerable evolution of interventional procedures, and there remains center-specific practice, depending on means and expertise. Initially, balloon angioplasty was the only interventional procedure available, and therefore most series reflect the much longer history of angioplasty than of stenting. The advent of stenting and more recently the availability of covered stents have substantially changed practice. There is a wide range of permutations of coarctation of the aorta that reflects the size and age of the patient and expected remaining growth of the aorta, whether the coarctation is native or previously repaired, anatomic aspects of the coarctation lesion (such as how long the segment is and how far it extends into the arch), associated vascular lesions (such as a patent ductus arteriosus), and associated cardiac lesions. Hence, treatment is highly individualized.

Balloon angioplasty is generally accepted as first-line treatment of recurrent coarctation. Surgery for recurrent coarctation is more difficult than it is for native coarctation and of higher risk because of adhesions and other technical factors; therefore, balloon angioplasty may be more favorable in this setting. Balloon angioplasty is considered a first-line treatment of some infantile cases if there are no other vascular malformations that need repair, the isthmus before the coarctation is well formed, the coarcted segment is short, and the infant is older than 12 months (or older than 6 months at some centers).

Potential complications of angioplasty include aortic rupture (<1%), aortic dissection, stroke, femoral access complications, aneurysm and false aneurysm formation (5%), and restenosis, which affects up to 50% of infants younger than 1 year.

The long-term outcome of balloon angioplasty of discrete native coarctation of the aorta in adolescents and adults suggests enduring hemodynamic success, fair clinical success in reducing blood pressure, but aneurysm and false aneurysm development in a significant number of patients, necessitating follow-up. Among 49 patients (an average of 22 ± 7 years of age initially) followed up to 15 years, there were no early or late deaths, successful reduction of the peak gradient (decreased from 66 mm Hg to 11 ± 7 mm Hg), and no restenosis (follow-up catheterization 12 months later demonstrated an average 6 ± 6 mm Hg gradient). Aneurysms developed at the site of coarctation in 7.5% of patients;

no new aneurysms developed, nor did size increase in existing ones. Blood pressure normalized in a majority (63%) of patients.[3]

Stenting for Coarctation of the Aorta

Stenting is increasingly performed for older children and adults (Fig. 16-20). Stenting is inappropriate in infants and small children because stent:body size mismatch will occur as the child grows. Percutaneous endovascular repair of aneurysms after previous coarctation surgery has been performed with considerable success. A small series of six patients (average of 49 ± 12 years of age) reported successful percutaneous placement of customized stent grafts, without interventional or 30-day complications. Follow-up during 11 to 47 months demonstrated optimal reconstruction of the aorta.[4] A larger series of 30 patients treated with covered Cheatham-platinum stents achieved nearly complete resolution of translesional gradients (36 mm Hg to 4 mm Hg; $P < .0001$) and increases in the diameter from 6 to 17 mm ($P < .0001$), with good short-term and intermediate-term clinical and radiographic stability rates and an ability to reduce or to eliminate antihypertensive medications in more than 40% of cases.[4] Covered stents are increasingly used for dilation of coarctation and for management of more complicated cases, such as with associated false aneurysms (Fig. 16-21).

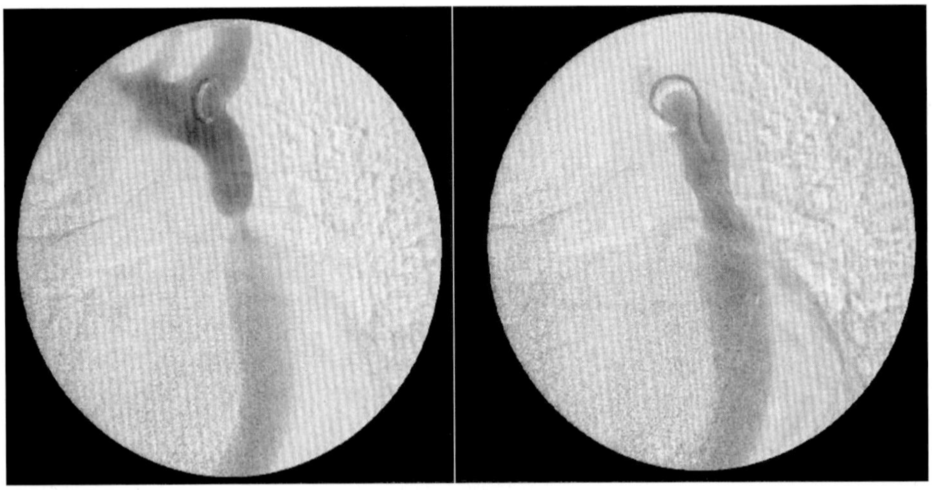

Figure 16-20. Angiographic views before (LEFT) and after (RIGHT) stenting of coarctation in an adult. The gradient has been abolished. Successful and complication-free stenting of coarctation often leaves a residual waist.

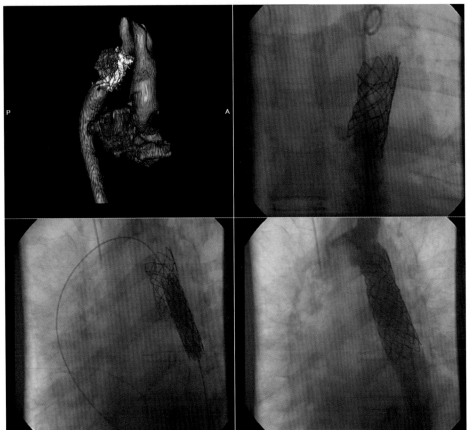

Figure 16-21. Exclusion of a false aneurysm that complicated a previous stenting of coarctation (uncovered stent). TOP LEFT, A 3D reconstruction of a contrast-enhanced CT scan. The stent is obvious. The body of the false aneurysm is apparent as the enhanced mass outside the stent. TOP RIGHT, Aortography dimly outlines the body of the false aneurysm. BOTTOM LEFT, Deployment of the covered stent. BOTTOM RIGHT, Aortography after covered stent deployment shows that the false aneurysm has been excluded. (Courtesy of Eric Horlick, MD, Toronto, Canada.)

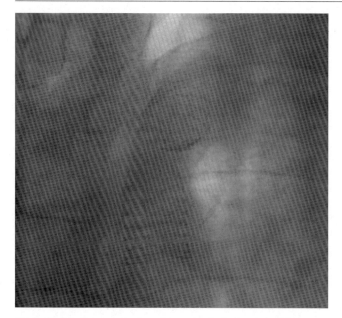

Figure 16-22. Fluoroscopic view of a previously deployed stent for coarctation that has fractured and separated. (Courtesy of Eric Horlick, MD, Toronto, Canada.)

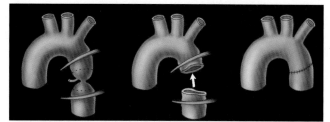

Figure 16-23. Surgical repair: end-to-end anastomosis.

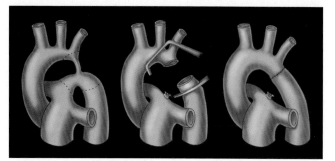

Figure 16-24. Surgical repair: extended end-to-end anastomosis.

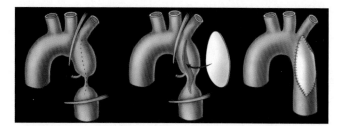

Figure 16-25. Surgical repair: prosthetic patch repair.

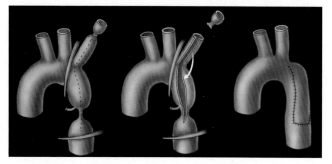

Figure 16-26. Surgical repair: left subclavian patch repair.

16

Dilation of the aorta is intended to alleviate the hemodynamic effect; it is not usually intended to quite normalize the coarcted segment to the diameter of the usually aneurysmal aorta distal to the site of coarctation. In adolescents, a stent is often oversized for the size of the patient, so that repeated dilations of the stent can be performed as needed over time until full growth of the patient and his or her aorta has occurred. Complications specific for stenting versus balloon angioplasty include stent fracture (Fig. 16-22), stent perforation of the aorta, and stent migration. Because the aorta distal to the coarctation site is usually dilated, the distal margin of the stent is often less well anchored, facilitating migration. In addition, covered stents may obstruct the true lumen of the distal arch if they are deployed too proximally. Ischemia due to left subclavian artery coverage by a covered stent is surprisingly uncommon. Stent design is under rapid evolution, and stents can be custom-made.

Surgery for Coarctation of the Aorta

Surgery is generally accepted as first-line treatment of native coarctation, especially in infants and children, but not for recurrent coarctation. Surgical techniques depend on the length of coarctation encountered, the state of the isthmus, and whether there is ductal patency. In addition to early perioperative risks, surgery is also associated with restenosis, recurrent coarctation, and late aneurysm formation.

Commonly used surgical techniques include excision of the coarcted segment with an end-to-end anastomosis (Fig. 16-23) or extended end-to-end anastomosis (Fig. 16-24) and incision across the coarcted segment with prosthetic patch insertion to increase the aortic diameter for cases in which the coarctation involves a longer segment (e.g., up into the arch). The aorta can be clamped between the left subclavian and left common carotid and obliquely along its length to enable incision along the length of the aorta and insertion of a patch along the length of the aorta.

This patch will not grow (Fig. 16-25). Uncommon techniques include left subclavian (autologous) patch aortoplasty (Fig. 16-26) and bypass technique.

Surgery for coarctation of the aorta is subject to significant complications, both early and late. Early complications include bleeding, spinal cord ischemia with paralysis, vocal cord paralysis, diaphragmatic paralysis, and paradoxical hypertension. Late complications include recurrence of coarctation as well as aneurysm and false aneurysm formation in 5% to 17% of cases (Fig. 16-27).

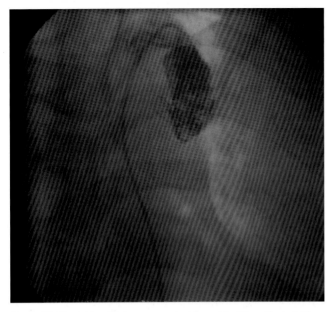

Figure 16-27. A large false aneurysm had formed in this patient at the site of previous surgical repair of coarctation. The body of the false aneurysm has been filled with coils in an attempt to embolize it and to obliterate it. Although it was largely successful, some portion of the body of the false aneurysm remained. The patient subsequently underwent exclusion of the body of the false aneurysm by deployment of a covered stent. (Courtesy of Eric Horlick, MD, Toronto, Canada.)

The mortality of surgery for coarctation of the aorta is heavily influenced by the clinical profile of the patient. In infants, surgical mortality for simple coarctation is less than 1%; coarctation with large VSD, more than 10%; and coarctation with complex cardiac anomalies, more than 15%. In older children, mortality associated with surgical correction of coarctation of the aorta is 3% to 5%.

CASE 1

History and Physical Examination

- A 5-day-old infant presented with tachypnea and poor feeding.
- There was evidence of left-sided heart failure.
- The patient was shocky and acidotic.

Management and Outcome

- There was no evidence of ductal flow.
- Closure of the ductus had resulted in poor flow to the lower body and hemodynamic distress.
- The patient was resuscitated with prostaglandin and underwent surgery the next day.

- The surgical procedure was an extended end-to-end anastomosis and ligation of the ductus.
- The patient was discharged 5 days later.

Comments

- A neonatal isolated coarctation case with a typical course, medical resuscitation, surgery, and outcome
- In neonatal coarctation, ductal flow is critical to maintain lower body perfusion, and closure of the ductus results in acidosis and shock.

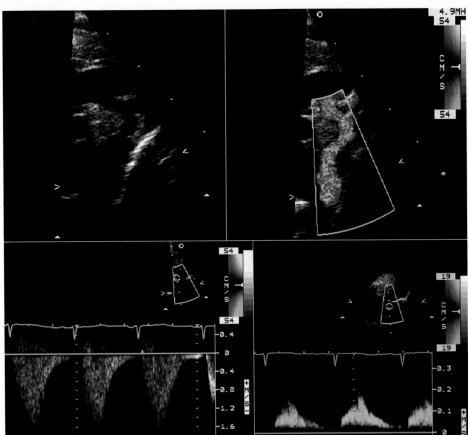

Figure 16-28. TTE suprasternal views. TOP LEFT, The aortic arch has normal diameter, but there is narrowing of the proximal descending aorta, with resumption of normal diameter. TOP RIGHT, Color Doppler flow mapping reveals turbulence along the length of narrowed aorta and continuing down into the normal segment beyond. BOTTOM LEFT, Spectral display of Doppler interrogation of the narrowed segment of the aorta. There is a diastolic tail of spectral dispersion. BOTTOM RIGHT, Spectral display of Doppler interrogation of the abdominal aorta. The upslope of the spectral profiles is delayed (tardus), consistent with upstream obstruction from the coarctation. (Courtesy of Fraser Golding, MD, Toronto, Canada.)

CASE 2

History and Physical Examination

▸ A 6-day-old infant presented with tachypnea.
▸ There was evidence of severe left-sided heart failure.
▸ TTE demonstrated severe left ventricular systolic dysfunction and preserved right ventricular systolic function.

Management and Outcome

▸ The patient underwent surgery, which consisted of an extended end-to-end anastomosis and ligation of the ductus.
▸ The patient was discharged 5 days later.

Comments

▸ An unusual hemodynamic pattern due to the combination of severe left ventricular systolic dysfunction, severe coarctation and a large ductus arteriosus, and normal right ventricle
▸ In neonatal coarctation, ductal flow is critical to maintain lower body perfusion and, in this case, also some upper body perfusion.
▸ Surgery to address the coarctation and ductus in neonatal cases

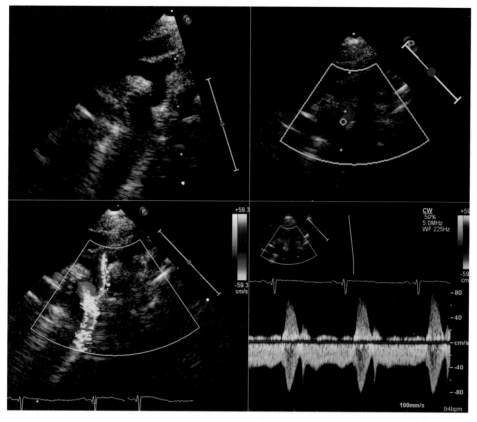

Figure 16-29. TTE suprasternal views. TOP LEFT, The aortic arch has reduced diameter, and there is a shelf in the proximal descending aorta, with resumption of normal diameter beyond. TOP RIGHT, Color Doppler flow mapping reveals anterograde flow in diastole proximal to the waist in the aorta. BOTTOM LEFT, Color Doppler flow mapping reveals systolic flow upward through the descending aorta. BOTTOM RIGHT, Spectral display of Doppler interrogation of the narrowed segment of the aorta. There is systolic flow reversal (upward) and diastolic flow downward. (Courtesy of Fraser Golding, MD, Toronto, Canada.)

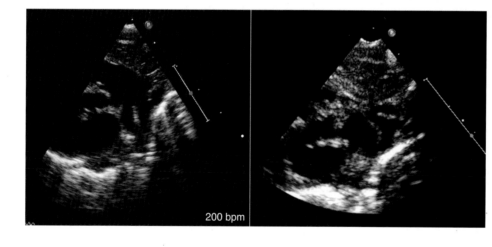

Figure 16-30. Views of the large ductus arteriosus and shelf of the coarctation. In this patient, a large ductus arteriosus (and the right ventricle) not only was sustaining flow to the lower body past the coarctation but, because of the severe left ventricular systolic dysfunction, also was delivering blood in reverse through the coarctation in systole, given the relative dominance of the right ventricle over the weakened left ventricle in this case. (Courtesy of Fraser Golding, MD, Toronto, Canada.)

CASE 3

History and Physical Examination

- A 17-year-old was found to be hypertensive (160/60 mm Hg).
- No precordial systolic ejection murmur or ejection click; no murmur of aortic insufficiency.

- There was a systolic ejection murmur between the scapulae.
- The upper body pulses had normal upslope and increased volume, and the femoral pulses were reduced and delayed.

Comments

- Stenting was elected because of the patient's adult body size.

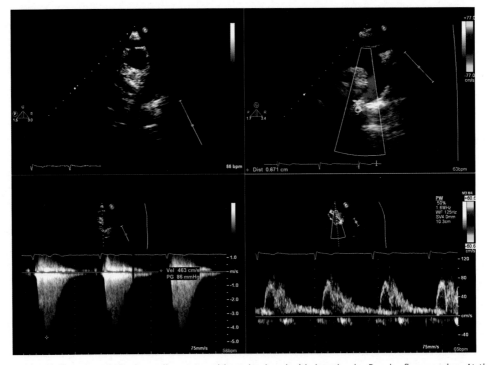

Figure 16-31. TOP, Suprasternal views toward the descending aorta, without (LEFT) and with (RIGHT) color Doppler flow mapping. At the site where there appears to be a narrowing, there is flow convergence and a proximal isovelocity surface area (PISA). BOTTOM LEFT, Continuous wave Doppler interrogation across the site of narrowing. There is spectral dispersion and a diastolic tail. The peak gradient is 86 mm Hg. BOTTOM RIGHT, Spectral profile of pulsed wave Doppler interrogation of the abdominal aortic flow demonstrates a reduced upslope and velocity, consistent with upstream fixed obstruction from the coarctation. (Courtesy of Fraser Golding, MD, Toronto, Canada.)

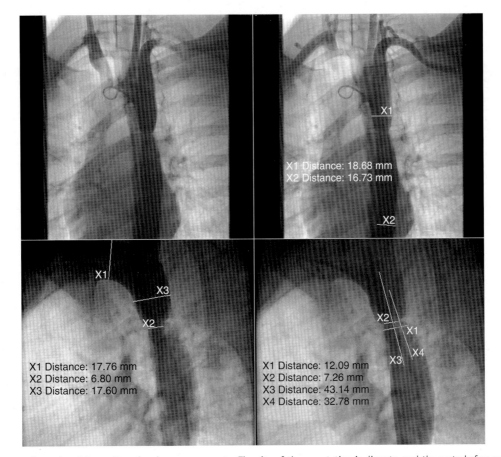

Figure 16-32. Aortography and preintervention planning measurements. The site of the coarctation is discrete, and the aorta before and after has normal caliber and appearance. (Courtesy of Fraser Golding, MD, Toronto, Canada.)

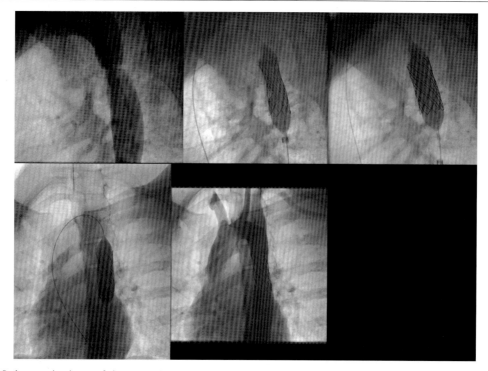

Figure 16-33. TOP, Preintervention image of the coarctation. BOTTOM, Balloon inflation and stenting of the coarctation, alleviating the obstruction (gradient) and nearly restoring normal aortic diameter. (Courtesy of Fraser Golding, MD, Toronto, Canada.)

CASE 4

History and Physical Examination

▸ A 41-year-old patient presented with atypical chest pains.
▸ Past medical history is significant for coarctation repair in childhood.
▸ BP 160/90 mm Hg, HR 67 bpm
▸ No murmurs or gallops

Comments

▸ Mild hypertension due to residual coarctation
▸ Hypertension was easily controlled with two additional antihypertensive medications.
▸ Chest pains were noncardiac and nonaortic.

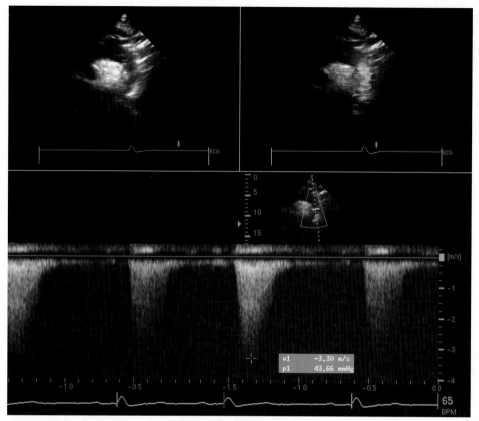

Figure 16-34. TTE suprasternal views show a largely unremarkable appearance of the arch and descending aorta by 2D imaging but turbulence suggested by color flow mapping. Continuous wave Doppler interrogation detects an approximately 45 mm Hg peak instantaneous gradient, without spectral widening or diastolic anterograde flow.

16

CASE 5

History and Physical Examination

▸ 64-year-old man presenting with chest pains of a severe but atypical nature
▸ Past medical history is significant for hypertension, dyslipidemia, and smoking.
▸ Coarctation and VSD repairs in childhood
▸ BP 175/95 mm Hg, HR 70 bpm
▸ Pulses increased; normal (not diminished) femoral pulses
▸ No murmurs
▸ S_4

Comments

▸ Mild residual gradient in the descending aorta after remote coarctation repair
▸ No dissection or rupture
▸ Three days later, shingles (herpes zoster) erupted, explaining the chest pain.
▸ With more antihypertensive medications, the BP has been controlled.

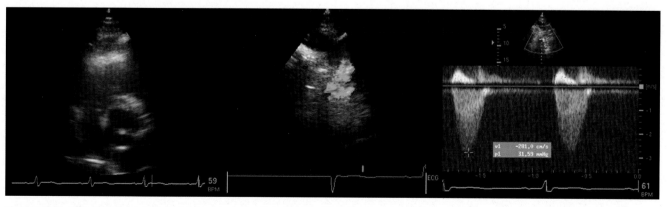

Figure 16-35. TTE. LEFT, Parasternal short-axis view demonstrates a bicuspid aortic valve. MIDDLE, Suprasternal view with color Doppler flow mapping suggests turbulence in the proximal descending aorta. RIGHT, Continuous wave Doppler interrogation down the proximal descending aorta from the suprasternal position demonstrates a 32 mm Hg peak instantaneous gradient without spectral broadening or anterograde diastolic flow.

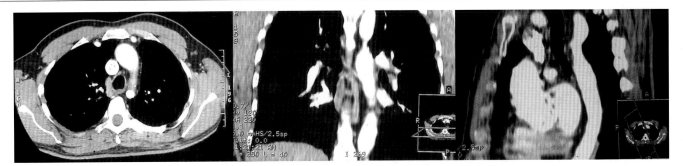

Figure 16-36. Contrast-enhanced CT scans. LEFT, Axial view shows a mild dilation of the ascending aorta and definite narrowing of the proximal descending aorta, consistent with coarctation. MIDDLE, Coronal view depicts the short waist of the coarctation site. RIGHT, Sagittal view again depicts the short waist, but it has a different appearance than in the coronal view. The basis of the figure-of-3 sign can be appreciated. The 3D complexity of coarctation lesions does not lend itself to uniplanar imaging; multiplanar imaging depictions are superior.

CASE 6

History and Physical Examination

▸ 61-year-old man with angina
▸ Hypertensive for decades
▸ Myocardial perfusion scan scintigraphically positive
▸ Renal insufficiency (variable)
▸ BP 120/80 to 180/90 mm Hg (variable), HR 70 bpm
▸ Brisk upper extremity pulses, nearly absent femoral pulses; no bruits
▸ 2/6 SEM at base without aortic insufficiency murmur

Evolution and Management

▸ Clinical impression was that of a bicuspid aortic valve, dilation (not aneurysm) of the ascending aorta, two-vessel coronary artery disease, and complete coarctation of the aorta.

▸ Percutaneous coronary intervention was performed successfully.
▸ The patient declined surgical repair of the aorta, concerned by risks of spinal ischemia.

Comments

▸ Although there is luminal discontinuity of the aorta, there is no anatomic discontinuity of the aorta. Therefore, the lesion is better described as coarctation rather than as interruption.
▸ Hypertension for decades and noted in early adulthood, but seemingly no prior consideration of coarctation as a cause
▸ Aggressive control of the BP in the upper extremities was leading to intervals of hypoperfusion of the kidneys beyond the coarctation and some part of the renal insufficiency.
▸ Associated well-functioning bicuspid aortic valve

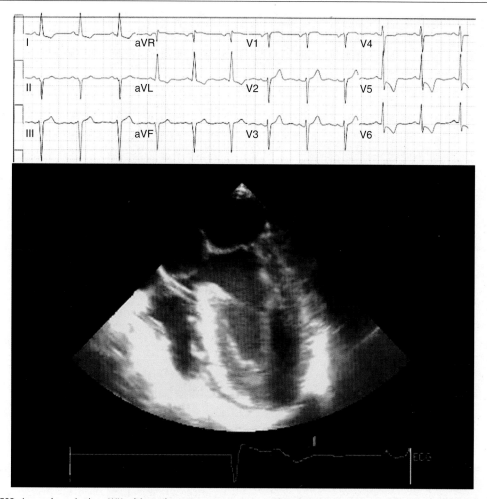

Figure 16-37. TOP, ECG shows sinus rhythm, LVH with strain pattern versus nonspecific repolarization abnormalities. BOTTOM, The TEE view corroborates the LVH.

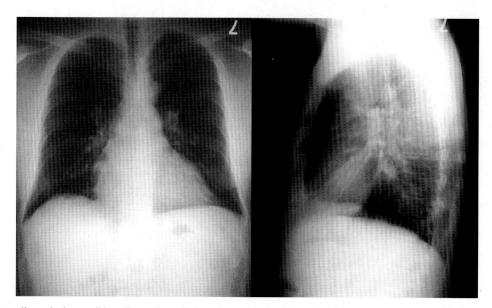

Figure 16-38. Chest radiograph shows mild cardiomegaly, an indentation on the lateral aspect of the proximal descending aorta (possible figure-of-3 sign), and rib notching.

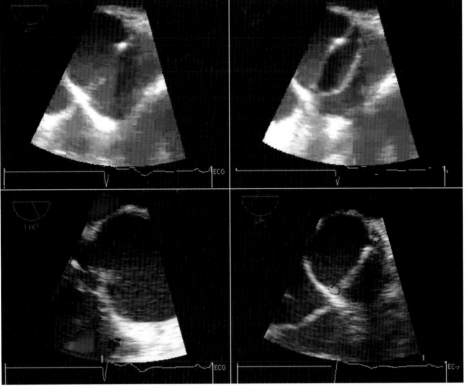

Figure 16-39. TEE views of the bicuspid aortic valve depict a two-sinus, two-cusp pattern. The systolic orifice configuration is elliptical, and the closure is symmetric on the cross-sectional views, although it appears to be eccentric on the long-axis view. There is mild aortic insufficiency, arising from the lateral aspects of the commissure.

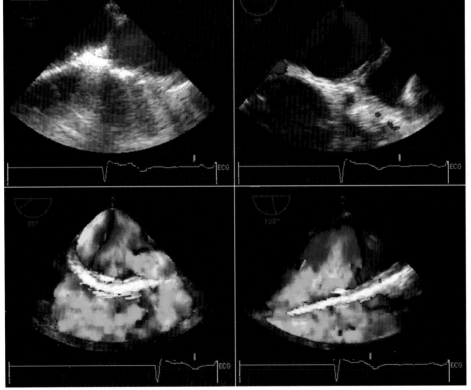

Figure 16-40. TEE. TOP LEFT, Long-axis view of the proximal descending aorta. There is a ridge across the aorta in the middle of the field, consistent with coarctation. TOP RIGHT, Color Doppler flow mapping does not demonstrate acceleration across the lesion; in fact, the flow is inconspicuous on the proximal side. BOTTOM LEFT, Color flow mapping reveals a large inflow of blood through a collateral distal to the coarctation site. BOTTOM RIGHT, There is an unusual finding of flow upward in the mid descending thoracic aorta due to the combination of a complete obstruction of the aorta and atresia (complete coarctation).

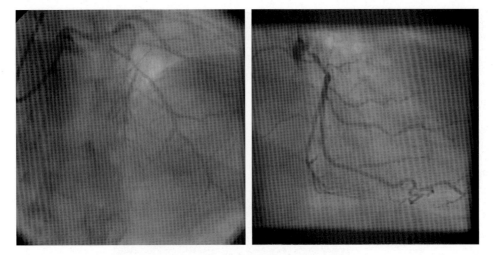

Figure 16-41. Coronary angiography shows severe disease in the left anterior descending coronary artery and proximal left circumflex artery, which is dominant.

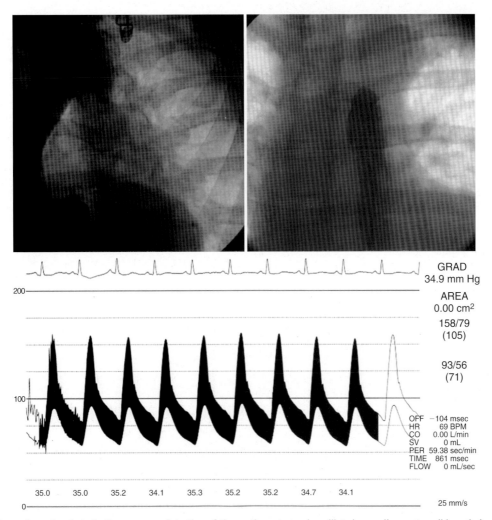

Figure 16-42. Aortography and catheterization. TOP LEFT, Injection of the aortic root reveals a dilated ascending aorta, mild aortic insufficiency, and probably complete occlusion of the proximal descending aorta. Large collaterals were apparent in the late-phase images. TOP RIGHT, Injection of the mid descending thoracic aorta reveals complete obstruction of the aorta. BOTTOM, Catheterization. Aortic pressure is 158/79 mm Hg above the site of coarctation and 93/56 mm Hg beneath the site of coarctation. Note that there is still pulsatile pressure distal to the coarctation and the rapid pressure upstroke in the proximal aorta and the delayed pressure upstroke in the distal aorta beyond the coarctation.

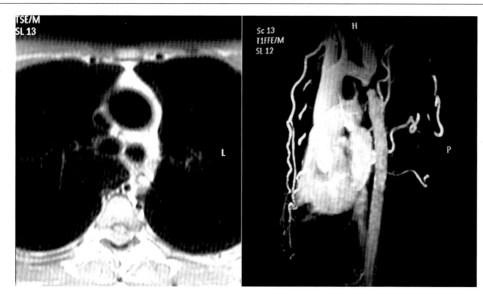

Figure 16-43. LEFT, MRI spin echo sequence. The mild dilation of the ascending aorta is apparent, as is the lack of a lumen in the proximal descending aorta. RIGHT, Gadolinium contrast–enhanced MRA. The obstruction to the aorta and its length and position are apparent, as are the large internal thoracic artery and subscapular collateral vessels.

CASE 7

History and Physical Examination

▸ 55-year-old man with chest pain on exertion, fatigue on exertion, and ankle edema
▸ Known to be hypertensive for only the last 3 years
▸ Six years before, he had undergone TEE, prompted by concerns of aortic dissection: negative for dissection.
▸ BP 150/80 to 230/50 mm Hg (variable if not volatile), HR 70 bpm
▸ Apex enlarged and sustained
▸ Brisk upper extremity pulses, reduced femoral pulses; left scapular pulsations and systolic bruit
▸ 2/6 SEM at base with 3/4 aortic insufficiency murmur; ejection click

Evolution and Management

▸ Clinical impression was that of a bicuspid aortic valve with severe aortic insufficiency, aneurysm of the ascending aorta, and significant coarctation of the aorta.
▸ Confirmed by surgical findings

▸ Management consisted of a Bentall procedure (composite aortic valve replacement + tube graft + coronary reimplantation), aortocoronary bypass grafting, and stenting of the coarctation.

Comments

▸ Bicuspid aortic valve with associated severe aortic insufficiency, aortopathy, aneurysm of the ascending aorta, and coarctation of the descending aorta
▸ The bicuspid valve dominated awareness until hypertension was obvious and a more resolved effort to pursue the possibility of a coarctation was made, underscoring the need to do so.
▸ The systolic hypertension was the result of the large volume of aortic insufficiency overtaxing the cushioning ability of the proximal aorta; the reflection of the pulse wave off the coarctation, which by being near to the heart returns the reflection in systole; and the higher pressure in the proximal aorta due to the coarctation gradient, which renders it stiffer, reducing available compliance for the aortic insufficiency and increasing the pulse wave velocity.
▸ Alleviation of the aortic insufficiency and the coarctation had a prominent effect on blood pressure.

Figure 16-44. ECG shows sinus rhythm and LVH with abnormal repolarization pattern.

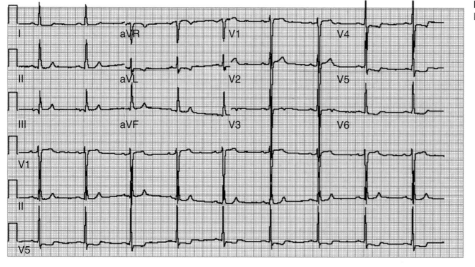

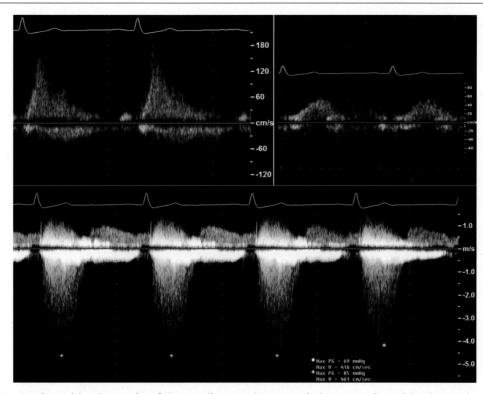

Figure 16-45. TTE. TOP LEFT, Spectral Doppler mapping of the ascending aorta (pre-coarctation). TOP RIGHT, Spectral Doppler mapping of the abdominal aorta (post-coarctation). Notice the striking delay in the upstroke of the abdominal aorta distal to the coarctation—a tardus upstroke consistent with an upstream fixed obstruction. BOTTOM, Continuous wave Doppler recording of flow from the suprasternal position across the coarctation; the peak instantaneous gradient is approximately 85 mm Hg. There is no increase or anterograde diastolic flow.

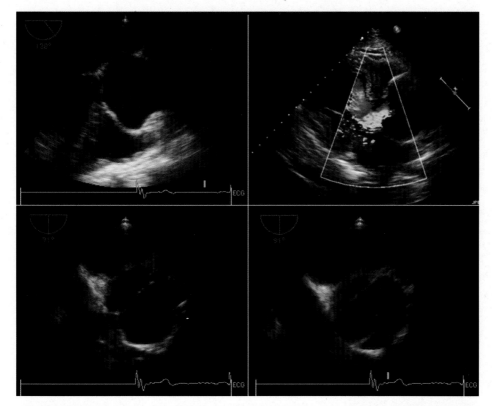

Figure 16-46. TOP LEFT, TEE longitudinal view of the aortic root. There is dilation of the root and ascending aorta and no intimal flap. TOP RIGHT, The corresponding TTE view with color Doppler mapping demonstrates moderate aortic insufficiency. BOTTOM, TEE cross-sectional views of the bicuspid aortic valve (two cusps and two sinuses) in diastole (LEFT) and systole (RIGHT). The systolic orifice configuration is elliptical or triangular.

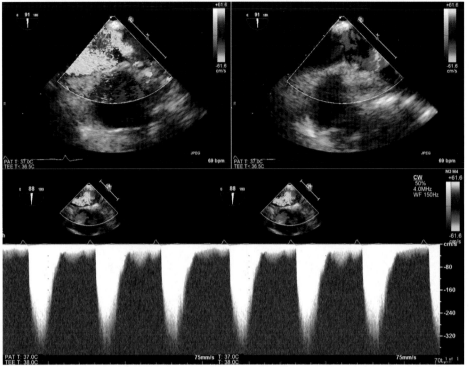

Figure 16-47. TEE views of the proximal descending aorta and spectral profile. There is a ridge across the aorta in the middle of the field, consistent with coarctation. TOP LEFT, Systole. TOP RIGHT, Diastole. There is prominent systolic flow acceleration (PISA variance) but none in diastole. The spectral profile reveals the same pattern and a peak instantaneous gradient of approximately 55 mm Hg.

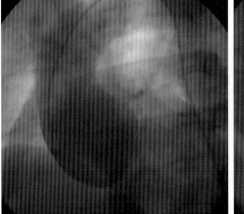

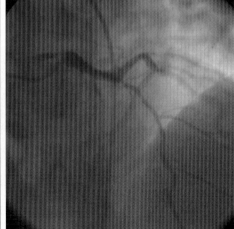

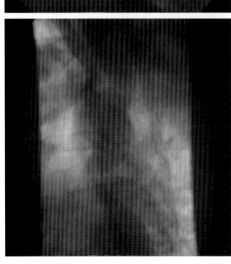

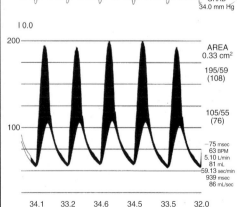

Figure 16-48. Aortography and catheterization. Injection of the aortic root reveals the dilation of the aortic root and ascending aorta. No intimal flap is imaged. Injection of the distal arch reveals a short waist-like shelf of coarctation. The appearance helps understand the figure-of-3 sign on the chest radiograph, when it is present in coarctation. Significant left anterior descending coronary artery disease is present. The aortic pressure is 195/59 mm Hg above the site of coarctation and 105/55 mm Hg beneath the site of coarctation. The gradient is systolic predominant—there is little diastolic gradient. Note the elevated pulse pressure before the coarctation as a result of the aortic insufficiency and coarctation and the delayed pressure upstroke in the distal aorta beyond the coarctation.

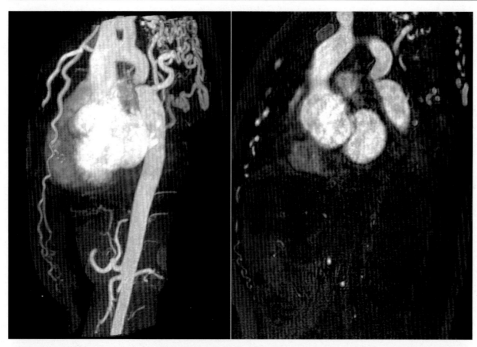

Figure 16-49. Gadolinium contrast–enhanced MRA. The waist of the coarctation is obvious as is its short length, as are the internal thoracic and subscapular collateral vessels, but the specific nature of the coarctation lesion is still somewhat unclear. Neither image distinguishes the lesion from the lumen sharply.

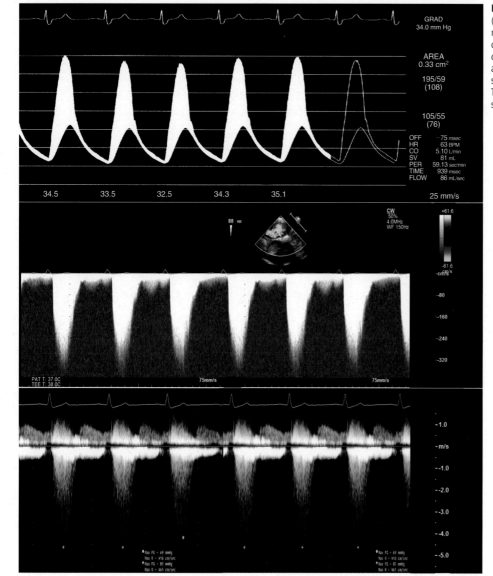

Figure 16-50. Catheterization (TOP), TEE (MIDDLE), and TTE suprasternal (BOTTOM) recordings. All reveal essentially systolic-only gradients. The transthoracic and catheterization gradients are the closest, as suprasternal Doppler sampling, although sometimes difficult, is usually well aligned. TEE undersampled the gradient because of significant misalignment.

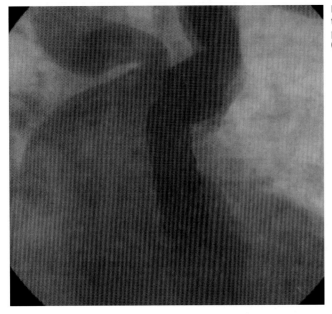

Figure 16-51. Angiography after the stenting procedure. Note the dilation of the left subclavian artery and the left common carotid artery as well as the post-coarctation dilation of the aorta. (Courtesy of Eric Horlick, MD, Toronto, Canada.)

References

1. Davutoglu V, Soydinc S, Sirikci A, et al: Interrupted aortic arch in an adolescent male. Can J Cardiol 2004;20:1367-1368.
2. Oliver JM, Gallego P, Gonzalez A, et al: Risk factors for aortic complications in adults with coarctation of the aorta. J Am Coll Cardiol 2004;44:1641-1647.
3. Fawzy ME, Awad M, Hassan W, et al: Long-term outcome (up to 15 years) of balloon angioplasty of discrete native coarctation of the aorta in adolescents and adults. J Am Coll Cardiol 2004;43:1062-1067.
4. Tzifa A, Ewert P, Brzezinska-Rajszys G, et al: Covered Cheatham-platinum stents for aortic coarctation: early and intermediate-term results. J Am Coll Cardiol 2006;47:1457-1463.

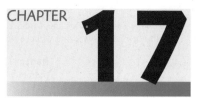

Marfan Syndrome

Marfan syndrome is a hereditary disorder affecting 1:5,000 to 1:10,000 people of all ethnicities and both genders. The transmission pattern is autosomal dominant (50%:50% transmission rate), but a prominent 30% of cases reflect a new mutation. The International Registry of Aortic Dissection established that 5% of acute aortic dissections are due to Marfan syndrome and that although acute aortic dissection patients with Marfan syndrome are much younger than those without, their acute mortality is simply no better (Table 17-1).[1]

HISTORICAL CONSIDERATIONS

Marfan syndrome was eponymously named after the French pediatrician Antonin Bernard Jean Marfan (1858-1942), who provided the first description of the condition when he remarked on one aspect of the skeletal abnormalities of the disorder in a 4-year-old child—long limbs that he termed *dolidochenostenome-lie*.[2] E. C. Achard coined the term *spider fingers (arachnodactylie)* in 1902 to further describe the skeletal abnormality. A decade later, the first cardiac associations (mitral valve prolapse, mitral regurgitation, death) of the disorder were recognized, as was lens dislocation, and shortly after that, the first vascular association (aortic rupture in a child) was described. In 1931, the autosomal dominant pattern of transmission typical of the disorder was recognized. In 1943, Helen Taussig described the great frequency

of aortic aneurysms that typifies the disorder and that underlies its mortality. Therapeutic advances were achieved by the demonstration of reduction of aortic root dilation and of rupture by the use of beta-blockers in 1994[3] and the benefit of surgical replacement of the aneurysmal aortic root in 1968.[4] Standardization of diagnostic criteria was advanced by the publication of the Berlin nosology in 1986[5] and the revised Ghent nosology in 1996.[6]

The first great challenge in understanding Marfan syndrome was recognizing the variable phenotypes. This challenge endures as the need to recognize cases of Marfan syndrome before acute and high-risk presentations occur. The second great challenge has been to unravel the responsible genotype, which has proven more complicated than anticipated.

GENETIC CONSIDERATIONS

Initially believed to be due to a defect of the fibrillin 1 (*FBN1*) gene alone, Marfan syndrome is now recognized to be caused by defects of the *TGFBR2* gene in some cases. Marfan syndrome cases due to defective *FBN1* are termed Marfan syndrome type 1 (MFS1), and cases due to defects in the gene for *TGFBR2* are termed Marfan syndrome type 2 (MFS2).

The very large (65-exon) *FBN1* gene (15q21.1, base pairs 46,489,478 to 46,724,390), also known as *FBN, FBN1_HUMAN,* fibrillin 1 (Marfan), *MASS, MFS1, OCTD, SGS,* and *WMS,* encodes

Table 17-1. Comparison of Age, Cardiovascular Pathology, and Mortality in Patients with and without Marfan Syndrome

	Marfan Syndrome	Non–Marfan Syndrome	P Value
Age (years)	35 ± 12	64 ± 13	<.001
Hypertensive	27%	74%	<.001
Atherosclerosis	0%	32%	<.001
Prior aneurysm	33%	13%	<.001
Prior cardiac surgery for aortic dissection	27%	8%	.001
Prior aortic valve surgery	19%	4%	<.001
Congestive heart failure	10%	5%	.09
Systolic BP >140 mm Hg	27%	44%	.001
Diastolic BP >90 mm Hg	19%	23%	<.001
Aortic insufficiency	64%	42%	.002
Mortality			
Overall (types A and B)	21%	23%	NS
Type A	25%	30%	NS
Type B	8%	13%	NS

Table 17-2. Genetic Syndromes That Share Marfan Syndrome–Like Findings

Syndrome	Comments
Ehlers-Danlos syndrome type IV	Ehlers-Danlos syndrome type IV (vascular type) is notable for rupture of the aorta and its branches, often without antecedent aneurysms. The incidence is greater than that of Marfan syndrome (1:500), and the pattern of transmission is autosomal dominant. The responsible gene is located on 2q31 and encodes a type III protocollagen. The clinical criteria are easy bruisability, thin skin with visible veins, characteristic facial features, and ruptured arteries or viscera. The median survival is 48 years; 20% have a complication by the age of 20 years and >80% by the age of 40 years. There are no proven medical or surgical preventive treatments. Surgical interventions are notable for poor results.
Beals syndrome	Congenital contractural arachnodactyly
Shprintzen-Goldberg syndrome	Arachnodactyly, craniosynostosis, hypotonia, hernias
Weill-Marchesani syndrome	Brachydactyly, stiff joints, short stature
MASS phenotype	Mitral valvulopathy, Aortopathy, Skeletal malformation, Skin
Cutis laxa	
Loeys-Dietz syndrome (types 1 and 2)	Wide-set eyes, cleft palate or split uvula, convoluted arrangement of blood vessels, and agressive swelling of the aorta. Patients are at high risk for aortic dissection or rupture at an early age (Fig. 17-1).
Noonan syndrome	
Turner syndrome	
Polycystic kidney disease	
Stickler syndrome	
XYY syndrome	
Homocysteinuria	
Osteogenesis imperfecta	
Familial ectopia lentis	
Familial arachnodactyly	
Familial cardiovascular syndromes	Familial thoracic aortic aneurysm syndrome, familial aortic dissection syndrome, familial mitral valve prolapse syndrome, familial bicuspid aortic valve, and thoracic aortic aneurysm syndrome

the glycoprotein fibrillin 1 that multimerizes into microfibrils and, with tropoelastin, forms elastic tissue. Fibrillin 1 also inactivates transforming growth factor beta (TGF-beta) by binding to its receptor, thereby suppressing inhibition of cell growth, differentiation, and extracellular matrix formation. The production of abnormal fibrillin 1 by the abnormal gene leads to suppression of production by the other allele, a phenomenon named positive-negative regulation. Marfan syndrome is characterized by markedly reduced overall production of fibrillin 1 and the production of small and defective fibrillin 1. Defective and reduced fibrillin 1 leads to availability and activation of *TGFBR2*, resulting in inhibited cell growth, differentiation, and extracellular matrix formation. The *TGFBR2* gene (also known as tumor suppressor, *AAT3*, *FAA3*, *HNPCC6*, *MFS2*, *RIIC*, *TAAD2*, TGF-beta receptor type IIB, TGFbeta-RII, TGF-beta type II receptor, *TGFR2*, *TGFR2_HUMAN*) is located on the short arm of chromosome 2 at location 21:3p21, base pairs 30,622,97 to 30,710,637.

Other type 1 fibrillinopathies (e.g., familial ectopia lentis, Shprintzen-Goldberg syndrome, Weill-Marchesani syndrome, MASS phenotype) share some phenotypic similarities to Marfan syndrome (Table 17-2); therefore, detection of simply any *FBN1* gene abnormality does not establish Marfan syndrome. Only detection of a specific mutation known to be associated with Marfan syndrome is useful as a diagnostic criterion.

MARFAN SYNDROME PHENOTYPES

Approximately 70% of cases of Marfan syndrome are associated with aortic root dilation. Complications of aortic root dilation clinically dominate Marfan syndrome and remain the principal cause of death. Aortic root size is the only consistent independent predictor of aortic complications in Marfan syndrome.[7]

Marfan syndrome is a prominent cause of aortic dissection in patients younger than 40 years, as are bicuspid aortic valves. In the International Registry of Aortic Dissection, the incidence of Marfan syndrome was 50% among acute aortic dissection patients younger than 40 years and only 2% among patients older than 40 years.[1,8]

CARDIOVASCULAR ABNORMALITIES IN MARFAN SYNDROME

Aortic abnormalities in Marfan syndrome include the following:

1. aortic root (sinuses of Valsalva) and ascending aorta dilation, which is seen in approximately 70% of Marfan cases, and aortic root complications, which account for the majority of mortality;

2. aortic aneurysms (thoracic and abdominal);

3. aortic dissection (predominantly type A; only 10% are type B, and rarely abdominal aortic dissections may occur); and

4. aortic intramural hematoma.

    Valvular abnormalities associated with Marfan syndrome include mitral valve, aortic valve, and tricuspid valve abnormalities. Mitral valve disorders (mitral valve prolapse and mitral regurgitation) occur in 60% to 80% of Marfan syndrome patients. Leaflet prolapse, chordal rupture, and annular dilation are common. Ten percent of cases have prominent submitral calcification (mitral annular calcification). Aortic valve prosthesis dehiscence occurs more often in Marfan syndrome patients. The risk of aortic valve insufficiency (dilation of the sinuses, annulus) correlates in incidence and severity with aortic root size and increases the mortality from Marfan syndrome. Tricuspid valve abnormalities include tricuspid valve prolapse.

DIAGNOSIS OF MARFAN SYNDROME

Diagnosis of Marfan syndrome cannot be made by a single test, even genetic testing. Therefore, it is necessary to use composite clinical and imaging criteria. Comprehensive testing for Marfan syndrome is summarized in Table 17-3. Imaging modalities most useful in diagnosis of Marfan syndrome include echocardiography (for dilation or dissection of the ascending aorta), chest radiography, cardiac computed tomography (Figs. 17-2 and 17-3), and subtraction aortography (Fig. 17-4).

Table 17-3. Comprehensive Testing for Marfan Syndrome

Family history

Medical history (for a history of spontaneous pneumothorax)

Physical examination

Ophthalmologic examination (slit lamp test, keratometry)

Echocardiography (for dilation or dissection of the ascending aorta)

Chest radiography (for apical blebs or dilation of the main pulmonary artery)

Cardiac magnetic resonance or cardiac computed tomography (for dilation of the ascending aorta and pulmonary artery or dural ectasia)

Genetic testing

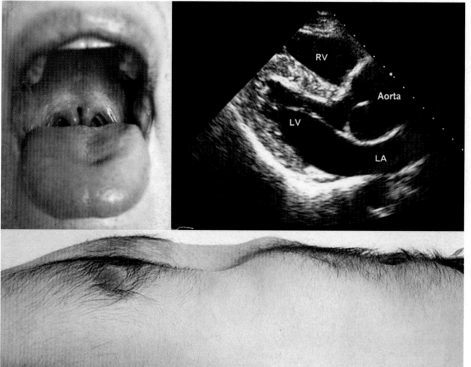

Figure 17-1. A 24-year-old man was hospitalized for evaluation of an aortic root aneurysm. He had a family history of aortic disease. Physical examination revealed proptosis, retrognathia, bifid uvula (TOP LEFT), and pectus excavatum (BOTTOM). Transthoracic echocardiography showed a 50 mm by 50 mm aortic-root aneurysm (TOP RIGHT). The presence of the classic triad of craniofacial abnormalities, aortic aneurysm, and bifid uvula, as well as the family history of aortic disease, strongly suggested a diagnosis of Loeys-Dietz syndrome type 1, which was confirmed by genetic analysis showing a mutation in exon 7 of the *TGFBR2* gene. Patients with this autosomal dominant syndrome are at high risk for aortic dissection or rupture at an early age; the aortic diameter may not be predictive of rupture. The patient underwent successful aortic root replacement and remains well at one year of follow-up. (From Vilacosta I, Cañadas Godoy V: Images in clinical medicine: Bifid uvula and aortic aneurysm. N Engl J Med 2008;359;e2, with permission.)

Genetic Testing

The more recent diagnostic criteria are the Ghent nosology (criteria),[6] revised from the Berlin criteria.[5] The Ghent diagnostic criteria include major criteria (features likely to occur in Marfan syndrome that seldom occur in the general population, thereby conferring specificity) and minor criteria (features seen in both Marfan syndrome and the general population, thereby conferring sensitivity) and organ involvement criteria, either major or minor (Table 17-4).[6] The Ghent major criteria include (1) family history, (2) genetic defect, (3) enlarged or aneurysmal aorta, (4) dissection of the ascending aorta, (5) lens dislocation, (6) dural ectasia, and (7) four or more skeletal criteria (chest deformities, long thin extremities, flat feet, scoliosis). The Ghent criteria are viewed as an improvement on the Berlin criteria but also as being possibly too stringent; approximately 20% of cases positive by Berlin criteria are negative by the Ghent criteria.

The single most useful determination is positive family history. Family history is positive if a consanguineous family member (parent, sibling, or child) is independently determined to have Marfan syndrome. If an independent family history is established, then only *one major and one minor criterion* or involvement of another organ system is needed to establish the diagnosis. If a family history is negative or unavailable, then *two major criteria involving two different organ systems and involvement of another organ system* are required by the Ghent criteria to establish a diagnosis of Marfan syndrome.

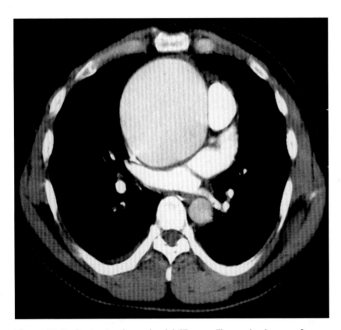

Figure 17-2. Contrast-enhanced axial CT scan. The predominance of ascending aortic involvement in Marfan syndrome can be seen in this image of a 9-cm aneurysm of the ascending aorta, with a normal-size descending aorta.

Genetic (Molecular) Testing

The result of a genetic test for Marfan syndrome is considered positive if it detects (1) presence of a mutation in *FBN1* known to cause Marfan syndrome or (2) presence of a haplotype around *FBN1*, inherited by descent known to be associated with unequivocably diagnosed Marfan syndrome in the family. The most prominent problem with gene testing beyond its cost and limited availability is that 25% to 30% of Marfan cases involve new mutations. Hence, gene testing may not corroborate an unequivocal clinical case of Marfan syndrome.

Genetic testing for Marfan syndrome does not by itself establish the diagnosis of Marfan syndrome. There are more than

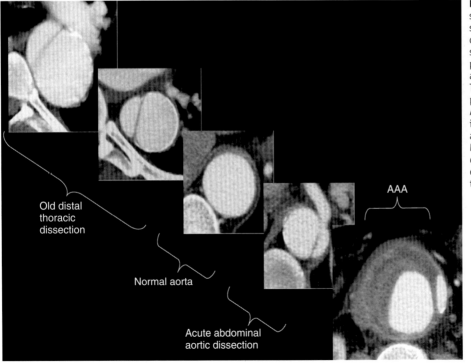

Old distal thoracic dissection

Normal aorta

Acute abdominal aortic dissection

AAA

Figure 17-3. Contrast-enhanced CT axial scan at several levels of the aorta in the same patient. The recurrent nature of complications of the aorta in Marfan syndrome is exemplified in this case. The patient previously had a type B dissection and an abdominal aortic aneurysm (AAA). This time, he presented with abdominal pain and a new acute dissection of the AAA was found, extending above the AAA into what had previously been a normal-appearing aorta. The familial nature of Marfan syndrome is also exemplified by this case—three siblings had five aortic dissections and three aneurysms between them.

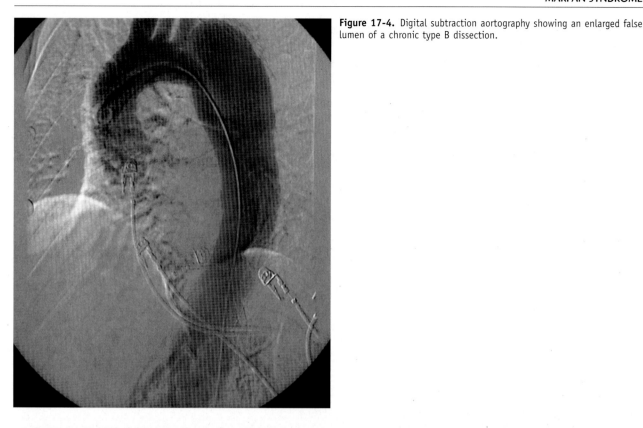

Figure 17-4. Digital subtraction aortography showing an enlarged false lumen of a chronic type B dissection.

Table 17-4. Ghent Diagnostic Criteria for Marfan Syndrome

System	Major Criteria	Minor Criteria	"Involvement"
Skeletal	Presence of *at least four* of the following manifestations Pectus carinatum Pectus excavatum requiring surgery Reduced upper to lower segment ratio or arm span to height ratio greater than 1.05 Wrist (Walker) sign: when the wrist is encircled by the thumb and little finger, the little finger overlaps by >1 cm in 80% of patients with Marfan syndrome.[9] Thumb sign: when a fist is made over an apposed thumb, the thumb does not normally extend beyond the ulnar aspect of the hand (false-positives occur in 1% of white and 3% of black children).[10] Scoliosis >20 degrees or spondylolisthesis (prevalence: 60%) Reduced extensions at the elbows (<170 degrees) Medial displacement of the medial malleolus causing pes planus Protrusio acetabuli of any degree (ascertained on radiographs) (prevalence: 50%)	Pectus excavatum of moderate severity Joint hypermobility Highly arched palate with crowding of teeth Facial appearance (dolichocephaly, malar hypoplasia, enophthalmos, retrognathia, down-slanting palpebral fissures)	At least 2 major criteria *or* 1 major criterion plus 2 minor criteria must be present.
Cardiovascular	Dilation of the ascending aorta with or without aortic regurgitation and involving at least the sinuses of Valsalva *or* Dissection of the ascending aorta	Mitral valve prolapse with or without mitral valve regurgitation (prevalence: 55%-70%) Dilation of the main pulmonary artery, in the absence of valvular or peripheral pulmonic stenosis or any other obvious cause, before the age of 40 years Calcification of the mitral annulus before the age of 40 years Dilation or dissection of the descending thoracic or abdominal aorta before the age of 50 years	A minor criterion must be present.

Table 17-4. Ghent Diagnostic Criteria for Marfan Syndrome—cont'd

System	Major Criteria	Minor Criteria	"Involvement"
Ocular	Ectopia lentis (dislocated lens). The dislocation is usually superior (ectopia lentis superioris) and temporal. (prevalence: 50%)	Flat cornea (measured by keratometry)	At least 2 minor criteria must be present.
		Increased axial length of the globe (measured by ultrasound)	
		Cataract (nuclear sclerotic) in patients younger than 50 years	
		Hypoplastic iris or hypoplastic ciliary muscle that causes decreased miosis	
		Nearsightedness regardless of whether the lens is in place: the most common refraction error is myopia due to elongated globe and amblyopia.	
		Glaucoma (patients <50 y)	
		Retinal detachment	
Pulmonary	None	Spontaneous pneumothorax (prevalence: 5%)	A minor criterion must be present.
		Apical blebs (ascertained by chest radiography)	
Skin and integument	None	Stretch marks (striae atrophicae) not associated with marked weight changes, pregnancy, or repetitive stress	A minor criterion must be present.
		Recurrent or incisional hernias	
Dura	Lumbosacral dural ectasia by CT or MR; an enlargement of the neural canal or ballooning of the dural sac, usually lumbosacral, often associated with herniation of the nerve root sleeves through their foramina. The prevalence is 65%-92%. The severity increases with age.	None	
	Less than 20% of patients have serious dural ectasia. Dural ectasia may also be associated with		
	Ehlers-Danlos syndrome		
	Neurofibromatosis type 1		
	Ankylosing spondylitis		
	Trauma		
	Scoliosis		
	Tumors		
Family history, genetics	Having a parent, child, or sibling who meets these diagnostic criteria independently	None	
	Presence of a mutation in *FBN1* known to cause the Marfan syndrome		
	Presence of a haplotype around *FBN1*, inherited by descent, known to be associated with unequivocally diagnosed Marfan syndrome in the family		

From De Paepe A, Devereux RB, Dietz HC, et al: Revised diagnostic criteria for the Marfan syndrome. Am J Med Genet 1996;62:417-426.

500 described mutations of fibrillin 1 gene (*FBN1*) on chromosome 15, and not all of them are specific for Marfan syndrome, as many Marfan-like disorders share the same gene. Cost and availability are limiting factors, as is the incomplete understanding of the Marfan phenotype and genotypes. However, several uses of genetic testing are irrefutable, including the testing of children of patients diagnosed with Marfan syndrome. Children of Marfan syndrome patients without the same genotype do not have to be observed throughout growth.

Multidisciplinary Marfan clinics afford a depth of assistance, including recognition of significant Marfan-related lesions, counseling of affected individuals and their families, and proficiency in recognizing the multiple genetic syndromes that share Marfan syndrome–like findings (see Table 17-2).

Aortic Root Surveillance

Because the aortic root is the principal anatomic segment of disease, transthoracic echocardiography (TTE) is usually adequate to observe root size. A starting frequency of once a year is reasonable.

MANAGEMENT OPTIONS

Medical Therapy

Long-term beta-adrenergic blockade in Marfan syndrome reduces the rate of aortic root dilation. The 1994 landmark study, although neither randomized nor unblinded, by Pyeritz and colleagues followed up 70 patients with Marfan syndrome treated with propranolol (n = 32; mean dose, 212 ± 68 mg/day; follow-up, 10.7 years) or control (n = 38; follow-up, 10 years).[3] The rate of root dilation was significantly less in the beta-blocker treatment group. Clinical endpoints (aortic insufficiency, acute aortic dissection, cardiovascular surgery, congestive heart failure, death) were reached in 5 patients in the treatment group and 9 patients in the control group.[3] There was significantly less mortality in the treatment group.[3]

In 2007, a 24-week randomized controlled trial of 17 patients with Marfan syndrome observed that the ACE inhibitor perindopril reduced both aortic stiffness and root dilation as well as TGF-beta levels.[11]

Similarly, another small, short-term cohort study of 18 pediatric patients followed for 12 to 47 months demonstrated that the addition of losartan or irbesartan to standard beta-blocker therapy reduced aortic root dilation by 2.75 mm/year, after age and sex adjustment.[12] A National Heart, Lung, and Blood Institute study is ongoing and recruiting, which randomizes patients to losartan versus atenolol, and is anticipated to yield particularly needed information.

Elective Surgical Repair

The optimal dimension of the aortic root on which to perform elective replacement is not firmly established in Marfan syndrome or non–Marfan syndrome patients. The low mortality of elective repair (1% to 2%)[13] and the good results of valve-sparing surgery (repair mortality of 0% to 1%)[14-16] at experienced centers are influencing the diameter thresholds, as are the 10-year data of 80% to 88% survival and 87% freedom from moderate or severe aortic insufficiency.[15,16] The reimplantation technique is emerging as the superior technique.[17]

Once the root diameter has exceeded 1.3 times normal, surveillance should occur more frequently (every 6 months). Once the root is dilated to 1.5 times normal, elective root repair should be considered. More rapid root dilation is associated with more events. Among 89 patients observed for 4 years, there were more events in patients with an initial aortic root size of 1.3 times or more of predicted (relative risk, 2.7) and among patients with annular diameter changes of 5% or more (relative risk, 4.3).[18] The upper limit of normal for the aortic root dimension is approximately 1.9 times the body surface area. Elective aortic root replacement may also be considered when the primary indication for surgery is mitral insufficiency (Figs. 17-5 and 17-6).

Size alone does not discriminate the risk of dissection in Marfan syndrome. The notion of threshold of risk is compromised by the observation that dissection occurs across a wide range of diameters (Fig. 17-7). Despite the fact that most dissections occur at aneurysm diameters of more than 5 cm, some occur at lesser

17

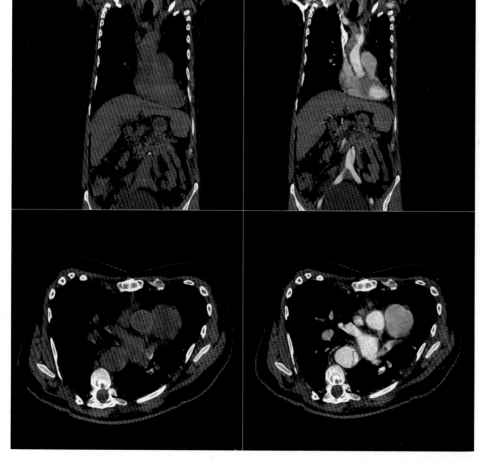

Figure 17-5. This patient with Marfan syndrome previously underwent concurrent elective repair of the mitral valve because of severe mitral insufficiency and valve-sparing aortic root replacement with a Dacron graft because of aortic root diameter of 5.3 cm. He presented 16 months later with severe chest pains due to acute aortic dissection. The primary entry tear was detected in the proximal descending aorta—extensive retrograde dissection had occurred right to the distal margin of the tube graft used to replace the aortic root. TOP, Non–contrast-enhanced (LEFT) and contrast-enhanced (RIGHT) coronal images. The Dacron tube graft is evident in the aortic root. The dissection has extended back to the distal margin of the root tube graft. BOTTOM, Axial non–contrast-enhanced and contrast-enhanced images revealing the Dacron tube graft in the ascending aorta and the intimal flap and false lumen in the descending aorta. The elective replacement of the aortic root spared catastrophic cardiac compromise by the dissection.

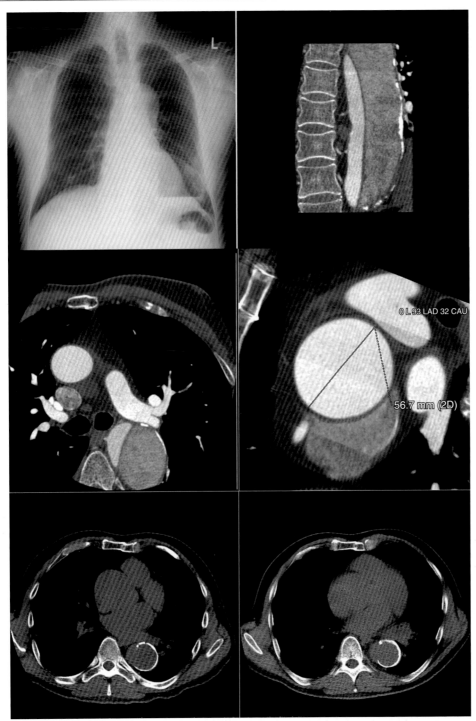

Figure 17-6. TOP LEFT, Posteroanterior chest radiograph demonstrating enlargement of the aortic arch and descending aorta. The ascending aorta is typically obscured on the posteroanterior radiograph. TOP RIGHT, Coronal CT image revealing definite calcification of the lateral false lumen of the descending aorta. MIDDLE LEFT, The ascending aorta is dilated, but the descending aorta is even more dilated, and there is calcification of the outer wall of the false lumen of a chronic dissection. MIDDLE RIGHT, The ascending aorta is dilated to 57 mm. BOTTOM, Non-contrast-enhanced CT images showing calcification of the outer wall of the false lumen. The patient was referred for and underwent elective successful replacement of the ascending aorta.

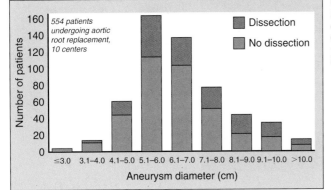

Figure 17-7. Size alone does not discriminate the risk of dissection in Marfan syndrome. The notion of threshold of risk is compromised by the observation that dissection occurs across a wide range of diameters. (From Gott VL, Greene PS, Alejo DE, et al: Replacement of the aortic root in patients with Marfan's syndrome. N Engl J Med 1999;340:1307-1313. Copyright © [2001] Massachusetts Medical Society. All rights reserved.)

diameters (Table 17-5).[19,20] Because of a higher risk of rupture in Marfan syndrome (for any size of the aorta), the threshold for surgical intervention is lower than in non-Marfan cases.

The recent (2007) observation that most patients with type A acute aortic dissection have an aortic root–ascending aorta size of less than 5.5 cm challenges the safety of using this threshold in non–Marfan syndrome patients and also adds to the debate as to what the Marfan syndrome threshold should be.[21]

Overall, the threshold to electively replace the aortic root in Marfan syndrome has been falling because of low and often very favorable early risk profiles (Table 17-6). For composite valve and root replacement, Gott and coworkers[13] published mortality of 1.5% (0.7%-3.3%) for elective repair, 2.6% (0.7%-7.9%) for urgent repair (1 to 7 days), and 11.7% (6.4%-20%) for emergency repair (<24 hours). For valve-sparing repair, mortality of less than 1%, even 0%, has been published.[14-16] The 10-year survival of patients undergoing valve-sparing surgery is 80% to 88%, and absence of moderate or severe aortic insufficiency is 87% ± 6% (reimplantation 94% ± 4% and remodeling 75% ± 10%), with 86% to 98% of patients being NYHA class I or II.[15,16]

Thresholds for elective aortic surgical repair also tend to be center specific and also may be lowered in consideration of other factors, such as (1) whether composite graft replacement is planned (>5.5 cm), (2) if valve sparing is anticipated (>5.0 cm), (3) in cases with higher risk of dissection or rupture (>4.5 cm), and (4) in female patients contemplating pregnancy (>4.0 cm).

The life expectancy of patients with Marfan syndrome is clearly increasing and reflects better prevention (beta-blockade and composite aortic valve and ascending aortic repair) and probably better treatment of complications. In 1972, the mean age at death for Marfan patients was 32 ± 16 years. In 1995, the mean age at death for Marfan syndrome patients was 41 ± 18 years ($P = .0023$).[22] Marfan patients are accordingly currently living into their sixth and seventh decades.

The long-term course of Marfan patients with aortic dissection is subject to ongoing cardiovascular events (Fig. 17-8). In a series of 40 patients with Marfan syndrome with aortic dissection followed up for 15 years, survival rates were 71% ± 8% at 5 years, 54% ± 10% at 10 years, and 22% ± 11% at 15 years.[23] There were 20 late operations performed in 14 patients. Causes of late mortality in 15 patients were as follows:

- Acute type B dissection (operative death, intestinal infarction), 1
- Chronic type A dissection (operative death, postoperative myocardial infarction), 1
- Thoracoabdominal aneurysm (operative death sepsis), 1
- Ruptured sinus of Valsalva aneurysm, 1
- Ruptured thoracoabdominal aneurysm, 1
- Congestive heart failure, 3
- Stroke, 2
- Cardiac allograft rejection, 1
- Nonaortic, noncardiovascular cause, 2

At least one third of patients with Marfan syndrome undergo extensive aortic reconstruction.[24,25] The need for ongoing clinical and imaging follow-up of patients with Marfan syndrome is critical to increase the rate of prophylactic and lower risk elective interventions rather than high-risk emergent interventions.

Table 17-5. Location and Size Comparison of Aortic Aneurysms in Marfan Syndrome Versus Non–Marfan Syndrome Cases

Location of Aneurysm	Non–Marfan Syndrome	Marfan Syndrome
Ascending aorta	>5.5 cm	>5.0 cm
	>5.0-5.5 cm	>4.5 cm
Aortic arch	>5.5-6.0 cm	
Descending aorta	>6.5 cm	>6.0 cm
Thoracoabdominal	>5.0-6.0 cm	

Table 17-6. Recommended Threshold for Elective Surgical Repair

Aortic Root Size	Study
>6.5 cm	Gott (1999)[13]
>5.5-6.0 cm	Coady (1997), Pyeritz (1994), Emory and Rimoin (1997), Shores (1994)
>5.5 cm	Baumgartner (1999)
>5.0 cm	Gott (2002)
>4.5 cm	de Oliviera (2003)

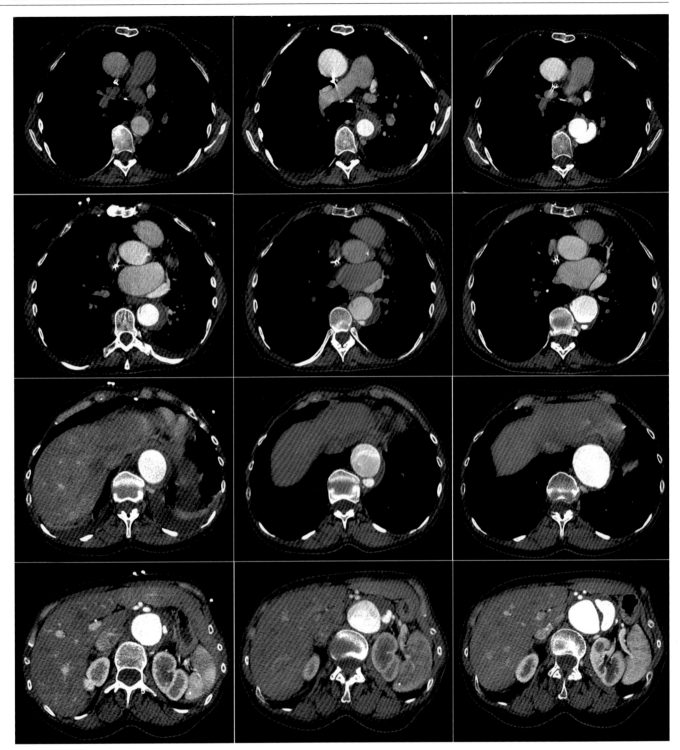

Figure 17-8. A 35-year-old woman with Marfan syndrome. LEFT IMAGES, At the time of an acute aortic syndrome (distal aortic intramural hematoma). MIDDLE IMAGES, Two months later, revealing breakdown of the distal aorta, with contrast enhancement of both thoracic and abdominal areas of the false lumen. RIGHT IMAGES, Four months later, revealing rapid and extensive false lumen formation of the thoracic and abdominal aorta.

CASE 1

History

▸ A 27-year-old man presented with shortness of breath for 6 months.
▸ He had two previous retinal detachments.
▸ Negative family history

Physical Examination

▸ BP 130/40 mm Hg, HR 60 bpm
▸ Corrigan's pulses
▸ Decrescendo aortic insufficiency murmur, displaced + dynamic apex
▸ Austin Flint murmur and 2/6 SEM at base

Management and Outcome

▸ Dissection of the upper ascending aorta and arch
▸ Surgery revealed dissection of the upper ascending aorta and arch, with the dissection flap extending into the carotid arteries.

▸ Composite (mechanical aortic valve replacement + tube) graft inserted
▸ Arch repair (sewing of the intima back to the wall of the carotid ostia) performed with use of hypothermic circulatory arrest
▸ The patient had an uneventful postoperative course and has been taking a beta-blocker.

Comments

▸ Chronic limited dissection of the upper ascending aorta and arch
▸ Severe aortic insufficiency from root dilation, not from the dissection, which is well above and away from the aortic root
▸ No cerebral ischemic symptoms despite carotid involvement
▸ The full complexity of the dissection (extension into the carotid arteries) was not appreciated preoperatively, necessitating adaptation of the surgery.

17

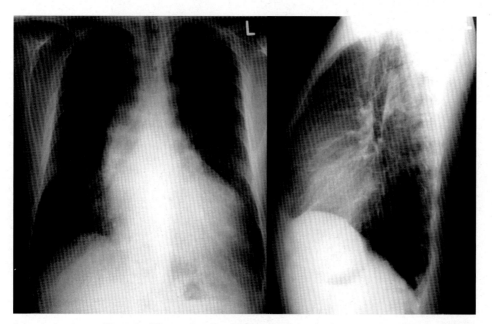

Figure 17-9. Chest radiograph showing cardiomegaly, hilar overlay sign of dilation of the ascending aorta, straight back, and pectus excavatum (seen as an inward depression on the lateral film).

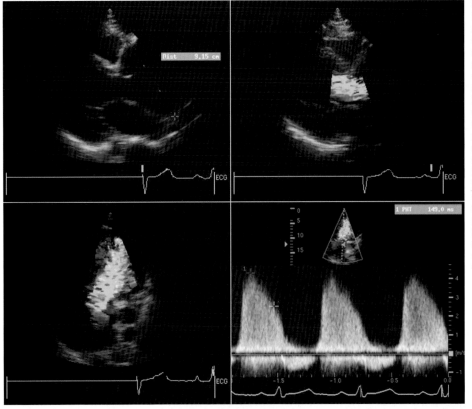

Figure 17-10. TTE. TOP LEFT, Parasternal long-axis view showing markedly dilated aortic root and ascending aorta (9.2 cm) with complete effacement of the sinotubular junction compatible with annuloaortic ectasia. The descending aorta does not appear enlarged, and there is no mitral valve prolapse. TOP RIGHT, Aortic insufficiency appears severe (occupies the entire height of the left ventricular outflow tract) by color Doppler flow mapping. BOTTOM LEFT, Apical 5-chamber axis view shows aortic insufficiency that appears severe by flow mapping. BOTTOM RIGHT, Steep deceleration time of aortic insufficiency waveform with low end-diastolic velocity, consistent with severe aortic insufficiency in which the aortic diastolic and left ventricular diastolic pressures nearly equilibrate by the end of diastole, reducing the diastolic aorta–left ventricle gradient and the end-diastolic velocity.

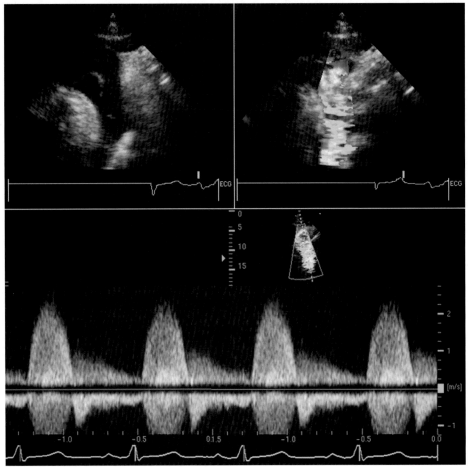

Figure 17-11. TTE. TOP LEFT, Suprasternal view. The distal arch does not appear dilated. There is a definite intimal flap starting in the distal arch and going down the aorta. TOP RIGHT, Color Doppler demonstrates the proximal isovelocity surface area (PISA), indicating flow into the intimal tear in the proximal descending aorta. BOTTOM, Spectral Doppler display of the flow in the proximal descending aorta shows increased anterograde and retrograde flow, consistent with severe aortic insufficiency. The sampling is confounded by the presence of the intimal flap and differential flows in the true and false lumens.

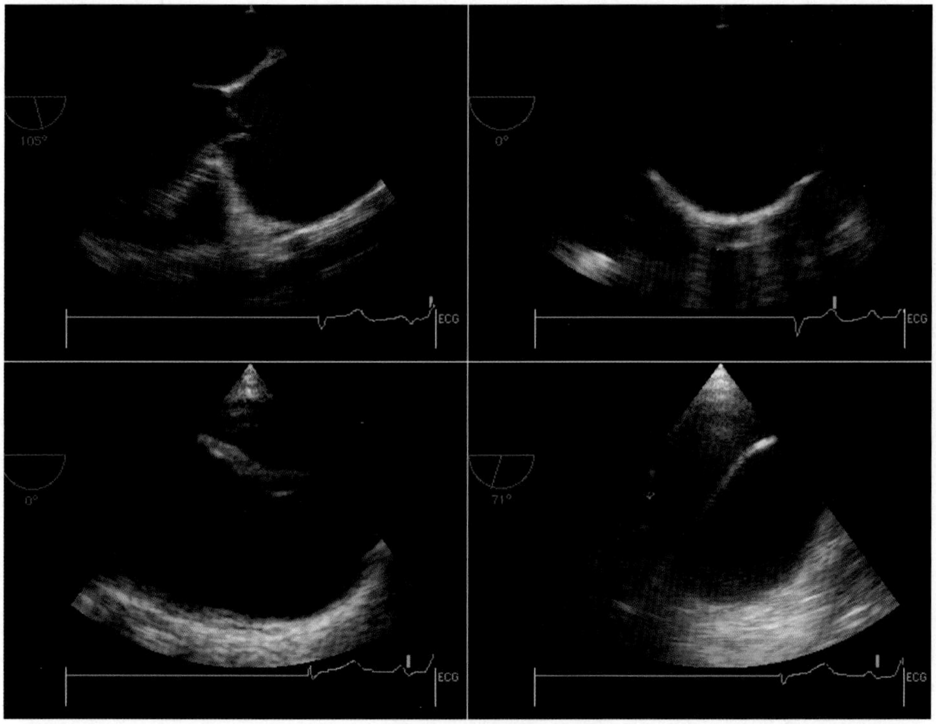

Figure 17-12. TEE. TOP LEFT, The aortic root in longitudinal axis. The root is severely dilated, as is the ascending aorta. There is complete effacement of the sinotubular junction. The root dilation has resulted in traction on the aortic valve leaflets and caused their " 'tenting" and failure of central coaptation. No intimal flap is present on this plane of imaging. TOP RIGHT, The mid descending aorta in cross section. There aorta is dilated, but without intimal flap or intramural hematoma. BOTTOM LEFT, The aortic arch in the horizontal plane. There is an intimal flap. BOTTOM RIGHT, The aortic arch in the vertical plane. The intimal flap is again seen, although with a thinner appearance than on the horizontal view. The variations in intimal flap orientation presumably influence its imaged thickness.

CASE 2

History

▸ A 44-year-old man experienced a severe, sudden-onset of midabdominal pain with some radiation into the back.
▸ He had a distal aortic dissection 5 years before that was managed medically, and he has been asymptomatic since.
▸ He has two brothers with Marfan syndrome; between them, they had two aortic dissections and one aneurysm.

Physical Examination

▸ BP 130/60 mm Hg, HR 90 bpm
▸ No pulse deficits
▸ No murmurs
▸ Midline abdominal tenderness

Evolution and Management

▸ Clinical impression was that of a stable old distal thoracic dissection and leakage of the AAA due to either its size or the dissection's extending into it.
▸ Surgery revealed a rupturing AAA with dissection.
▸ Aortoiliac tube graft was obtained.
▸ Uneventful outcome

Comments

▸ The case of this patient and his siblings illustrates the ongoing nature of aortic disease in the patient with Marfan syndrome and the need for regular follow-up of the entire aorta, including the abdominal aorta.
▸ Arguably, this patient had experienced three syndromes of aortic disease—distal thoracic dissection, AAA, and abdominal aortic dissection (aortic rupture).

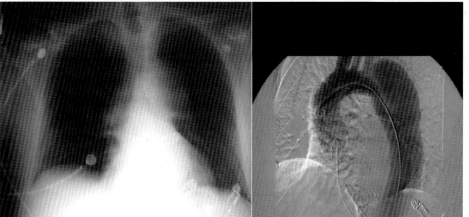

Figure 17-13. LEFT, Chest radiograph shows normal heart size, enlarged mediastinum, and transverse aortic width at the arch level. RIGHT, Digital subtraction angiography reveals the false lumen on the outside curvature of the aorta that begins just distal to the left subclavian artery, which accounts for the abnormal aortic contour on the anteroposterior chest film.

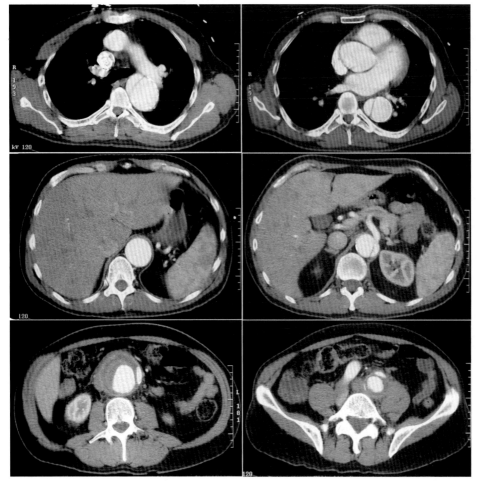

Figure 17-14. Contrast-enhanced axial CT images. TOP LEFT, Intimal flap in the descending aorta at the level of the left pulmonary artery, with equal opacification of both the true and false lumens. No intimal flap in the aortic root, which has normal dimensions. TOP RIGHT, Intimal flap in the descending aorta behind the left side of the heart, with equal opacification of both the true and false lumens. MIDDLE LEFT, Other than mild dilation, the abdominal aorta above the renal arteries appears normal. The thoracic dissection ended at the level of the diaphragm. MIDDLE RIGHT, Intimal flap in the abdominal aorta, below the normal segment of aorta. Splanchnic vessel being supplied by the false lumen. BOTTOM LEFT, Abdominal aortic aneurysm (AAA) with mural thrombus, but also with flow in a separate channel at the 3-o'clock position. There is some streaking and haziness to the tissue adjacent to the posterior wall of the aorta. This suggests inflammation or leakage. BOTTOM RIGHT, AAA with mural thrombus but also with flow in a separate channel at the 2-o'clock position. There is streaking and haziness circumferential to the aorta, more suggestive of leakage.

CASE 3

History

▸ 57-year-old man with obvious marfanoid features (unusual height, unusually low body fat percentage, very long limbs, myopia, prior retinal detachment) and positive family history

Physical Examination

▸ Class II-III shortness of breath
▸ Normal BP and HR
▸ Normal venous pressures
▸ Loud S_1, increased P_2
▸ 4/6 pansystolic murmur heard at the apex but radiating to the base, not the axilla

▸ No aortic insufficiency murmur; normal pulses
▸ No AAA by palpation

Management and Outcome

▸ Clinical impression was that of Marfan-related mitral valve prolapse, flail mitral leaflet, mitral regurgitation, and root dilation.
▸ Surgical repair of the mitral valve was obtained.
▸ Surgery revealed a flail posterior mitral leaflet.
▸ The patient had a long postoperative course marred by a stroke that left residual motor and speech deficits.

Comments

▸ Aortic and cardiac abnormalities associated with Marfan syndrome
▸ Mitral disease presenting earlier than aortic disease

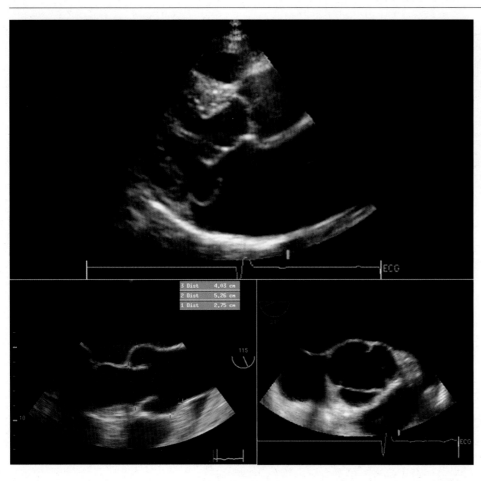

Figure 17-15. TOP, TTE parasternal long-axis view shows posterior mitral leaflet prolapse, and dilated left atrium and left ventricle portend severe mitral regurgitation. BOTTOM LEFT, Transesophageal echocardiography (TEE) longitudinal plane view of the ascending aorta shows enlarged aortic root and mildly enlarged ascending aorta (root: 53 mm; sinotubular junction: 40 mm). BOTTOM RIGHT, TEE cross-sectional view of the aortic root shows dilated sinuses of Valsalva; the posterior noncoronary sinus is the largest.

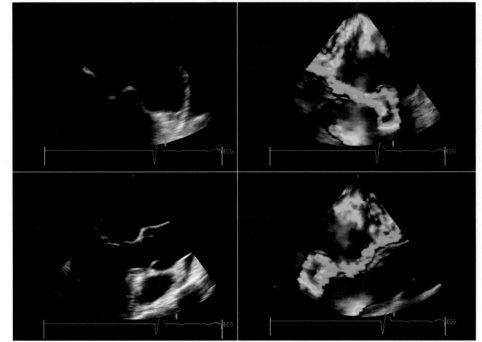

Figure 17-16. TEE. LEFT IMAGES, 2D. RIGHT IMAGES, With color Doppler flow mapping. TOP IMAGES, P$_2$ scallop prolapse with leftward-directed jet of mitral insufficiency. BOTTOM IMAGES, Left ventricular outflow tract longitudinal view shows P$_2$ scallop prolapse and anteriorly directed jet of mitral insufficiency. The PISAs are large, indicative of significant mitral regurgitation volume.

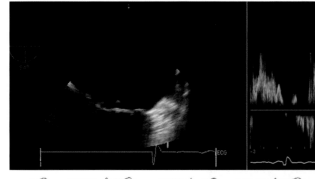

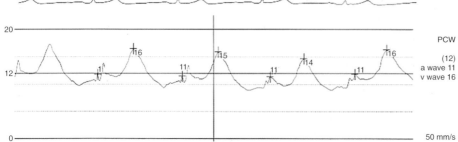

Figure 17-17. TOP LEFT, TEE vertical plane view of the mitral valve shows a small thread-like flail element of the mitral valve consistent with torn chordae tendineae. TOP RIGHT, Pulmonary venous sampling demonstrates systolic flow reversal indicative of severe mitral regurgitation. BOTTOM, Pulmonary capillary wedge (PCW) tracing. Although the mean pressure is only borderline elevated (the ventricular function was normal), there is a significant V wave, consistent with significant mitral regurgitation.

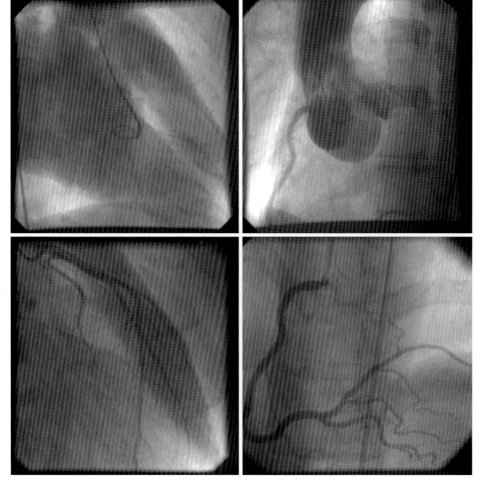

Figure 17-18. TOP LEFT, Right anterior oblique contrast ventriculogram: dilated and dynamic. Severe mitral regurgitation (fills the left atrium in one cardiac cycle and opacifies the left atrial appendage). TOP RIGHT, Aortography: prominent sinuses of Valsalva; no aortic insufficiency. BOTTOM, Normal coronary angiography, as is usually the case in Marfan syndrome patients.

CASE 4

History

▶ A 19-year-old man developed severe sudden-onset chest pain while playing basketball. He endured the pain and was seen 3 days later by his family physician, who noted a widened mediastinum and referred him that day to a cardiologist, who diagnosed aortic dissection by transthoracic echocardiography.

Physical Examination

▶ Marfanoid appearance
▶ Nonhypertensive (BP 120/70 mm Hg), no pericardial rub, no signs of tamponade, no pulse deficits or BP differential

▶ A murmur of aortic insufficiency was present as well as a murmur of mitral regurgitation, but no signs of left-sided heart failure

Comments

▶ Classic case of aortic dissection occurring during athletic activity in a young patient with Marfan syndrome
▶ Bentall procedure (composite aortic valve replacement–tube graft) performed with coronary reimplantation

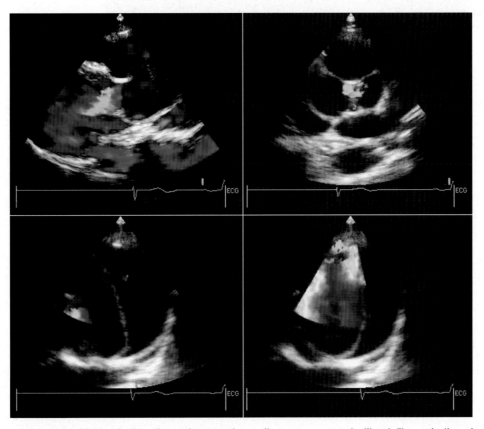

Figure 17-19. TTE. TOP LEFT, Parasternal long-axis view. The aortic root and ascending aorta are severely dilated. The aortic dimensions rival those of the left ventricle. There is aortic insufficiency, which on this view appears to be due to dilation of the root and sinuses. There is no pericardial effusion. The aortic insufficiency is approximately moderate. It is central and again appears to be due to asymmetric dilation of the sinuses. An intimal flap is present in the low ascending aorta. TOP RIGHT, Parasternal short-axis view of the aortic valve. The aortic insufficiency arises from the center of the aortic valve, probably indicating poor coaptation from root enlargement. BOTTOM, TTE views of the low ascending aorta in diastole (LEFT) and systole (RIGHT). The intimal flap is well seen, as is the intimal tear. There is flow across the intimal tear into the false lumen in systole.

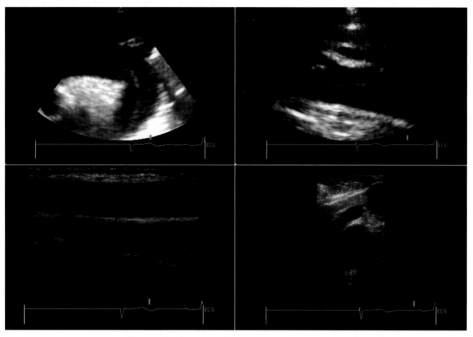

Figure 17-20. TTE. TOP LEFT, Suprasternal view clearly shows the intimal flap in the distal arch and descending aorta. It is not seen in the mid arch, possibly because it is off the plane of imaging. TOP RIGHT, Long-axis view of the subcostal abdominal aorta also shows the intimal flap. BOTTOM LEFT, Vascular ultrasound image of the common carotid artery. No flap is present. BOTTOM RIGHT, Vascular ultrasound image of the abdominal aorta in cross section. The intimal flap is again seen.

References

1. Januzzi JL, Marayati F, Mehta RH, et al: Comparison of aortic dissection in patients with and without Marfan's syndrome (results from the International Registry of Aortic Dissection). Am J Cardiol 2004;94:400-402.

2. Marfan AB: Un cas de déformation congénitale des quatre membres plus prononcée aux extrémités caractérisée par l'allongemont des os avec un certain degré d'amincissement. Bull Mem Soc Med Hop Paris 1896; 13:220.

3. Shores J, Berger KR, Murphy EA, Pyeritz RE: Progression of aortic dilatation and the benefit of long-term beta-adrenergic blockade in Marfan's syndrome. N Engl J Med 1994;330:1335-1341.

4. Bentall H, De Bono A: A technique for complete replacement of the ascending aorta. Thorax 1968;23:338-339.

5. Beighton P, De Paepe A, Danks D, et al: International Nosology of Heritable Disorders of Connective Tissue, Berlin, 1986. Am J Med Genet 1988;29:581-594.

6. De Paepe A, Devereux RB, Dietz HC, et al: Revised diagnostic criteria for the Marfan syndrome. Am J Med Genet 1996;62:417-426.

7. Roman MJ, Rosen SE, Kramer-Fox R, Devereux RB: Prognostic significance of the pattern of aortic root dilation in the Marfan syndrome. J Am Coll Cardiol 1993;22:1470-1476.

8. Hagan PG, Nienaber CA, Isselbacher EM, et al: The International Registry of Acute Aortic Dissection (IRAD): new insights into an old disease. JAMA 2000;283:897-903.

9. Walker BA, Murdoch JL: The wrist sign: a useful physical finding in the Marfan syndrome. Arch Intern Med 1970;126:276-277.

10. Steinberg I: A simple screening test for the Marfan syndrome. Am J Roentgenol Radium Ther Nucl Med 1966;97:118-124.

11. Ahimastos AA, Aggarwal A, D'Orsa KM, et al: Effect of perindopril on large artery stiffness and aortic root diameter in patients with Marfan syndrome: a randomized controlled trial. JAMA 2007;298:1539-1547.

12. Brooke BS, Habashi JP, Judge DP, et al: Angiotensin II blockade and aortic-root dilation in Marfan's syndrome. N Engl J Med 2008;358:2787-2795.

13. Gott VL, Greene PS, Alejo DE, et al: Replacement of the aortic root in patients with Marfan's syndrome. N Engl J Med 1999;340:1307-1313.

14. Karck M, Kallenbach K, Hagl C, et al: Aortic root surgery in Marfan syndrome: comparison of aortic valve–sparing reimplantation versus composite grafting. J Thorac Cardiovasc Surg 2004;127:391-398.

15. Kallenbach K, Baraki H, Khaladj N, et al: Aortic valve–sparing operation in Marfan syndrome: what do we know after a decade? Ann Thorac Surg 2007;83:S764-S768.

16. David TE, Feindel CM, Webb GD, et al: Long-term results of aortic valve–sparing operations for aortic root aneurysm. J Thorac Cardiovasc Surg 2006;132:347-354.

17. Miller DC: Valve-sparing aortic root replacement in patients with the Marfan syndrome. J Thorac Cardiovasc Surg 2003;125:773-778.

18. Legget ME, Unger TA, O'Sullivan CK, et al: Aortic root complications in Marfan's syndrome: identification of a lower-risk group. Heart 1996;75: 389-395.

19. Elefteriades JA: Thoracic aortic aneurysm: current approach to surgical timing. ACC Curr J Rev 2002;11:82-88.

20. Faxon DP, Creager MA, Smith SC Jr, et al: Atherosclerotic Vascular Disease Conference: Executive summary: Atherosclerotic Vascular Disease Conference Proceeding for Healthcare Professionals from a Special Writing Group of the American Heart Association. Circulation 2004;109:2595-2604.

21. Pape LA, Tsai TT, Isselbacher EM, et al: Aortic diameter greater than or equal to 5.5 cm is not a good predictor of type A aortic dissection: observations from the International Registry of Acute Aortic Dissection (IRAD). Circulation 2007;116:1120-1127.

22. Silverman DI, Burton KJ, Gray J, et al: Life expectancy in the Marfan syndrome. Am J Cardiol 1995;75:157-160.

23. Smith JA, Fann JI, Miller DC, et al: Surgical management of aortic dissection in patients with the Marfan syndrome. Circulation 1994;90: II235-II242.

24. Detter C, Mair H, Klein HG, et al: Long-term prognosis of surgically-treated aortic aneurysms and dissections in patients with and without Marfan syndrome. Eur J Cardiothorac Surg 1998;13:416-423.

25. Carrel T, Beyeler L, Schnyder A, et al: Reoperations and late adverse outcome in Marfan patients following cardiovascular surgery. Eur J Cardiothorac Surg 2004;25:671-675.

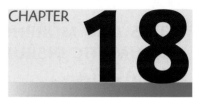

Traumatic Disruption of the Aorta

Traumatic disruption of the aorta (TDA) is a major injury complicating blunt chest trauma. Approximately 13% of injury-related fatalities have traumatic injury to the thoracic aorta or its branches. There are an estimated 7500 fatal cases per year in the United States. Typically, TDA arises from abrupt deceleration injury (>50 km/h [30 mph]), such as head-on motor vehicle collisions (car, motorcycles, or snowmobile), usually without the buffering effect of a seat belt restraint ("un–seat-belted"). A driver or passenger ejected from a car is twice as likely to experience TDA as is a nonejected victim. In the cases of pedestrians or cyclists, abrupt acceleration may result in the same lesions. The mortality is dominant—approximately 80% mortality at the site of the accident; 20% survive long enough to receive treatment of the TDA and other traumatic injuries.

Penetrating injury to the aorta is likely to result in death before hospitalization.[1]

COMPLETE AND PARTIAL TRAUMATIC DISRUPTION OF THE AORTA

Complete disruption of the aortic wall is catastrophic and leads to immediate exsanguination. Partial disruption may occur when the intima and media are disrupted but part of the media or the adventitia retains its integrity and contains rupture. Such patients may survive to be admitted but may proceed to experience dilation and rupture of the remaining wall of the aorta. Thus, timely diagnosis of TDA may be lifesaving.

Mechanisms of Disruption

Abrupt acceleration or deceleration results in forces being applied unevenly to the aorta, which thereby subjects its wall to mechanical stress. The aorta is tethered by ligaments at the arch level, by the pericardium, and by its foramen through the diaphragm. Abrupt acceleration or deceleration forces are therefore applied at these sites of tethering. Elsewhere, particularly through the length of the descending portion, the aorta is not directly tethered and hence is subject to considerable flexing when strong forces are applied to the chest. The aorta, being a large structure with considerable weight because of the large volume of blood it contains, is susceptible to its own inertia. At the sites where applied forces and inertial forces are in proximity, the aortic wall may be disrupted. The isthmus portion of the descending aorta and the supradiaphragmatic portion of the descending aorta are the sites where aortic attachment and the descending aorta's inertia subject the aorta to shearing forces, bending forces, and torsional forces.

The ascending aorta is subject to complex forces because of the local influence of the large mass and inertia of the heart, the attachments to the heart, and the sternum, which may be depressed far into the chest with trauma.

Another proposed mechanism of aortic disruption is the osseous pinch, which proposes that the anterior thoracic structures (manubrium, first rib) are forced posteriorly and inferiorly to impact on the vertebral column, damaging the proximal descending aorta in particular. Models support the concept, as does the similarity of TDA intimal lesions to those produced by the traumatic pinching of vascular clamps.[2] Vertebral displacement may frankly lacerate the aorta.

SITES AND MORPHOLOGY OF TRAUMATIC DISRUPTION OF THE AORTA

The sites of TDA are adjacent to points of attachment and flexing (Fig. 18-1). A large majority (95%) of cases occur at the proximal descending aorta, just distal to the left subclavian artery origin (the isthmus), at the site of the ligamentum arteriosum. The remaining 5% of cases involve the ascending aorta (seen more often at autopsy than in alive patients) and the supradiaphragmatic aorta.

TDA of the ascending aorta is less common than TDA of the descending aorta but is nevertheless a high-risk lesion. Presentations include postmortem identification, pseudoaneurysm, sinus of Valsalva fistula, subadventitial hematoma, and intimal and medial tears. Aortic valve disruption is commonly associated with TDA of the ascending aorta.[3]

From a series using aortography to detect TDA among 50 patients, typical lesion morphology was well described.[4] Mean distance from the left subclavian artery to the superior aspect of the injury was 5.8 mm along the lesser curvature and 14.9 mm along the greater curvature.[4] Mean length of the injury was 17.0 mm along the lesser curvature and 26.0 mm along the greater curvature.[4] Mean degree of curvature along the injury was 27 degrees.[4]

CLINICAL FINDINGS THAT SHOULD PROMPT CONSIDERATION OF TRAUMATIC DISRUPTION OF THE AORTA

Clinical findings that should prompt consideration of TDA include severe deceleration; midline chest pain (caveat: head injuries or rib fractures may obscure aortic chest pain); multiple rib fractures, especially high ribs (first and second), indicating severe forces inflicted on the chest; sternal fractures, indicating severe forces applied to the chest in an anteroposterior direction; pulse deficits, which may indicate disruption of the aortic continuity; upper extremity hypertension; and interscapular murmur, indicating turbulent flow in the descending aorta.

DIAGNOSIS OF TRAUMATIC DISRUPTION OF THE AORTA

Clinical suspicion is imperative. The chest radiograph can be suggestive, but not diagnostic, of TDA. Any of the following can make the diagnosis: computed tomography (CT), aortography, transesophageal echocardiography (TEE), magnetic resonance, and surgical inspection.

Chest Radiography in Traumatic Disruption of the Aorta

Widened superior mediastinum (>8 cm) and mediastinal hematoma may be surrogate signs of aortic injury. Haziness of the aortic knob contour and obliteration of the aorticopulmonary window have a good negative predictive value for TDA.[5] Rightward deviation of a nasogastric tube at the T4 level of more than 1 or 2 cm also has a very good negative predictive value.[6] Rightward deviation of the trachea or depression of the right main bronchus, apical cap, haziness of the medial left upper lobe due to hematoma, and fracture of the sternum or high ribs have also been shown to be associated with TDA.

At least one third and possibly two thirds of older patients with TDA may not have an initial chest radiograph with findings that would support the diagnosis of TDA.[7] Any abnormal finding in the context of suspected TDA requires further evaluation with aortography, CT, or TEE.

Computed Tomography in Traumatic Disruption of the Aorta

CT findings in TDA (Figs. 18-2 to 18-4) include direct findings such as abnormal aortic contour, pseudocoarctation, pseudoaneurysm (97% of cases), focal bulge (5% of cases), diffuse aneurysmal enlargement (32% of cases), and intimal flap or disruption (91% of cases).[8,9] The most commonly seen indirect finding is periaortic hematoma (91% of cases). Aortic injury occurred without periaortic hematoma in only 9% of cases, of which 6% had a pseudoaneurysm and 3% an intimal flap.

The sensitivity and specificity of CT for the detection of TDA depend on the criteria used and probably also on the equipment used. The use of mediastinal hematoma as a surrogate of TDA entails potential false-positives (as mediastinal hematoma may be due to injury of another vessel) and false-negatives (approximately 10% of cases do not have mediastinal hematoma).

Successful use of direct signs of aortic injury is dependent on sufficiently high resolution and artifact-free quality imaging.

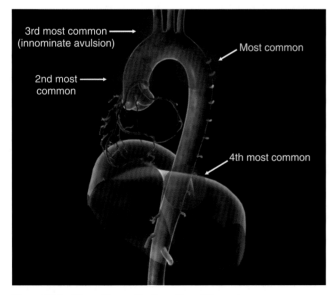

3rd most common (innominate avulsion)

Most common

2nd most common

4th most common

Figure 18-1. Sites of traumatic disruption of the aorta.

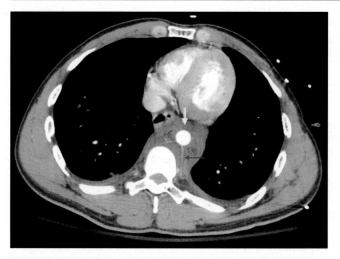

Figure 18-2. CT findings in TDA. Contrast-enhanced axial CT scan of a 30-year-old man found unconscious beside a building, presumed to have fallen 50 feet. Note the periaortic hematoma *(yellow arrow)*. Repeated examinations of the aorta (CT and TEE) failed to demonstrate signs of disruption. Although there was concern of occult TDA, a tear of an intercostal (or other branch) artery *(red arrow)* was presumed to be the cause of the hematoma. It resolved in 6 days.

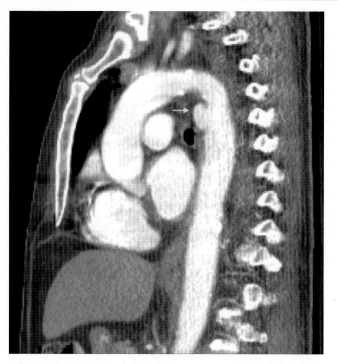

Figure 18-4. CT findings in TDA. Note mushroom cap–shaped disruption of the proximal descending aorta *(arrow)*.

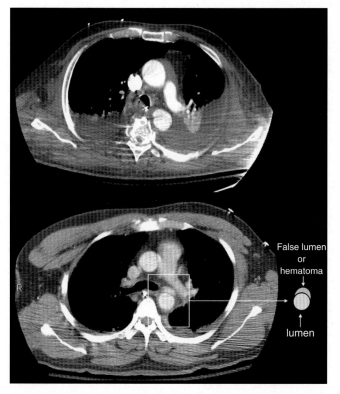

Figure 18-3. CT findings in TDA. Contrast-enhanced axial CT scans at the level of the pulmonary artery show typical findings of an intimal flap and a false lumen (pseudoaneurysm) cap.

Comparisons of CT with aortography and surgical findings for the detection of TDA show that direct signs of injury are superior. Mirvis and colleagues[9] analyzed 677 suspected cases of TDA and found that the sensitivity and specificity of CT were 90% and 99%, respectively, for signs of aortic injury and 100% and 87%, respectively, for mediastinal hematoma. Comparison studies, admittedly using older equipment, have not always dem-

onstrated results as good as those of the traditional test—aortography.[10-14] In those studies, CT had sensitivity of 67% to 100%, specificity of 96%, and negative predictive value of 100% (compared with 100%, 92%, and 100%, respectively, for aortography).

Given concerns about sensitivity, CT is not universally considered definitive for exclusion of TDA. Current generation (64-slice) CT scanning is likely to have greater sensitivity and specificity than reported in older studies. However, CT scanning clearly offers enormous versatility to assess, in the same session, head, other chest, abdominal, and limb injuries. Its diagnostic role in trauma is incontrovertible, and its use in emergent trauma is well incorporated into practice. CT scanning is increasingly used as a screening test or definitive test for TDA, depending on institutional expertise. In general, CT is used as a screening test. The cost of CT scanning may be less than that of aortography.[13]

Aortography in Traumatic Disruption of the Aorta

Aortography is the traditional initial "gold standard." Whether other tests have succeeded it is debated. It is generally accepted that aortography should be performed on any patient if there is even a small chance of aortic or major vessel injury, unless refractory shock or rapidly enlarging mediastinal contour is occurring.

Aortographic findings of TDA include pseudoaneurysm, intimal flap, abnormal aortic contours, and branch vessel involvement (Figs. 18-5 to 18-8). Branch vessel rupture is seen in up to 20% of TDA cases.

The ability to image the ascending aorta well is favorable compared with CT or TEE. CT may have artifact arising from superior vena cava dye streaking and from cardiac motion, and

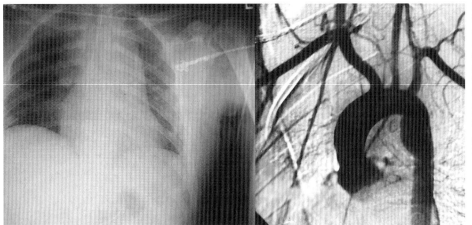

Figure 18-5. An 18-year-old man was involved in a motor vehicle accident and suffered polytrauma, pelvic fracture, and bladder disruption. LEFT, Chest radiograph shows a widened mediastinum and displaced endotracheal tube, suggesting, in this context, aortic enlargement. There are signs of a left superior vena cava. RIGHT, Aortogram shows a bulbous dilation of the proximal descending aorta starting immediately after the left subclavian artery, consistent with an adventitial hematoma from TDA.

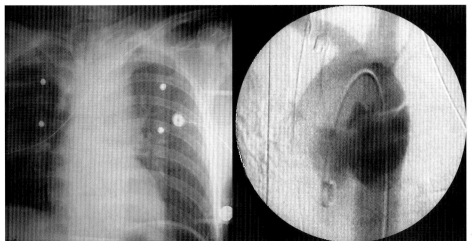

Figure 18-6. A 26-year-old man suffered closed head trauma, extremity trauma, lacerated spleen, and hematuria as a result of a motor vehicle accident. LEFT, Chest radiograph shows a widened mediastinum and displaced endotracheal tube. RIGHT, Aortogram shows a false aneurysm around the proximal descending aorta and a linear ridge at the superior margin. At surgery, an adventitial hematoma and an intimal flap were found. Surgery was successful.

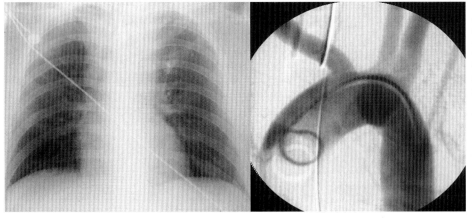

Figure 18-7. LEFT, Chest radiograph shows a widened mediastinum and displaced endotracheal tube, suggesting aortic enlargement. RIGHT, On the aortogram, a false aneurysm and a linear oblique ridge in the proximal descending aorta can be seen. At surgery, a spiral tear was found starting at the left subclavian artery. Hemorrhage was uncontrollable, and exsanguination ensued.

TEE does not image the ascending aorta in all patients because the tracheal air column interposed between the esophagus and the part of the ascending aorta precludes complete interrogation.[15]

Issues concerning aortography include the need for transport away from critical care environments, contrast infusion with its potential risks, puncture-related risks, additional time to obtain aortography, motion artifacts, dye streaming artifacts, poor opacification, poor image projection, confusion about ductal diverticulum versus disruption, and thrombosis of the false lumen. Less than 10% of aortograms yield positive results.

Transesophageal Echocardiography in Traumatic Disruption of the Aorta

The TEE findings of TDA are complex and numerous (Figs. 18-9 and 18-10).[16-18] Direct signs include intimal disruption, free-edge intimal flap, thick stripes, false lumen, aortic dissection, fusiform aneurysm, complete aortic obstruction, and aortic wall mural or adventitial hematoma. Indirect signs include minor increase in aortic diameter, impairment in aortic color Doppler flow (turbulent flow distal to intimal disruption), increase in aorta:TEE probe distance (indicating hemomediastinum), blurring of the aortic outline (in 20% of cases), and intraluminal artifacts (in 36% of cases).

Different studies have shown different sensitivity and specificity of TEE for detection of TDA. Although some studies have seen more findings on TEE than were seen with aortography, suggesting greater sensitivity, other studies have shown the reverse (Table 18-1).[19-21] TEE findings of TDA differ from those of aortic dissection (Table 18-2).[19,21]

Other issues concerning TEE are its variable availability depending on the institution, operator experience in imaging the aorta, and feasibility in trauma patients. Unlike CT and aortography, TEE study may not be feasible in some patients (8%).[19]

TREATMENT OF TRAUMATIC DISRUPTION OF THE AORTA

Surgical repair of the aorta is the traditional definitive treatment of TDA with substantial wall disruption. Blood pressure control with a beta-blocker is often instituted if it is feasible preoperatively and borrows it rationale from the traditional treatment of aortic dissection, but it is not proven.

Surgery of the isthmus portion of the aorta is performed through left thoracotomy and therefore requires that ventilation intraoperatively be maintained by right single-lung ventilation. As pulmonary contusion and aspiration are common in TDA cases, single-lung ventilation may not be feasible. Coagulopathy is common in trauma patients, also potentially confounding surgery. Required aortic cross-clamp time is generally 30 to 60 minutes, as is cardiopulmonary bypass time, if it is used.

Surgical repair of the descending aorta carries a 5% risk of paraplegia, 1% to 2% risk of stroke, and 1% to 2% risk of myocardial infarction. A common conundrum arises concerning the timing of surgical repair of TDA. If there is shock attributable to the TDA or if the aortic contour is expanding, emergent repair is appropriate. If the patient is stable, and particularly if there are major trauma-associated comorbidities, selective delay of surgery pending resolution of comorbidities (respiratory failure, coagulopathy, massive head injury, or sepsis) has been opted for, with acceptable outcomes.[22,23]

Endovascular stent grafting (TEVAR) has been performed successfully in cases of TDA. The role of nonsurgical (endovascular) repair of the aorta in TDA has yet to be clearly defined.[24] Certain technical challenges are actually greater for TEVAR in TDA cases than in aneurysmal disease, as TDA cases typically have a normal-caliber aorta with a tight arch curvature, whereas aneurysmal aortas have larger diameters and unfolded arches that are more amenable to TEVAR placement with current devices. Most EVAR devices are configured for aneurysmal disease, not traumatic disease of normal aortas.

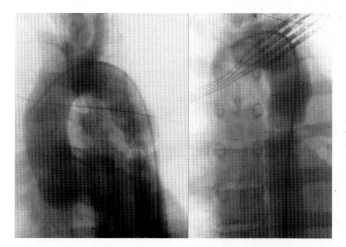

Figure 18-8. Aortography in TDA. A 24-year-old woman was involved in a motor vehicle accident (broadside driver's door), suffering a fractured pelvis and left hemothorax. Note the annular defect in the proximal descending aorta, seen on both views. At surgery, a complete transection of the intima and media was found, with a 5-cm adventitial hematoma. A tube graft was inserted. Postoperatively, there was a gradient across the graft.

Table 18-1. Transesophageal Echocardiography Versus Aortography for Detection of Traumatic Disruption of the Aorta

Study	No. of Patients	Modality	Sensitivity	Specificity
Smith[19]	101	TEE	100%	98%
Goarin[20]	209	TEE	97%	100%
Goarin[20]	209	Aortography	97%	100%
Vignon[21]	32	TEE	91%	100%

TEE, transesophageal echocardiography.

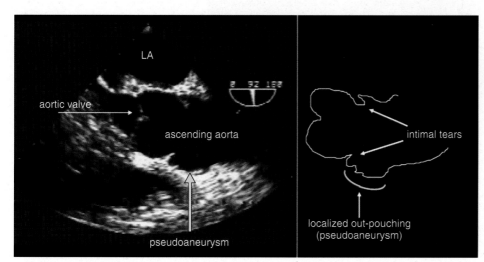

Figure 18-9. TEE long-axis view of the ascending aorta and aortic valve in a 42-year-old man involved in a motorcycle accident at 50 km/h (30 mph). Intimal tears are present on the posterior and anterior wall, as the disruption was circumferential. The aortic valve remained competent.

Table 18-2. Transesophageal Echocardiographic Findings of Traumatic Disruption of the Aorta Versus Aortic Dissection

		Subadventitial TDA	Aortic Dissection
Transverse imaging	Symmetry	Asymmetry	Symmetry
	Flap	Thick	Thin
	Highly mobile flap	Mobile	Less mobile
	Tears	No entry or re-entry tear	Entry ± re-entry tears
	Thrombus	None	Thrombus may form in the false lumen in a subacute or acute time period
	Mediastinal hematoma	Common	Uncommon
Longitudinal imaging		Oblique or vertical flap	Parallel flap
Color flow	Mosaic from turbulence	Mosaic from turbulence	No mosaic
	Flow on one side versus the other	Same on both sides	Different
Usual location		Isthmus	Originating in isthmus (type B) or in ascending aorta (type A)
Size		Small-medium	Large

TDA, traumatic disruption of the aorta.

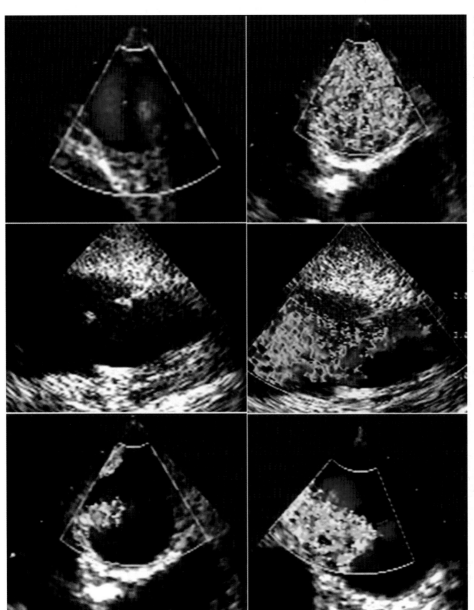

Figure 18-10. TEE. TOP LEFT, Cross-sectional view of the most proximal descending aorta. The appearance of the aorta and the flow within it are normal. TOP RIGHT, Cross-sectional view of the mid proximal descending aorta. There is no anatomic abnormality apparent of the aorta, but the flow pattern is entirely abnormal with variance indicative of turbulence that must arise more proximally. MIDDLE LEFT, Longitudinal view of the proximal descending aorta shows intimal irregularities. MIDDLE RIGHT, Color Doppler flow mapping reveals that the intimal irregularities initiate the turbulent flow. BOTTOM LEFT, Cross-sectional view of the proximal descending aorta. BOTTOM RIGHT, Longitudinal view of the proximal descending aorta. The turbulent flow is caused by intimal irregularities and is the clue in this case to localization of the problem.

CASE 1

History and Physical Examination

- 40-year-old man with polytrauma (splenic rupture, limb fractures) after a snowmobile accident
- Direct collision with a tree at 100 km/h (60 mph)
- Transferred for evaluation, as CT described hematoma around the aortic arch
- No murmurs, no pulse deficits

Management and Outcome

- Clinical impression was that of a small, localized intimal tear.
- The patient was managed conservatively and continues beta-blocker therapy.
- Follow-up CT scans did not show changes.

Comments

- Whether TDA occurred in this case is not certain. TEE offered the only evidence of this. If there was disruption, it was small, superficial, and localized.
- The aberrant left subclavian artery complicated the interpretation of the appearance of the aorta on the CT scan and the TEE and underscores the need to have familiarity with aortic arch vessel variants.

18

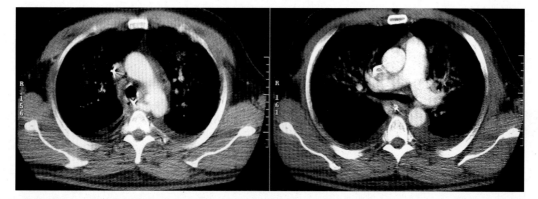

Figure 18-11. Contrast-enhanced axial CT scans. The appearance of the ascending aorta is normal. There is an abnormal appearance of the posterior distal arch and proximal descending aorta. There is a button-sized protrusion and a tubular protrusion that is presumably an aberrant right subclavian artery. The button anterior to it on the posterior wall of the arch may be the ostium of the left subclavian artery or possibly a traumatic defect. What appears to be crescentic thickening of the wall of the descending aorta may just be the pleural effusion running up onto the aorta.

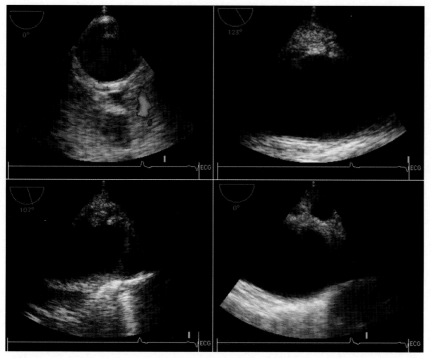

Figure 18-12. TEE. TOP LEFT, The appearance of the mid and proximal descending aorta is normal, and there is no sign of disruption of flow. TOP RIGHT, The proximal descending aorta in longitudinal plane. The near wall has a shallow cap-like luminal extension into it. BOTTOM LEFT, Proximal descending aorta immediately distal to the left subclavian artery. The appearance is complex and ambiguous. There is a linear tissue shelf from the 12-o'clock to the 3-o'clock position; this may represent an intimal disruption. BOTTOM RIGHT, An aberrant right subclavian artery courses between the transducer and the aorta. The short linear intimal line or disruption is seen from the 12-o'clock to the 1-o'clock position; the origin of the left subclavian artery is at the 3-o'clock position.

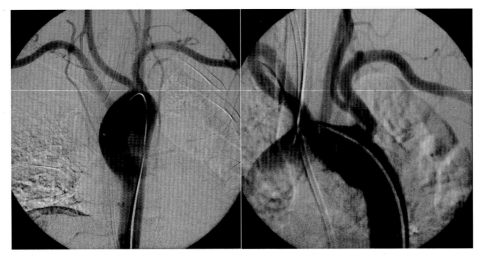

Figure 18-13. Aortography. LEFT, Normal appearance of the aorta in this projection, but abnormal arch vessel configuration. RIGHT, Irregular appearance to the proximal descending aorta—ductal diverticulum versus traumatic disruption of the aorta. Abnormal common origin to the left great arch vessels.

CASE 2

History

▸ 21-year-old woman with polytrauma suffered in a motor vehicle accident
▸ Ejected un–seat-belted passenger found on the road
▸ No known or obtainable history

Management and Outcome

▸ Clinical impression was that of a traumatic intimal disruption.
▸ There was no evidence of external bleeding from the aorta.
▸ Given the small size of the tear and its stability on repeated imaging, it was observed during the hospitalization for polytrauma and then subsequently on an outpatient basis. It has remained stable.
▸ The patient is taking beta-blockers and avoiding traumatic activities.
▸ Strategy is watchful waiting and CT follow-up, with a plan to intervene only in a case of worsening lesion.

Comments

▸ A small and initially stable tear of the intima
▸ Will need to be observed

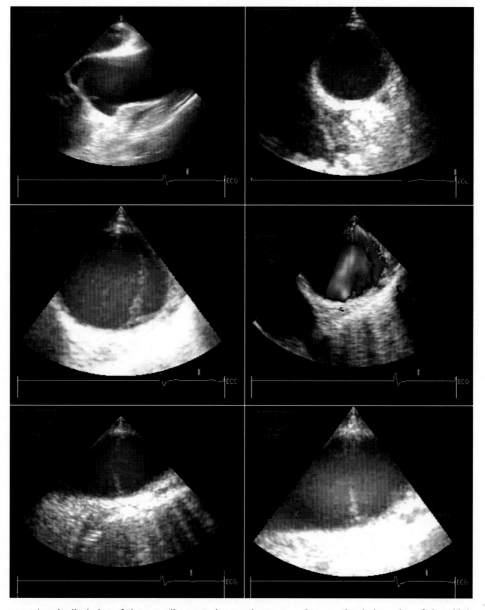

Figure 18-14. TEE. TOP LEFT, Longitudinal view of the ascending aorta is normal. TOP RIGHT, Cross-sectional plane view of the mid descending aorta is also normal. MIDDLE LEFT, View of the proximal descending aorta shows an intimal flap. MIDDLE RIGHT, There is flow partitioning by the intimal flap, but no turbulent flow in the true lumen. BOTTOM, Proximal descending aorta in longitudinal axis. The intimal flap is short and transverse.

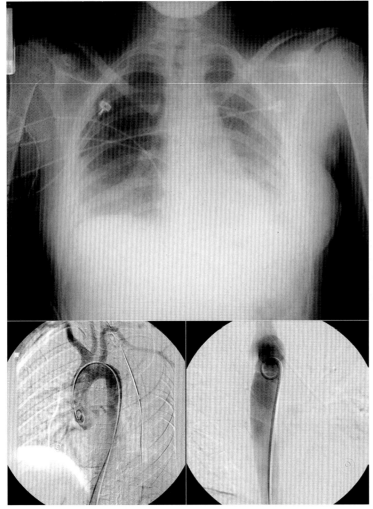

Figure 18-15. TOP, Chest radiograph shows a normal cardiopericardial silhouette. No definite widening of the aorta. Pulmonary infiltrates. BOTTOM, Aortography shows a transverse line across the proximal descending aorta, consistent with an intimal tear.

CASE 3

History

- 31-year-old man in a motor vehicle accident with polytrauma (liver laceration, limb fractures)
- Ejected un–seat-belted driver; combined vehicle collision speed >100 km/h (60 mph)
- Obvious aortic trauma seen on the CT scan
- No murmurs or pulse deficits

Management and Outcome

- Clinical impression was that of a disruption of the aorta at the isthmus with hematoma.

- Surgery found a 90-degree tear through the intima with adventitial hematoma.
- Primary repair with the heart on left ventricular assist device bypass (left atrium to descending aorta) was performed.
- Uneventful outcome

Comments

- Typical unequivocal TDA
- Partial circumferential tear with limited hematoma and therefore survival into the hospital and through surgery

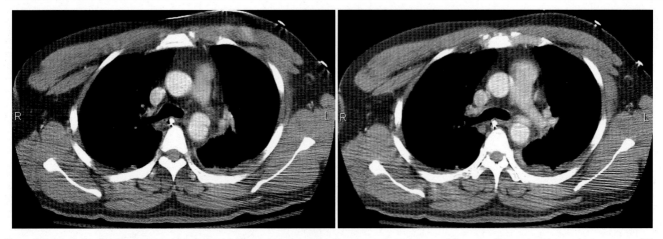

Figure 18-16. Both of these contrast-enhanced axial CT scans show normal diameter and appearance of the ascending aorta. Abnormal appearance of the proximal descending aorta, with a tear and false lumen. Soft tissue around the descending aorta and under the arch—possibly a hematoma.

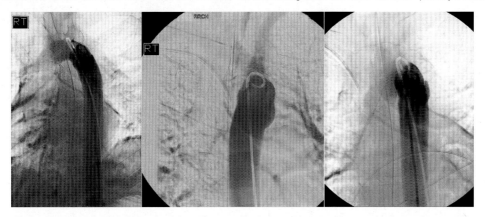

Figure 18-17. Aortography shows a tear and false lumen seen on the posterior wall of the descending aorta. Dye density is greater around the area of the tear, consistent with retention of dye in a localized pocket. The lateral view (LEFT) best reveals the abnormal contour of the posterior wall of the proximal descending aorta.

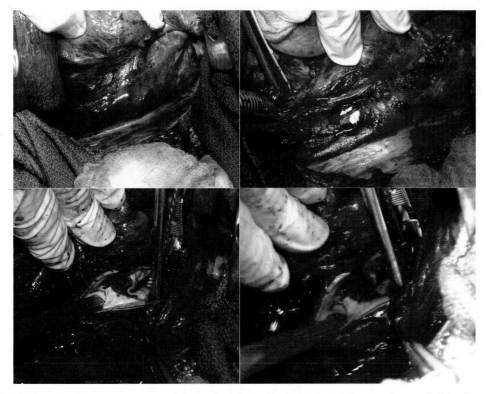

Figure 18-18. Surgical findings. TOP, Hematoma seen around the proximal descending aorta. BOTTOM, The aorta is opened with a long-axis incision and accessed through a left thoracotomy. The transverse intimal tear is obvious, and the pocket behind it.

CASE 4

History

▸ A 27-year-old un–seat-belted male driver was involved in an unwitnessed motor vehicle accident and ejected.
▸ He suffered polytrauma (pelvic and long bone fractures, skull fracture).
▸ Obvious aortic trauma seen on the CT scan

Management and Outcome

▸ Clinical impression was that of a disruption of the aorta at the isthmus with hematoma.
▸ Management was focused on the ongoing major medical and surgical complications.
▸ TDA remained stable during 4 months.
▸ The plan is to observe the lesion and to intervene only if significant enlargement occurs.

Comments

▸ Typical unequivocal TDA
▸ Partial tear with limited hematoma and characteristic cap
▸ Major ongoing medical and surgical issues

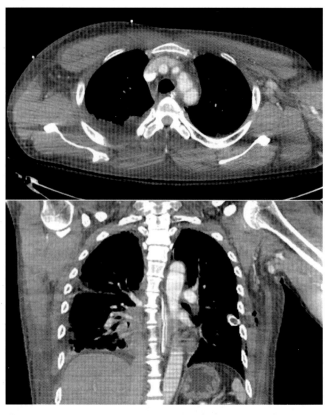

Figure 18-19. Contrast-enhanced CT scans. TOP, Axial view shows a mushroom cap–shaped hematoma over the distal aortic arch and proximal descending aorta. BOTTOM, Coronal view shows the mushroom cap over the distal aorta.

CASE 5

History

▸ A 65-year-old un–seat-belted male driver was involved in a head-on high-speed motor vehicle accident.
▸ He suffered polytrauma (pelvic fractures, long bone fractures, spinal fractures) and massive neurologic deficits.
▸ Obvious aortic trauma seen on the CT scan

Management and Outcome

▸ Clinical impression was that of a disruption of the aorta at the isthmus with hematoma.

▸ Management was conservative, given the neurologic comorbidity.
▸ The TDA remained stable for months.

Comments

▸ Typical unequivocal TDA
▸ Typical mushroom cap appearance of a partial circumferential tear
▸ Comorbidities dominated the clinical course.

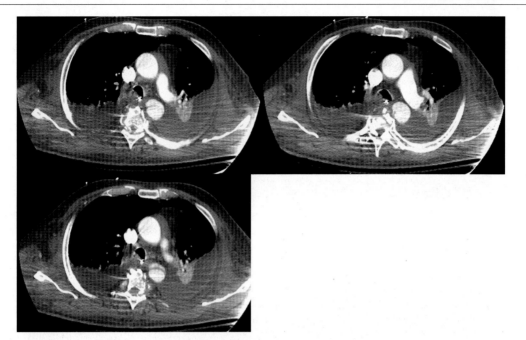

Figure 18-20. Contrast-enhanced axial CT scan shows prominent streaking off the vertebral column. In the top left image, this confuses the assessment of the descending aorta, as the line across the aorta appears to be artifact. The top right image reveals an intimal flap, and the bottom left image reveals a false lumen anteriorly. The line in the top left image was a true flap with an artifact superimposed on it.

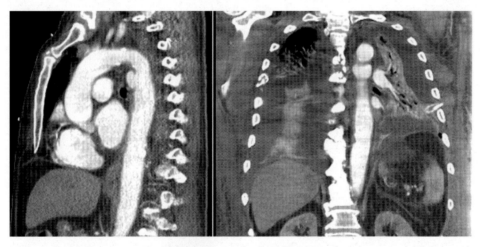

Figure 18-21. Contrast-enhanced axial CT scans. LEFT, Sagittal view shows a localized false lumen (pseudoaneurysm) off the anterior wall of the proximal descending aorta. RIGHT, On the coronal view, the body of the false lumen is seen anterior to the descending aorta.

CASE 6

History

▸ An 18-year-old un–seat-belted man was involved in an unwitnessed motor vehicle collision.
▸ He was intubated at the scene.
▸ He suffered multiple long bone fractures, pelvic fracture, and abdominal and neurologic injuries.

Management and Outcome

▸ Transthoracic echocardiography (TTE) revealed abnormally turbulent flow in the retrocardiac and abdominal aorta. The heart itself was normal.

▸ TEE revealed disruption of the proximal descending aorta over several centimeters of length.
▸ CT confirmed a complex disruption of the aorta over several centimeters and periaortic-mediastinal hematoma.
▸ 10 days after the accident, the patient underwent uncomplicated and uneventful TEVAR of the disrupted aorta.

Comments

▸ Un–seat-belted driver in a high-speed collision
▸ Aortic disruption as one of numerous polytrauma injuries
▸ Typical imaging findings
▸ Successful TEVAR

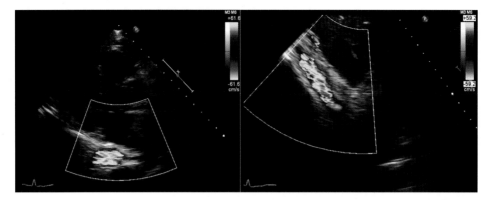

Figure 18-22. TTE. LEFT, Parasternal long-axis view. RIGHT, Subcostal view of the aorta. In both images, there is an abnormal turbulence to flow in the aorta.

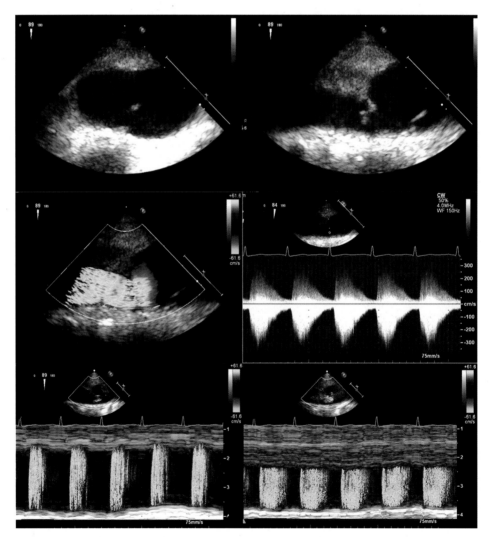

Figure 18-23. TEE. TOP, Long-axis views of the proximal descending aorta reveal intimal irregularities, with mobility, abrupt narrowing of the lumen, and increased soft tissue between the TEE probe and the aorta, consistent with periaortic hematoma. MIDDLE LEFT, Color Doppler flow mapping reveals convergence at the site of narrowing and turbulence of flow in the ongoing descending aorta. MIDDLE RIGHT, Continuous wave Doppler sampling demonstrates a significant spectral dispersion and velocity increase at the site of disruption and narrowing. BOTTOM, Color M-mode study before (LEFT) and after (RIGHT) the narrowing depicts the abrupt thickening of the periaortic tissue and abrupt narrowing of the aorta as well as flow acceleration and dispersion.

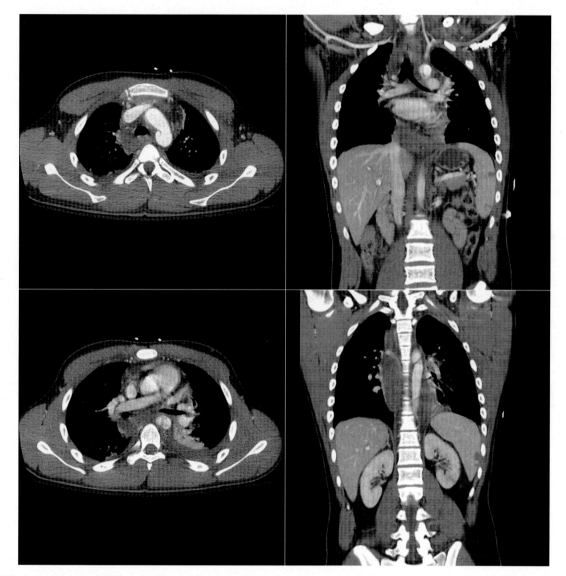

Figure 18-24. Contrast-enhanced CT scans in the axial (LEFT COLUMN) and coronal (RIGHT COLUMN) planes. An intimal flap is present in the distal arch–proximal descending aorta. In the proximal descending aorta, the appearance of the lumen becomes complex, with two channels separated by an oblique ridge. There is periaortic or mediastinal hematoma.

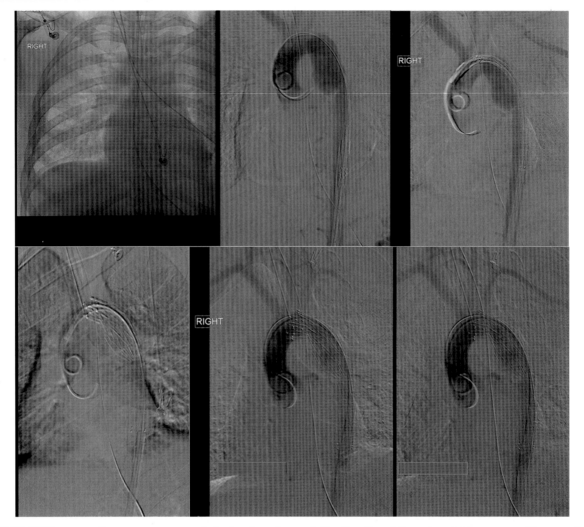

Figure 18-25. TEVAR. TOP LEFT, Fluoroscopy. TOP MIDDLE, Contrast aortography reveals the disruption of the aorta and false aneurysm. The covered stent is being advanced. Other images show the deployment of the TEVAR covered stent. Although the stent covers the left subclavian ostium, there is still flow in the left subclavian artery. There is no leak.

References

1. Dosios TJ, Salemis N, Angouras D, Nonas E: Blunt and penetrating trauma of the thoracic aorta and aortic arch branches: an autopsy study. J Trauma 2000;49:696-703.

2. Crass JR, Cohen AM, Motta AO, et al: A proposed new mechanism of traumatic aortic rupture: the osseous pinch. Radiology 1990;176:645-649.

3. Pretre R, LaHarpe R, Cheretakis A, et al: Blunt injury to the ascending aorta: three patterns of presentation. Surgery 1996;119:603-610.

4. Borsa JJ, Hoffer EK, Karmy-Jones R, et al: Angiographic description of blunt traumatic injuries to the thoracic aorta with specific relevance to endograft repair. J Endovasc Ther 2002;9(Suppl 2):II84-II91.

5. Marnocha KE, Maglinte DD, Woods J, et al: Blunt chest trauma and suspected aortic rupture: reliability of chest radiograph findings. Ann Emerg Med 1985;14:644-649.

6. Gerlock AJ Jr, Muhletaler CA, Coulam CM, Hayes PT: Traumatic aortic aneurysm: validity of esophageal tube displacement sign. AJR Am J Roentgenol 1980;135:713-718.

7. Exadaktylos AK, Sclabas G, Schmid SW, et al: Do we really need routine computed tomographic scanning in the primary evaluation of blunt chest trauma in patients with "normal" chest radiograph? J Trauma 2001;51:1173-1176.

8. Cleverley JR, Barrie JR, Raymond GS, et al: Direct findings of aortic injury on contrast-enhanced CT in surgically proven traumatic aortic injury: a multi-centre review. Clin Radiol 2002;57:281-286.

9. Mirvis SE, Shanmuganathan K, Miller BH, et al: Traumatic aortic injury diagnosis with contrast-enhanced thoracic CT: five-year experience at a major trauma center. Radiology 1996;200:413-422.

10. Fenner MN, Fisher KS, Sergel NL, et al: Evaluation of possible traumatic thoracic aortic injury using aortography and CT. Am Surg 1990;56:497-499.

11. Madayag MA, Kirshenbaum KJ, Nadimpalli SR, et al: Thoracic aortic trauma: role of dynamic CT. Radiology 1991;179:853-855.

12. Miller FB, Richardson JD, Thomas HA, et al: Role of CT in diagnosis of major arterial injury after blunt thoracic trauma. Surgery 1989;106:596-602.

13. Parker MS, Matheson TL, Rao AV, et al: Making the transition: the role of helical CT in the evaluation of potentially acute thoracic aortic injuries. AJR Am J Roentgenol 2001;176:1267-1272.

14. Tomiak MM, Rosenblum JD, Messersmith RN, Zarins CK: Use of CT for diagnosis of traumatic rupture of the thoracic aorta. Ann Vasc Surg 1993;7:130-139.

15. Ahrar K, Smith DC, Bansal RC, et al: Angiography in blunt thoracic aortic injury. J Trauma 1997;42:665-669.

16. Shapiro MJ, Yanofsky SD, Trapp J, et al: Cardiovascular evaluation in blunt thoracic trauma using transesophageal echocardiography (TEE). J Trauma 1991;31:835-839.

17. Karalis DG, Victor MF, Davis GA, et al: The role of echocardiography in blunt chest trauma: a transthoracic and transesophageal echocardiographic study. J Trauma 1994;36:53-58.

18. Goarin JP, Catoire P, Jacquens Y, et al: Use of transesophageal echocardiography for diagnosis of traumatic aortic injury. Chest 1997;112:71-80.

19. Smith MD, Cassidy JM, Souther S, et al: Transesophageal echocardiography in the diagnosis of traumatic rupture of the aorta. N Engl J Med 1995;332:356-362.

20. Goarin JP, Cluzel P, Gosgnach M, et al: Evaluation of transesophageal echocardiography for diagnosis of traumatic aortic injury. Anesthesiology 2000;93:1373-1377.

21. Vignon P, Gueret P, Vedrinne JM, et al: Role of transesophageal echocardiography in the diagnosis and management of traumatic aortic disruption. Circulation 1995;92:2959-2968.

22. Stiles QR, Cohlmia GS, Smith JH, et al: Management of injuries of the thoracic and abdominal aorta. Am J Surg 1985;150:132-140.

23. Maggisano R, Nathens A, Alexandrova NA, et al: Traumatic rupture of the thoracic aorta: should one always operate immediately? Ann Vasc Surg 1995;9:44-52.

24. Kato N, Dake MD, Miller DC, et al: Traumatic thoracic aortic aneurysm: treatment with endovascular stent-grafts. Radiology 1997;205:657-662.

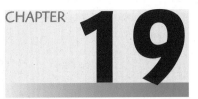

Tumors of the Aorta

KEY POINTS

- Malignant tumors of the aorta are rare.
- Essentially all are sarcomas:
  - Malignant endothelioma
  - Angiosarcoma
  - Epithelioid angiosarcoma
  - Intimal sarcoma
- Leiomyosarcoma
- Malignant fibrous histiocytoma
- Presentations of aortic tumors are numerous.
- Outcomes are almost uniformly poor because of massive (life-threatening) embolization of tumor at presentation, extensive local disease disadvantaging surgical repair, and metastases by the time of diagnosis.

Malignant tumors of the aorta are, fortunately, rare. Several different types of tumors of the aorta have been described. Essentially all are sarcomas: malignant endothelioma, angiosarcoma, epithelioid angiosarcoma, intimal sarcoma, leiomyosarcoma, and malignant fibrous histiocytoma.

Endothelial origin sarcomas grow into the lumen and wall and are prone to fragmentation into the lumen, with life-threatening embolization to the viscera and lower extremities. Leiomyosarcomas (smooth muscle cell sarcomas) tend to grow outward into the pleural or other adjacent spaces and are very large by the time of detection, with metastases already present. Some have been reported to cause frank aortic obstruction and thereby hypertension, and some have been reported to cause intramural hematomas and dissection or to have an appearance mimicking dissection.

The presentations of aortic tumors are numerous. The outcomes are almost uniformly poor because of massive (life-threatening) embolization of tumor at presentation, extensive local disease disadvantaging surgical repair, and metastases by the time of diagnosis.

It is hoped that surgical intervention may benefit a rare patient, but this remains more hope than experience.

Some primary aortic malignant neoplasms have been observed to cause hematoma and dissection of the aorta, and an occasional tumor has been erroneously diagnosed as being a dissection. Therefore, consideration of this rare possibility in atypical cases of dissection is reasonable.[1]

CASE 1

History

- A 35-year-old woman was incidentally found to have an abnormal chest radiograph.
- No complaints by history, and normal physical examination findings

Management

- A percutaneous biopsy established that the mass was a sarcoma, believed to have arisen from the aorta.
- Thorascopic surgery was unable to address the mass, so the patient underwent open thoracotomy, excision, and replacement of the involved aorta.

Evolution and Outcome

- The patient convalesced from surgery, but the malignant neoplasm recurred, causing death within a year.

Comments

- Leiomyosarcoma of the aorta, which silently grew to a very large size, as it grew predominantly into the left pleural space
- Unfortunately, most malignant neoplasms of the aorta have similarly poor outcomes.

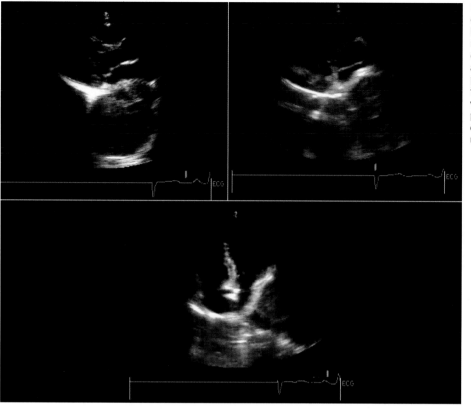

Figure 19-1. Transthoracic echocardiography. TOP LEFT, Parasternal long-axis view shows a large soft tissue mass posterior to the left atrium, compressing it. TOP RIGHT, Parasternal short-axis view shows a large soft tissue mass posterior to the left ventricle, compressing it anteriorly. BOTTOM, Apical 4-chamber view. There is a large soft tissue mass posterior and lateral to the left atrium, compressing it and pushing the lateral mitral annulus apically.

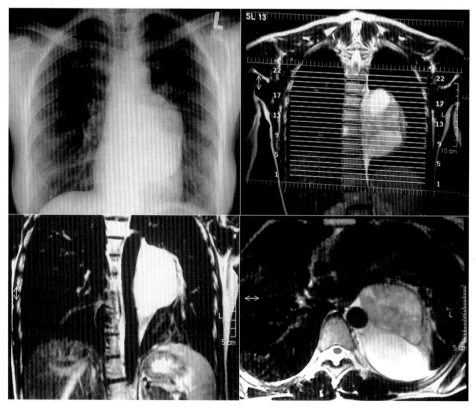

Figure 19-2. TOP LEFT, Chest radiograph shows a large left-sided soft tissue mass. No lung masses. No pleural effusions. TOP RIGHT, T1-weighted MR image (scout view) shows a large posterior mass beside the spine. There is a probable smaller but similar mass in the vertebral column. BOTTOM LEFT, T1-weighted MR image (coronal view) shows a large soft tissue mass adjacent to the aorta. BOTTOM RIGHT, T1-weighted MR image (axial view) shows a large soft tissue mass adjacent to the aorta. No narrowing of the aorta.

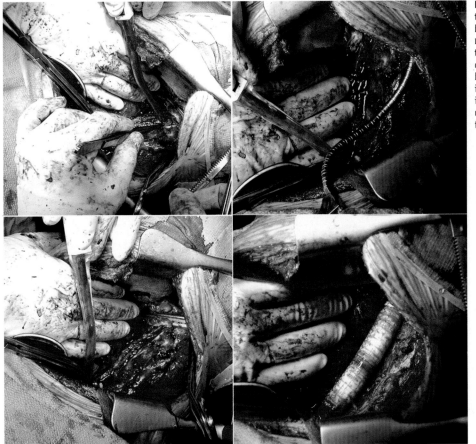

Figure 19-3. Surgery. TOP LEFT, Left thoracotomy. TOP RIGHT, Soft tissue mass bulging into the left pleural cavity. BOTTOM LEFT, Soft tissue mass is being excised, and the aorta has been clamped. The segment of the aorta that had been involved has been resected. BOTTOM RIGHT, An interposition Dacron tube graft has been inserted. The graft is pressurized as the upper clamp has been released, allowing flow through the graft.

Reference

1. Borislow DS, Floyd WL, Sane DC: Primary aortic sarcoma mimicking aortic dissection. Am J Cardiol 1989;64:549-551.

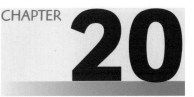

Infectious and Mycotic Aneurysms

Infection of the aorta may occur through several mechanisms: direct spread of infection from contiguous spaces or structures; direct seeding of the wall from blood-borne infection; septic embolism to the aorta; infection of the vasa vasorum by blood-borne pathogen (e.g., syphilis); and infection of a damaged segment of aorta by blood-borne infection.

Agents that may potentially infect the aorta include bacteria (most commonly *Staphylococcus aureus, Salmonella* species, and *Clostridium* species), mycobacteria, fungi, and syphilitic treponemes.[1,2]

AORTIC BACTERIAL INFECTION

Bacterial infection has a predilection for preexisting damage of the aortic wall, such as aneurysm, false aneurysm, old dissection or traumatic disruption, instrumentation site, or repair site. Infection into the wall of the aorta (endovascular infection) through an infected aortic graft may occur, with a profile of organisms similar to that of endocarditis. *Salmonella* species have proclivity to adhere to vascular endothelium, particularly if it is abnormal.

Clinical Presentation and Management

Fevers and leukocytosis are common. Unless the infection has become sequestered, cases will have bacteremia. Complications are common and may be complex. They include septicemia, breakdown of the aorta, aneurysm and false aneurysm formation (may be rapid), dissection of the aorta, fistulization of the aorta (especially aortoenteric fistula), rupture of the aorta, and vegetations that may occur on the luminal side and may be of size large enough to embolize.[3]

Intravenous antibiotics are rarely adequate to eliminate the infection, although they are essential and should be given before surgery to lessen reinfection.

Surgical revision of the infected segment according to the extent of involvement is preferred to avoid rupture of the aorta.

SYPHILITIC AORTITIS

About 10% of untreated tertiary syphilis cases develop clinical cardiovascular involvement. Syphilitic treponemes invade through the vasa vasorum, initiating inflammation, which secondarily damages the media, initiating aneurysmal dilation. As the abdominal aorta has little vasa vasorum, syphilitic involvement there is rare, whereas it is common in the ascending aorta and the arch.

On gross examination, the syphilitic aorta is described as having a characteristic tree bark appearance on the outside and wrinkling on the inside. Fine linear calcification may occur in the elderly. Three quarters of syphilitic aneurysms are saccular; one quarter are fusiform. Most syphilitic aneurysms are located in the proximal aorta (half in the ascending portion, one third in the arch). Only 10% are located in the descending aorta, and few occur in the abdomen. Branch vessel involvement may occur (innominate arteries, internal thoracic arteries). Aortic insufficiency may arise from either root dilation or sclerosis of the aortic valve, or both.

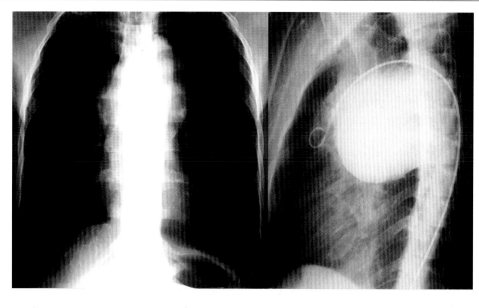

Figure 20-1. A 41-year-old Haitian man presented with a 2-month history of fatigue, respiratory distress on lying supine, and systolic ejection murmur. Past medical history was significant for venereal diseases and soccer-related chest trauma. Chest radiograph was uniformly interpreted as bihilar adenopathy. Aortography conclusively identified a large aneurysm of the ascending aorta without aortic insufficiency. Given VDRL positivity, the etiology was presumed to be syphilitic. The patient underwent uncomplicated surgical aortic repair. (Courtesy of Andrew Common, MD, Toronto, Canada.)

Clinical Presentation and Diagnosis

Syphilitic aortitis can be asymptomatic. Aortic insufficiency and coronary ostial narrowing occur in one third of patients and commonly coexist. Aortic aneurysm occurs in 10% of cases (Fig. 20-1).

In patients younger than 50 years, in whom advanced atheromatous aortic disease and advanced hypertensive disease of the aorta are uncommon, syphilitic aortic disease is easier to diagnose as the etiology of aneurysms.

In patients older than 50 years, in whom advanced atheromatous aortic disease and advanced hypertensive disease of the aorta are common, syphilitic aortic disease is more difficult to distinguish and to diagnose. Serologic evidence is important; more than 50% have VDRL positivity, and more than 95% have FTA-ABS positivity.

CASE 1

History and Physical Examination

▸ A 66-year-old man presented 7 weeks after bioprosthetic aortic valve replacement for aortic stenosis and aortocoronary bypass surgery with shortness of breath, fatigue, and mild chest pains.
▸ No venous distention or edema
▸ Incisions well healed
▸ Normal heart sounds; no murmurs or rubs
▸ Chest clear
▸ 38° C, mild leukocytosis
▸ CT scan at community hospital excluded pulmonary embolism but revealed an abnormal ascending aorta.

Management and Outcome

▸ A false aneurysm of the cannulation site was suspected and proven at surgery.

▸ The surrounding soft tissue was ambiguous; leakage of the false aneurysm was suspected.
▸ Surgery found a rupturing false aneurysm at the cannulation site with pus around the aorta and within the false aneurysm due to *Staphylococcus aureus*.
▸ Drainage, débridement, and patch repair of the false aneurysm were performed.
▸ The patient had a somewhat longer but successful postoperative course.

Comments

▸ Infected false aneurysm of the cannulation site with leakage of blood
▸ The local infection appeared to be facilitating the breakdown of the aorta. How the infection became located there was unclear, but it was presumably by either hematogenous spread or incisional or mediastinal spread.

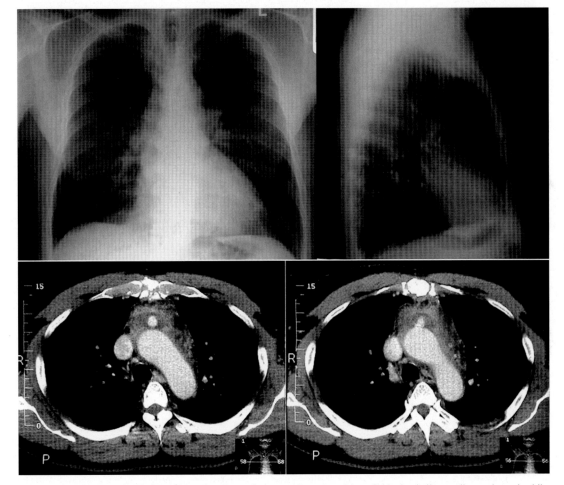

Figure 20-2. TOP, Chest radiographs taken before the aortic valve replacement show normal lung fields, borderline cardiomegaly, and a hilar overlay sign of dilation of the ascending aorta. BOTTOM, Contrast-enhanced axial CT scans show a small luminal extension anteriorly off the ascending aorta, surrounded by several centimeters of soft tissue. Because the mass is seen en face to the aorta on the posteroanterior view, it is not apparent here.

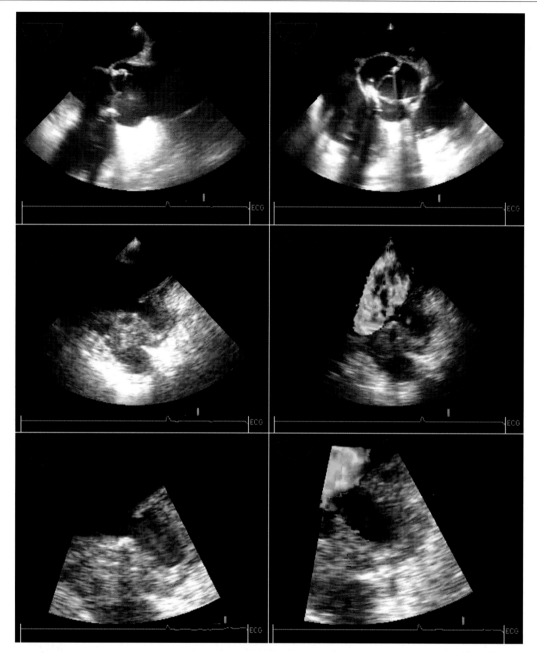

Figure 20-3. Transesophageal echocardiography. TOP, Longitudinal (LEFT) and cross-sectional (RIGHT) plane view of the ascending aorta and bioprosthetic aortic valve. Mildly dilated ascending aorta. Well-seated aortic bioprosthetic valve. MIDDLE, Two-dimensional imaging (LEFT) and color Doppler flow mapping (RIGHT) of an irregular, lobulated false aneurysm arising from the anterior wall of the ascending aorta, nearly entirely filled in with thrombus other than a small fingertip area, and with low flow (spontaneous contrast on two-dimensional imaging) within. BOTTOM, Better visualization of the communication of the aorta and the lumen of the false aneurysm. It is in the general area of the efferent bypass cannula insertion. The communication (or neck) is very narrow in relation to the width of the false aneurysm.

References

1. Zenati MA, Bonanomi G, Kostov D, Lee R: Images in cardiovascular medicine. Fulminant *Clostridium septicum* aortitis. Circulation 2002;105:1871.

2. Sugane T, Takahashi N, Koura T, et al: A case of tuberculous aneurysm of the aorta. Kekkaku 2000;75:589-593.

3. Bansal RC, Ashmeik K, Razzouk AJ: An unusual case of vegetative aortitis diagnosed by transesophageal echocardiography. J Am Soc Echocardiogr 2001;14:237-239.

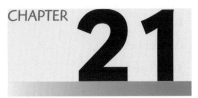

Noninfectious Aortitis: Takayasu's Disease

Takayasu's disease, or Takayasu's arteritis, was named after a Japanese ophthalmologist who first identified unusual wreath-like collateral vessels in the retina. Because arch vessel occlusions are so common in the disease, it has also been termed *pulseless disease* and *aortic arch disease*. Originally described in the Japanese population, it has subsequently been identified worldwide (Table 21-1). There is an initial pre-pulseless inflammatory phase of systemic constitutional symptoms and a later pulseless phase of chronic scarring.

The characteristic patient is female (90%) in her 20s (80% are first recognized in the second or third decade of life) and with an absent or diminished left radial pulse (narrowing of the left subclavian is present in 90%).

Hypertension is common, but the detection of it is confounded by the presence of stenoses of the subclavian arteries. Causes of hypertension in Takayasu's arteritis include stiffening of the aorta due to scarring, aortic narrowing or obstruction at the thoracic or abdominal level, and renal artery stenosis with secondary hypertension.

CLINICAL PRESENTATION

Arterial clinical presentations include occlusions (ischemic occlusions of the carotid, arm, leg, coronary, and visceral arteries), occlusions of the branch vessels of the aorta, and occlusions of the aorta; aneurysms (single or multiple) of the aorta or branch vessels, including coronary; dissection; hypertension due to aortic narrowing or renal ostial stenosis; and "porcelain" (calcified) aorta.

Angiographic Classification

Cases are classified according to the distribution of disease and are further subclassified as C+ or C−, depending on coronary involvement, and P+ or P−, depending on pulmonary artery involvement (Fig. 21-1).[1]

Cardiac clinical presentations (Table 21-2) include aortic insufficiency from aortic root dilation; angina, myocardial infarction, or sudden death from ostial coronary involvement (coronary involvement has been described in up to 10% of cases); congestive heart failure from hypertension ± aortic insufficiency; pericarditis (more commonly a postmortem finding); and myocarditis (more commonly a postmortem finding).

Ophthalmologic lesions commonly seen include retinal ischemia, wreath-like collateral anastomoses, cataracts, and corneal opacities.

The American College of Rheumatology identified six major diagnostic criteria for Takayasu's arteritis:

1. Onset by the age of 40 years (eliminates giant cell arteritis; Table 21-3)

Table 21-1. Characteristics of Patients at Diagnosis

Characteristic	N (%)
Sex distribution	
Men	17 (15.7)
Women	91 (84.3)
Age at disease onset (years)	
≤10	7 (6.5)
11-20	21 (19.4)
21-30	25 (23.1)
31-40	30 (27.8)
41-50	19 (17.6)
≥51	6 (5.6)
Systemic symptoms	
Malaise	70 (64.8)
Headache	61 (56.5)
Dizziness	49 (45.4)
Weight loss	11 (10.2)
Fever	10 (9.3)
Vascular manifestations	
Vascular bruit	78 (72.2)
Blood pressure difference	69 (63.9)
Claudication	41 (38.0)
Dyspnea on exertion	29 (26.9)
Chest pain	21 (19.4)
Carotodynia	15 (13.9)
Visual disturbance	5 (4.6)
Disease activity	
Active disease	91 (84.3)
Stable disease	17 (15.7)
Laboratory findings	
Elevated ESR	90 (83.3)
Elevated CRP	55 (50.9)

CRP, C-reactive protein; ESR, erythrocyte sedimentation rate.
From Park MC, Lee SW, Park YB, et al: Clinical characteristics and outcomes of Takayasu's arteritis: analysis of 108 patients using standardized criteria for diagnosis, activity assessment, and angiographic classification. Scand J Rheumatol 2005;34:284-292, with permission from Elsevier.

Table 21-2. Cardiac Clinical Presentations of Takayasu's Disease

Anatomic Distribution	Number of Involved Lesions		
	Right	Left	Total (%)
Site of involved aortic branches			
Subclavian artery	52	32	84 (33.7)
Renal artery	36	27	63 (25.3)
Common carotid artery	33	21	54 (21.7)
Coronary artery	7	3	23 (9.2)
Left main artery	2	1	3 (1.2)
Left anterior descending artery	1	1	9 (3.6)
Left circumferential artery			7 (2.8)
Right coronary artery			4 (1.6)
Vertebral artery			10 (4.0)
Superior mesenteric artery			5 (2.0)
Innominate artery			3 (1.2)
Celiac artery			3 (1.2)
Pulmonary artery			2 (0.8)
Inferior mesenteric artery			2 (0.8)
Total count of involved aortic branches			249 (100)
Site of involved portions of aorta			
Abdominal aorta			37 (37.4)
Descending thoracic aorta			30 (30.3)
Aortic arch			18 (18.2)
Thoracic ascending aorta			14 (14.1)
Total count of involved aorta			99 (100)

From Park MC, Lee SW, Park YB, et al: Clinical characteristics and outcomes of Takayasu's arteritis: analysis of 108 patients using standardized criteria for diagnosis, activity assessment, and angiographic classification. Scand J Rheumatol 2005;34:284-292, with permission from Elsevier.

Table 21-3. Giant Cell Arteritis Versus Takayasu's Arteritis

	Giant Cell Arteritis	Takayasu's Arteritis
Onset	Later in life, thus difficult to differentiate from atherosclerotic disease	Earlier in life, thus less likely to be confused with atherosclerotic disease
Predominant form of disease	Aneurysmal disease common, and secondary complications (dissection and rupture)	Occlusive disease is more common than aneurysmal; hence pulselessness
Other disease manifestations	AI and CHF are possible, as is branch vessel ischemia including LMCA	Aneurysms, dissection, and rupture are all possible, as are AI and CHF

AI, aortic insufficiency; CHF, congestive heart failure; LMCA, left main coronary artery.

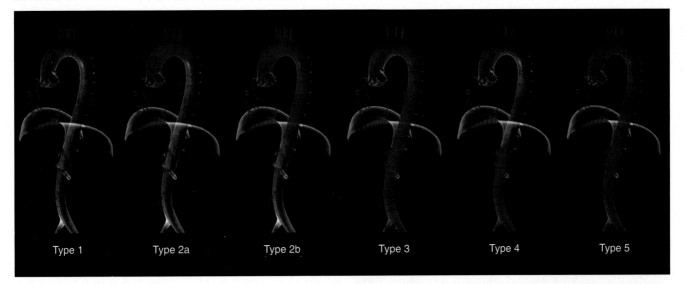

Figure 21-1. Angiographic classification of Takayasu's arteritis. Cases are classified according to the distribution of disease and are further subclassified as C+ or C−, depending on coronary involvement, and P+ or P−, depending on pulmonary artery involvement. Red denotes angiographic disease.

2. Upper extremity claudication
3. Diminished brachial pulses
4. Difference in arm blood pressure of 10 mm Hg
5. Subclavian or arm bruit
6. Identification of an arterial narrowing by imaging

IMAGING OF TAKAYASU'S ARTERITIS[2-5]

Magnetic resonance (MR) imaging is best suited for imaging of the aortic wall thickening (spin echo imaging). Gadolinium contrast delayed enhancement in and around the aorta and carotids is useful in the acute phase. In the chronic phase, gadolinium contrast delayed enhancement in the aorta is greater than in the myocardium and suggestive of disease activity. MR aortography (Fig. 21-2) is useful for imaging of the aortic luminal appearance and branch occlusions. Positron emission tomography (PET) scanning with [18F]-fluorodeoxyglucose ([18F]FDG-PET) is used for defining increased wall metabolism and for increased sensitivity of aortic wall involvement. Computed tomography (CT) scanning (Fig. 21-3) is useful for depiction of luminal narrowing and wall thickening. PET-CT scanning is useful for specific localization of disease. Conventional aortography is useful for imaging of the aortic luminal appearance and branch occlusions (Table 21-4).

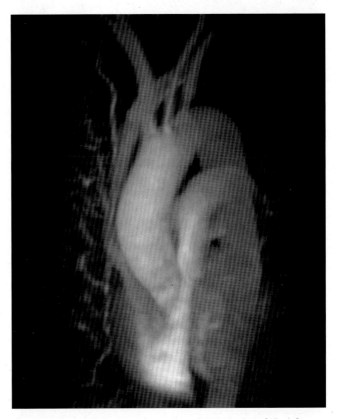

Figure 21-2. Gadolinium contrast aortography. Narrowing of the left subclavian artery ostium from Takayasu's arteritis is present—a usual finding in the disease.

TREATMENT

Glucocorticoids suppress the active inflammation phase, and immunosuppressives have also been used. Blood pressure control, obstetric management through pregnancy, and interventional and operative treatment as needed, depending on the specific complication, are the mainstays of management.

LONG-TERM MORBIDITY AND SURGICAL MORTALITY

Surgical vascular and aortic reparative procedures and aortic valve replacement in the setting of Takayasu's arteritis are frequently more challenging because of the poor quality of the tissues affected by aortitis. In a series of 90 patients who

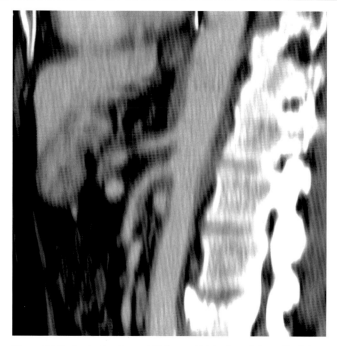

Figure 21-3. Contrast-enhanced CT image. Thickening of the wall of the abdominal aorta due to Takayasu's arteritis.

Table 21-4. Imaging of Takayasu's Disease

Mean age at presentation	25 years [14-66 years]
Female	75%
White	8%
Most common presentation	Hypertension
Central nervous system symptoms	20%
Involvement of the entire aorta	70%
Occlusions	93%
Aneurysms	46%
Vascular reconstructions performed	36%
No further progression during 5 years	25%
Principal cause of death	Congestive heart failure

From Mwipatayi BP, Jeffery PC, Beningfield SJ, et al: Takayasu arteritis: clinical features and management: report of 272 cases. ANZ J Surg 2005;75:110-117. Copyright Elsevier, 2005.

underwent cardiac surgery for aortic insufficiency from Takayasu's arteritis, aortic valve replacement (AVR) was performed in two thirds (n = 63), and composite graft repair was necessary in one third (n = 27). The overall 15-year survival was 76%. Notably, late AVR detachment occurred in 11% of patients undergoing AVR and 4% of patients undergoing composite grafting. Late aortic dilation was also greater in AVR versus composite graft patients (11% versus 4%). Active inflammation (seen on surgical specimen) was a risk factor for detachment.[6]

CASE 1

History

▶ A 30-year-old woman presented with left arm claudication.
▶ She had a protracted febrile illness 4 years before.

Physical Examination

▶ BP 130/50 right arm, 60/30 mm Hg left arm
▶ Other pulses normal; no bruits
▶ No murmurs

Comments

▶ Takayasu's arteritis with left subclavian ostial occlusion
▶ Presumed type 2b (left subclavian + descending aorta)

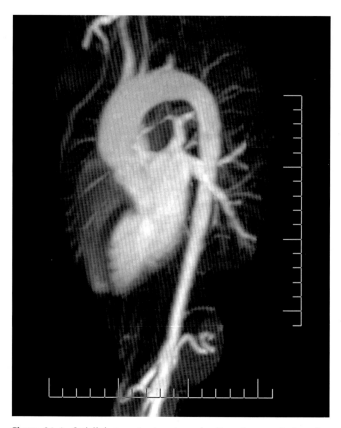

Figure 21-4. Gadolinium contrast aortography. There is an occlusion of the left subclavian artery, a common occurence in the disease. The descending aorta has a tapered appearance.

CASE 2

History

▸ 40-year-old woman
▸ Stable claudication of both legs since age 14

Physical Examination

▸ BP 160/50 mm Hg right arm, 75/– mm Hg left arm
▸ No murmurs
▸ Mid abdominal bruit
▸ Diminished femoral pulses (ankle-brachial index 0.5)

Comments

▸ Takayasu's arteritis with two arch vessel occlusions (left subclavian and right common carotid)
▸ Aortic occlusion (abdominal), classified as type 5

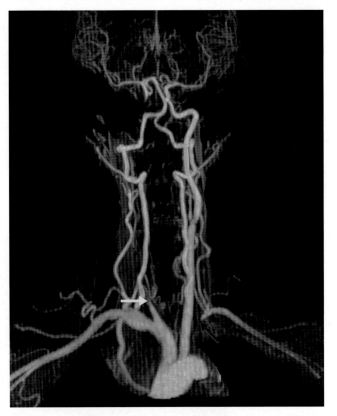

Figure 21-5. Gadolinium contrast aortography. Right common carotid occlusion *(yellow arrow)*. Left subclavian occlusion *(red arrow)*.

CASE 3

History

▸ A 24-year-old male student presented with 2 months of shortness of breath on exertion.
▸ Four years before, he had presented with a fever of unknown origin that was eventually determined to be Takayasu's arteritis.
▸ Known left subclavian ostial narrowing and arm BP differential for 3 years

Physical Examination

▸ BP 170/50 right arm, 90/40 left arm; HR 100 bpm
▸ Murmur of aortic insufficiency
▸ Dilated and dynamic apex

Impression and Management

▸ Clinical impression was that of aortic root degeneration with
  ▸ Nearly circumferential pseudoaneurysms of the root
  ▸ Aortic valve disruption with aortic insufficiency
  ▸ Fistulous flow through the false aneurysm into the left ventricle
  ▸ Congestive heart failure from the aortic insufficiency and fistulous flow into the left ventricle
▸ Surgery found tree bark appearance of the proximal aorta, which was fragile and friable.
▸ Bentall procedure (composite AVR + tube graft insertion)
▸ Postoperative bleeding, prolonged ICU stay, but discharged heart-failure free

Evolution

▸ 2 years later, presented with sudden-onset presyncope and dyspnea
▸ BP 100/60 right arm
▸ 1/6 SEM
▸ Crisp mechanical valve clicks
▸ No diastolic murmurs

Outcome

▸ Dehiscence and detachment of the proximal anastomosis of the Bentall composite graft
▸ Surgical reconstruction was attempted.
▸ Surgery found a large recurrent pseudoaneurysm beside the aortic root and ascending aorta.
▸ Great difficulty encountered working with the fragile and friable residual tissues
▸ Massive postoperative bleeding on several occasions
▸ Died in the ICU

Comments

▸ Fever of unknown origin presentation of Takayasu's aortitis
▸ Left subclavian artery ostial stenosis
▸ Late AVR detachment, root pseudoaneurysms
▸ Poor tissues (after acute inflammation and chronic scarring phase of the disease) haunted the surgery.
▸ Male gender (uncommon)

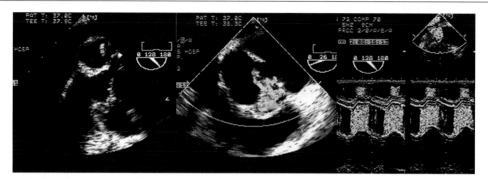

Figure 21-6. Aortic root pseudoaneurysms, aortic insufficiency: pseudoaneurysms nearly circumferentially at the root level, aortic valve annulus level. Flow within pseudoaneurysm. Aortic insufficiency.

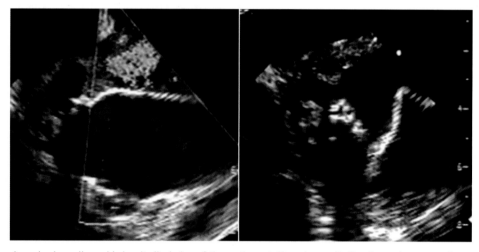

Figure 21-7. Transesophageal echocardiographic longitudinal view of the aortic root. There is systolic flow into a large posterior pseudoaneurysm. Blood entered into this recurrent pseudoaneurysm through a large dehiscence of the sewing margin of the composite graft at the aortic annular level. Pressurization of the false lumen compressed the true lumen, kinking the composite graft in systole.

References

1. Hata A, Noda M, Moriwaki R, Numano F: Angiographic findings of Takayasu arteritis: new classification. Int J Cardiol 1996;54(Suppl): S155-S163.
2. Choe YH, Kim DK, Koh EM, et al: Takayasu arteritis: diagnosis with MR imaging and MR angiography in acute and chronic active stages. J Magn Reson Imaging 1999;10:751-757.
3. Blockmans D: The use of (^{18}F)fluoro-deoxyglucose positron emission tomography in the assessment of large vessel vasculitis. Clin Exp Rheumatol 2003;21(Suppl 32):S15-S22.
4. Meller J, Strutz F, Siefker U, et al: Early diagnosis and follow-up of aortitis with [^{18}F]FDG PET and MRI. Eur J Nucl Med Mol Imaging 2003;30:730-736.
5. Kobayashi Y, Ishii K, Oda K, et al: Aortic wall inflammation due to Takayasu arteritis imaged with ^{18}F-FDG PET coregistered with enhanced CT. J Nucl Med 2005;46:917-922.
6. Matsuura K, Ogino H, Kobayashi J, et al: Surgical treatment of aortic regurgitation due to Takayasu arteritis: long-term morbidity and mortality. Circulation 2005;112:3707-3712.

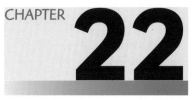

Noninfectious Aortitis: Giant Cell Aortitis, Systemic Lupus Erythematosus, and Other Aortitides

KEY POINTS

▶ Numerous systemic inflammatory disorders may result in aortitis.

▶ Aortic involvement may be recognized in the acute phase, but it is more likely to be recognized in the chronic phase.

▶ All known complications of aortic involvement may occur:

▶ Aneurysms, rupture

▶ Dissection

▶ Coronary ostial or other branch ostial involvement

▶ Aortic insufficiency

▶ Some consideration of aortitis should occur when aortic disease and aortic insufficiency are identified.

Multiple specific systemic inflammatory diseases may involve the aorta, resulting in aortic valve insufficiency and congestive heart failure, branch vessel ostial narrowing (including coronary), aortic or branch vessel aneurysm, aortic dissection, or aortic false aneurysm formation. The classification of noninfectious aortitis involves degrees of overlap (Table 22-1).

Noninfectious aortitides are treatable with immunosuppressive medications; hence, their specific identification is worthwhile as glucocorticoids suppress active inflammation. Vascular complications may independently need surgical or interventional treatment. Surgical repair of inflammatory aneurysms has been performed successfully in many cases but is often described as being more difficult than in the setting of atherosclerotic disease.[1]

GIANT CELL AORTITIS

Giant cell arteritis (temporal arteritis, polymyalgia rheumatica–associated arteritis) includes involvement of the aorta in approximately 10% of cases. The peak incidence is notably late in life (whereas with Takayasu's disease, it is much earlier). Giant cell aortitis only rarely involves the descending or abdominal aorta, again in contradistinction to Takayasu's disease (Table 22-2). Clinical presentations of giant cell aortitis include aneurysms and rupture, dissections, aortic insufficiency, and coronary ostial or other branch vessel involvement. A substantially elevated erythrocyte sedimentation rate is consistent with giant cell arteritis; biopsy proof of giant cells is pathognomonic (Fig. 22-1).

RHEUMATOID ARTHRITIS AND SYSTEMIC LUPUS ERYTHEMATOSUS

Non–giant cell aortitis may occur in cases of systemic lupus erythematosus (SLE) and be responsible for chest pains and aortic dissection (Fig. 22-2).[2] The "tree bark" appearance of the aorta, known from syphilis, may occur in SLE.[3] Aneurysms of the aorta from aortitis have been described in association with rheumatoid arthritis.[4,5]

Table 22-1. Noninfectious Aortitides

Giant cell aortitis

Takayasu's aortitis

HLA-B27–associated spondyloarthropathies

Crohn's disease–associated aortopathy

Behçet syndrome–associated aortopathy

Systemic lupus erythematosus–associated aortopathy

Rheumatoid arthritis–associated aortopathy

Sarcoidosis-associated aortopathy

Psoriasis-associated aortopathy

Table 22-2. Giant Cell Arteritis Versus Takayasu's Arteritis

	Giant Cell Arteritis	Takayasu's Arteritis
Onset	Later in life, thus difficult to differentiate from atherosclerotic disease	Earlier in life, thus less likely to be confused with atherosclerotic disease
Predominant form of disease	Aneurysmal disease common, and secondary complications (dissection and rupture)	Occlusive disease is more common than aneurysmal; hence pulselessness
Other disease manifestations	AI and CHF are possible, as is branch vessel ischemia including LMCA	Aneurysms, dissection, and rupture are all possible, as are AI and CHF

AI, aortic insufficiency; CHF, congestive heart failure; LMCA, left main coronary artery.

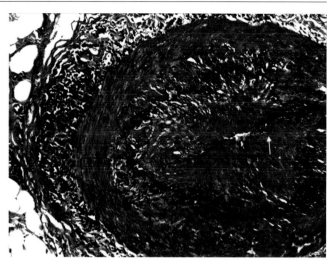

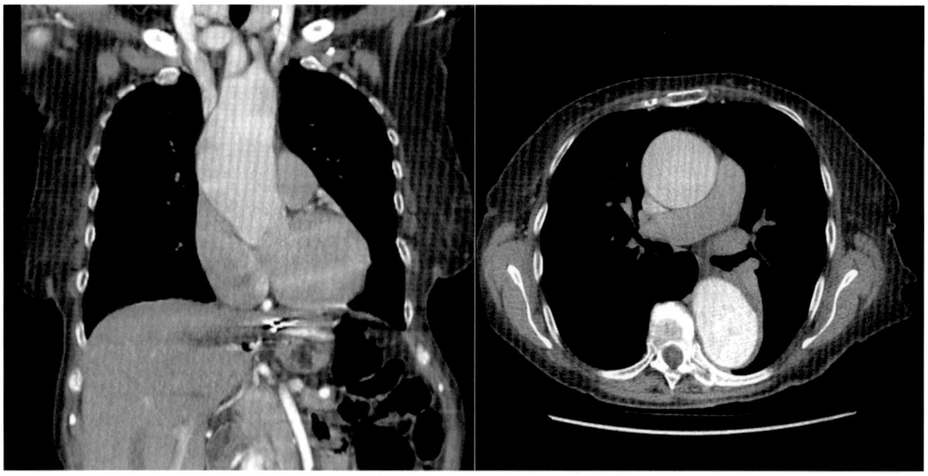

Figure 22-1. A photomicrograph showing thickening of the arterial wall (temporal artery) due to inflammation from giant cell arteritis.

Figure 22-2. Contrast-enhanced CT scans of a patient with long-standing SLE. There are aneurysms of the ascending and descending thoracic aorta.

ANKYLOSING SPONDYLITIS

Aortic root and left-sided heart valvular skeleton involvement may occur with ankylosing spondylitis. Aortic root involvement is seen in 25% of cases pathologically but surmised in less than 10% of cases clinically. Manifestations include thickening of the wall of the root, dilation of the root, and extension of the thickening along the annulus fibrosus onto the anterior mitral leaflet.

SERONEGATIVE AORTOPATHY–ASSOCIATED AORTITIS

Aortitis syndromes have been described in the setting of seronegative disorders, including Crohn's disease and Behçet syndrome.

CASE 1

History

▸ 52-year-old woman with long-standing SLE and renal failure, presenting with pain from the front chest through to her back
▸ Known saccular aneurysm of the aorta
▸ Prior ischemic chest pains: perfusion study low risk

Physical Examination

▸ BP 140/85 mm Hg, HR 90 bpm, RR 16/min
▸ Normal venous pressures
▸ Normal pulses, no deficits
▸ No rubs, clear chest
▸ Positive troponin results, lateral ST elevation, lateral wall motion abnormality

Clinical Impression

▸ Coronary ischemic presentation
▸ Unclear if thoracic false aneurysm was enlarging

▸ Consideration of percutaneous coronary intervention to responsible artery versus combined surgical procedure
▸ Very discordant opinions

Evolution and Outcome

▸ She abruptly deteriorated and experienced several cardiac arrests.
▸ She died of complications of the cardiac arrests.

Comments

▸ Extensive vascular disease in a patient with SLE
▸ Although not autopsy proven, likely to be SLE related
▸ Saccular aneurysm of the aorta filled with thrombus and concurrent coronary artery disease
▸ Succumbed to complications of coronary artery disease rather than to the aneurysm
▸ Much of the challenge of the case pertained to determination of which pathologic process to treat: the coronary artery disease or the aortic disease.

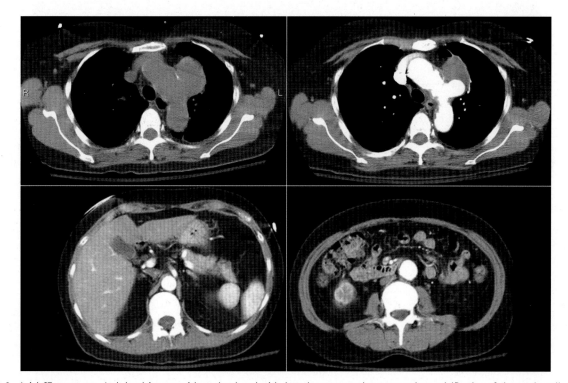

Figure 22-3. Axial CT scans. TOP, Arch-level images without (LEFT) and with (RIGHT) contrast enhancement show calcification of the aortic wall. There is a saccular blood-filled cavity extending off the right wall of the arch—saccular aneurysm or false aneurysm with mural thrombus. BOTTOM, There is a small abdominal aortic aneurysm as well. The image on the right is from a more inferior level of the abdomen, and the aortic diameter is larger (LEFT).

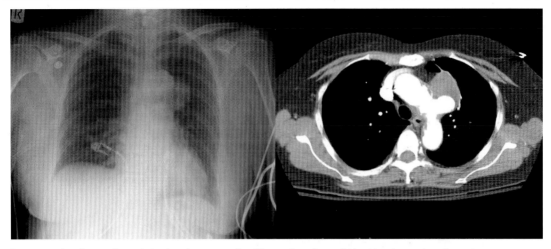

Figure 22-4. Posteroanterior chest radiograph (LEFT) and corresponding CT scan (RIGHT) correlating the abnormal aortic contour.

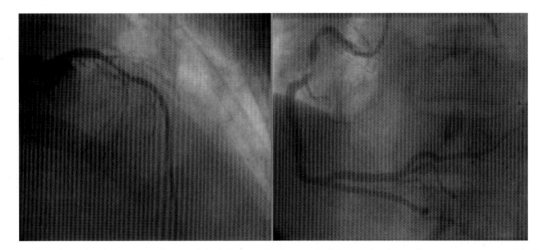

Figure 22-5. Coronary angiography shows severe disease of the left circumflex artery, the left anterior descending coronary artery and its first diagonal branch, and the right coronary artery.

References

1. Takagi A, Kajiura N, Tada Y, Ueno A: Surgical treatment of non-specific inflammatory arterial aneurysms. J Cardiovasc Surg (Torino) 1986;27: 117-124.
2. Guard RW, Gotis-Graham I, Edmonds JP, Thomas AC: Aortitis with dissection complicating systemic lupus erythematosus. Pathology 1995; 27:224-228.
3. MacLeod CB, Johnson D, Frable WJ: "Tree-barking" of the ascending aorta: syphilis or systemic lupus erythematosus? Am J Clin Pathol 1992;97: 58-62.
4. Gravallese EM, Corson JM, Coblyn JS, et al: Rheumatoid aortitis: a rarely recognized but clinically significant entity. Medicine (Baltimore) 1989; 68:95-106.
5. Reimer KA, Rodgers RF, Oyasu R: Rheumatoid arthritis with rheumatoid heart disease and granulomatous aortitis. JAMA 1976;235:2510-2512.

Index

Note: Page numbers followed by f indicate figures; those followed by t indicate tables.

A

Abdominal aorta, 6, 6f
  anatomy of, variant, 22
  disease involvement of, 6
  function of, 13t–14t
  imaging considerations for, 6
  structure of, 13t–14t
Abdominal aortic aneurysms, 215–235
  case studies of, 227–235
  clinical presentation of, 216
  growth rate of, beta-blockade and, 217
  identification of, 6
  imaging of, 219, 219f–223f, 220t
  infrarenal, 51f
  mural thrombus and, 218
  natural history of, 217, 217f
  pathogenesis of, 217
  pathology and morphology of, 216, 216f, 217f
  physical diagnosis of, 34, 216, 216t
  renal arteries and, 6
  rupture of, 217–218, 218f
    sites of, 218
  screening for, 218
  surgical findings in, 228f
  treatment of, 221, 223–227
    endovascular, 223, 226f, 227
    medical, 221, 224f
    surgical, 223, 224f, 225f, 225t
Abdominal coarctation, 159
Abdominal radiography, 35, 36f
  in abdominal aortic aneurysm, 219f, 232f
Abscesses, of aortic root, 251, 252f, 253f
Acute aortic dissection, 55–111
  case studies of, 80–111, 145, 146f, 153, 153f
  classification of, 60–61, 61f
  clinical presentation of, 62, 62t, 63t
  complications of, 56, 56f, 56t
  definition of, 55
  diagnosis of, 61–62, 62f
  diagnostic testing in, 64f, 64–72
    aortography for, 68, 71, 71f, 71t
    chest radiography for, 64–65, 65f, 65t
    computed tomography for, 65 67, 66f, 67f, 68t, 69f, 70f

Acute aortic dissection *(Continued)*
    echocardiography for, 64, 64t, 71–72, 72f–74f, 75t, 76t
    magnetic resonance imaging for, 67, 68t
  etiology of, 55–56
  follow-up of, 79–80, 131, 133f, 134, 134f
  incidence of, 55–56
  management of, 74, 76f, 77f, 77–79
    endovascular, 79, 79f
    medical, 74
    with pericardial tamponade, 79
    surgical, 74, 77f, 77–79
  natural history of, 56
  outcomes of, 79–80
  pathogenesis of, 56–57, 57f–60f
  physical examination findings in, 62–63, 63t
  risk factors for, 60, 60t
  Stanford type A, 61, 61f
    surgical repair of, 77–78, 78f, 78t
  Stanford type B, 61, 61f
    surgical repair of, 78–79
  terminology for, 55
  variants of, 61–62, 62f
Acute coronary syndromes, case study of, 152, 152f
Adventitia, histology of, 7–8
Anatomy, aortic, 1–6, 2f
  of abdominal aorta, 6, 6f
  of aortic arch, 4f, 4–5
  of aortic root, 1–3, 2f
  of ascending aorta, 3–4, 4f
  of descending aorta, 5f, 5–6
  of isthmus, 5f, 5–6
  normal, 24f
  of sinotubular junction, 3, 3f
Aneurysms
  of abdominal aorta. *See* Abdominal aortic aneurysms.
  of aortic root, 196–197, 299f
    annuloaortic ectasia and, 196–197, 197f
    sinus of Valsalva aneurysms as, 196, 251, 252f
    surgical treatment of, 251
  of ascending aorta, 197–198, 198f
    case study of, 201, 202f, 203f
  complications of, 195

Aneurysms *(Continued)*
  definition of, 55
  detection by chest radiography, 34
  false, 55
    case study of, 205, 205f
    in coarctation of the aorta, at site of surgical correction, 282f
  fusiform, 195
  infectious. *See* Infectious aneurysms.
  morphologic descriptive terms for, 195
  mycotic, 337
  saccular, 195
    case studies of, 206, 206f, 349–350
    of descending thoracic aorta, 199–200
  sinus of Valsalva, 196, 251, 252f
    case study of, 253–254
  syphilitic, 337–338
    clinical presentation and management of, 338, 338f
  of thoracic aorta. *See* Thoracic aortic aneurysms.
  thoracoabdominal, 51f, 195, 200f, 200–201, 201f
    case study of, 206, 207f
  tubular, 195
Angiography. *See also* Coronary angiography.
  in aortic atherosclerosis, 167f
  in coarctation of the aorta, 280f, 296f
  contrast, in coarctation of the aorta, 277, 278f, 279f
  in dissection, 147f
  in intramural hematoma, 118
  in thoracic aortic aneurysms, 210f
Angioplasty, balloon, for coarctation of the aorta, 279–280
Ankylosing spondylitis, aortitis and, 348
Antiatherogenic function, of aorta, 13t
Antithrombotic function, of aorta, 13t
Annuloaortic ectasia, 196–197, 197f
Aortic arch
  anatomy of, 4f, 4–5
    variant, 18f, 18–21
  aneurysms of, 198–199, 199f
    case study of, 201, 202f, 203f
    cervical, 21, 22f
    classification of, 20t

Aortic arch (Continued)
  disease involvement of, 5
  double, 21, 21f, 29f, 30f
  imaging considerations for, 5
  right-sided, 20–21, 21f, 30f–32f
  usual branch anatomy arising from, 19
Aortic arch disease. See Takayasu's disease.
Aortic insufficiency murmur, 33
Aortic pressure waveforms, 12, 12f, 12t, 14f, 15f
  in acute aortic dissection, 100f
Aortic pulse pressure contour, 11, 11f, 12f
Aortic pulse wave, 9–10, 10f
  hypertension and, 11, 11f
  reflected, 10t, 10–11, 11f
Aortic root, 251–258
  abscesses of, 251, 252f, 253f
  anatomy of, 1–3, 2f
    variant, 17–18
  aneurysms of, 196–197
    annuloaortic ectasia and, 196–197, 197f
    sinus of Valsalva aneurysms as, 196, 251, 252f
    surgical treatment of, 251
  aortic root to right atrium-right ventricle fistula and, case study of, 255–256
  bioprosthetic valve endocarditis and, 252f
  disease involvement of, 2
  imaging considerations for, 2–3
  mechanical valve replacement endocarditis and, case study of, 257–258
  sinus of Valsalva fistulas and, 251, 252f
    case study of, 253–254, 256–257
  sinuses of, variant anatomy of, 27–28
  surveillance of, for Marfan syndrome diagnosis, 300
Aortic valve, bicuspid. See Bicuspid aortic valve.
Aortography
  abdominal, in atheromatous disease, 179f
  in abdominal aortic aneurysm, 220t, 230f, 233f, 235f
  of aberrant right subclavian artery, 25f
  in acute aortic dissection, 68, 71, 71f, 71t
  in aortic root to right atrium-right ventricle fistula, 256f
  in aortic ulcers and penetrating ulcers, 183f, 187f
  in bicuspid aortic valve, 264f, 266f, 269f
  in coarctation of the aorta, 279f, 280f, 285f, 291f, 294f
  computed tomography. See Computed tomography.
  contrast. See Contrast aortography.
  in dissection, 239f
  of double aortic arch, 30f
  endovascular therapy and, 241f
  fluoroscopic, in atherosclerotic intimal calcification, 158f
  magnetic resonance. See Magnetic resonance imaging.
  in Marfan syndrome, 312f
  in mechanical valve endocarditis, 253f, 258f
  of normal aorta, 24f
  in thoracic aortic aneurysms, 198f, 213f
  in traumatic disruption of the aorta, 317–318, 318f, 319f, 322f, 325f
Aortoplasty, subclavian patch, for coarctation of the aorta, 281f

Arterial pulse wave, reflected, 10t, 10–11, 11f
Arthritis, rheumatoid, aortitis and, 347
Ascending aorta
  anatomy of, 3–4, 4f
    variant, 18
  aneurysms of, 197–198, 198f
    case study of, 201, 202f, 203f
  disease involvement of, 4
  imaging considerations for, 4
Atheroembolism, aortic, 171–172, 172f
Atheroma, aortic, 155
  intimal, calcified, as marker of intimal location, 159, 159f
Atheromatous disease, aortic, 169–180
  atheroembolism as, 171–172, 172f
  atherosclerotic, 155–167, 156f
    aortic obstruction in, 159
    case studies of, 160–167
    intimal calcification and, 155–157, 156f–158f
    surgical specimen in, 166f
  case studies of, 172–180
  thromboembolism as, 171
  ulcers and penetrating ulcers in, 181–193
    case studies of, 184–193
    imaging of, 181–182, 183f
    management of, 182, 183f
Atresia, aortic, 271

B

Bacterial infectious aneurysms, 337
  clinical presentation and management of, 337
Balloon angioplasty, for coarctation of the aorta, 279–280
Barium swallow study, of aberrant right subclavian artery, 25f
Beta-blocker therapy
  abdominal aortic aneurysm growth and, 217
  for Marfan syndrome, 302
Bicuspid aortic valve, 259–269, 260f, 260t
  as acute aortic dissection risk factor, 60, 60t
  case studies of, 261–269
  clinical presentation of, 259–260, 260f
  in coarctation of the aorta, 272
  progressive aortic dilation and, 261
Bioprosthetic valve endocarditis, 252f
Blood flow, arterial, 15, 15f
Blood pressure
  aortic pressure waveform and, 12, 12f, 12t, 14f, 15f
  aortic pulse wave and, 11, 11f, 12f
  arterial, 15, 15f
    age and, 9, 10f
  contrast-enhanced pulmonary capillary wedge pressure tracing and, in Marfan syndrome, 312f
  description of, 8–9, 9f, 10f
  pressure waveforms and, in acute aortic dissection, 100f
  pressure:volume relationships and, 8
Brachiocephalic artery
  anatomy of, 19
  common origin with left common carotid artery, 19, 19f, 20f
Brachiocephalic vein, on echocardiography, 37, 37f

Brain, emboli to, 169
Bronchial arteries, variant anatomy of, 22

C

Capacitor function, of aorta, 13t
Cardiac catheterization, in coarctation of the aorta, 291f, 294f, 295f
Cardiac surgery, aortic complications of, 141
  case studies of, 142–143, 145–146, 152–153
Carotid artery, left
  anatomy of, 19
  common, common origin with brachiocephalic artery, 19, 19f, 20f
  computed tomography of, 23f
Catheter-based interventions, aortic complications of, 141
  case studies of, 143–145, 147–151
Chest pain, acute aortic dissection and, 62
Chest radiography
  in abdominal aortic aneurysm, 230f, 231f
  of aberrant right subclavian artery, 25f
  in aortic atherosclerosis, 164f, 166f, 167f
  following aortic dissection, 132f, 135f
  in aortic dissection, 34
    acute, 64–65, 65f, 65t, 67f, 76t, 80f, 91f, 95f, 100f, 103f, 104f, 106f, 108f, 109f
  in aortic root to right atrium-right ventricle fistula, 255f
  in aortic ulcers and penetrating ulcers, 185f, 188f
  in atheromatous disease, 173f, 174f, 176f, 178f
  in atherosclerotic intimal calcification, 159f
  in bicuspid aortic valve, 261f, 263f, 266f, 268f
  in coarctation of the aorta, 273, 274f–276f, 289f
  of descending aorta, 30f, 31f
  of double aortic arch, 29f
  intimal calcification on, 34, 34f
  intimal displacement on, 34, 35f
  in intramural hematoma, 121f, 122f, 128f, 144f
  in Marfan syndrome, 304f, 307f, 309f
  pleural effusion on, 34
  of right-sided aortic arch, 30f, 31f
  in saccular aortic aneurysms, 349f
  in Staphylococcus aureus aneurysms, 339f
  in syphilitic aneurysms, 338f
  in thoracic aortic aneurysms, 198f, 202f, 203f, 205f, 206f, 207f, 209f, 211f
  in traumatic disruption of the aorta, 316, 318f, 324f
  in tumors of the aorta, 334f
  utility for detecting specific aortic diseases, 34, 35f
Coarctation of the aorta
  anomalies associated with, 272
  case studies of, 282–296
  definition of, 271
  etiology of, 271
  imaging of, 273, 273t, 274f–276f, 276–277
    contrast angiography for, 277, 278f, 279f
    echocardiography for, 273, 276, 276f, 277f
    magnetic resonance imaging for, 277, 277f, 278f
  management of, 279–282
    balloon angioplasty for, 279–280
    stenting for, 280f, 280–281, 281f
    surgical, 281f, 281–282, 282f

Coarctation of the aorta (Continued)
  physical findings in, 273
  prognosis of, 273
  types of, 271–272
Collateral vessel formation, in coarctation of the
    aorta, 273
Computed tomography, 38, 41
  in abdominal aortic aneurysm, 220t, 222f
  of aortic arch, 5
  of aortic root, 2
  in aortic ulcers and penetrating ulcers, 191f
  artifacts on, 66–67, 68t
    linear, 66
    motion, 66, 67f
    streak, 66–67, 67f
  of ascending aorta, 4
  comparison with other imaging modalities,
    52t
  contrast-enhanced, 41, 42f, 43f
    in abdominal aortic aneurysms, 221f, 226f,
      227f, 229f, 231f, 233
    of aberrant right subclavian artery, 26f
    in acute coronary syndrome, 152f
    in aortic atheromatous disease, 169
    following aortic dissection, 132f–134f, 137f,
      139f
    in aortic dissection, 143f, 149f, 151f
    in aortic dissection, acute, 65–67, 66f, 69f,
      70f, 83f, 85f, 101f–105f, 108f, 110f,
      111f, 153f
    in aortic ulcers and penetrating ulcers, 183f,
      184f, 186f, 190f
    in atheromatous disease, 173f, 175f, 180f
    in atherosclerotic intimal calcification, 159
    in bicuspid aortic valve, 261f
    in coarctation of the aorta, 272f, 280f, 288f
    of descending aorta, 30f–32f
    of double aortic arch, 29f
    endovascular therapy and, 246f–249f
    in intramural hematoma, 123f, 145f
    of left common carotid artery, 23f
    in Marfan syndrome, 309f
    of right-sided aortic arch, 23f, 30f–32f
    in Staphylococcus aureus aneurysms, 339f
    in systemic lupus erythematosus-associated
      aortitis, 348
    in Takayasu's disease, 344f
    in thoracic aortic aneurysms, 202f–204f,
      208f, 209f, 212f, 213f
    in traumatic aortic transection, 240f
    in traumatic disruption of the aorta, 321f,
      325f, 326f, 327f, 329f
  in dissection, 150f, 239f
    acute, 76t
  endovascular therapy and, 240, 240f, 241f
  in intramural hematoma, 117, 118f
  in Marfan syndrome, 304f
  non–contrast-enhanced, 41, 41f
    in abdominal aortic aneurysms, 219f, 220f,
      232f, 234f
    in aortic atherosclerosis, 165f
    following aortic dissection, 137f
    in aortic ulcers and penetrating ulcers, 190f
    in atherosclerotic intimal calcification, 157f,
      159
    in dissection, 148f, 149f, 151f
    in dissection, acute, 105f–107f
    in intramural hematoma, 126t, 128t

Computed tomography (Continued)
  in Marfan syndrome, 304f
  in thoracic aortic aneurysms, 206f, 207f,
    211f, 213
  post-processing and, 41, 45f–49f
  reconstructed
    endovascular therapy and, 247f
    after stent graft deployment, 239f
    in thoracic aortic aneurysms, 210f
  reformatted, 41, 43f, 44f
    endovascular therapy and, 245f, 246f
  in saccular aortic aneurysms, 349f, 350f
  in Takayasu's disease, 343, 344f
  technique for, 41
  of thoracic aorta, 6
  in thoracic aortic aneurysms, 202f
  in traumatic disruption of the aorta, 316–317,
    317f
Conduit function, of aorta, 13t
Contrast aortography, 51–52
  of aberrant right subclavian artery, 27f, 28f
  in acute aortic dissection, 76t
  in aortic ulcers and penetrating ulcers, 183f
  comparison with other imaging modalities,
    52t
  in Takayasu's disease, 344f, 345f
  technique of, 52, 53f
Cook Zenith TX2 graft, 243
Coronary angiography
  in abdominal aortic aneurysms, 225f
  in aortic dissection, 142f
  in bicuspid aortic valve, 267f, 269f
  in coarctation of the aorta, 291f
  in saccular aortic aneurysms, 350f
Coronary arteries, variant anatomy of, 18
Cushion function, of aorta, 13t
Cystic medial necrosis, 60, 197

D

Descending aorta
  anatomy of, variant, 21–22
  right-sided, 30f–32f
  thoracic, aneurysms of, 199f, 199–200
    saccular, 199–200
Dilation. See also Abdominal aortic aneurysms;
    Aneurysms.
  detection by chest radiography, 34, 35f
Dissection, 34
  acute. See Acute aortic dissection.
  case study of, 142, 142f, 143f, 147, 147f–151f
  late complications of, 131–139
    case studies of, 135–139
    follow-up recommendations and, 131, 133f,
      134, 134f
Distal aorta, obstruction of, 159
Ductus diverticulum, 22, 22f, 23f

E

Echocardiography
  in acute aortic dissection, 64, 64t, 108f
  of aortic arch, 5
  of aortic root, 3
  of ascending aorta, 4
  in bicuspid aortic valve, 260, 260f
  in coarctation of the aorta, 276
  of thoracic aorta, 6

Echocardiography (Continued)
  transesophageal. See Transesophageal
    echocardiography.
  transthoracic. See Transthoracic
    echocardiography.
Electrocardiography
  in acute aortic dissection, 80f, 83f, 87f, 90f, 93f,
    95f, 97f, 100f
  in aortic atherosclerosis, 163f, 167f
  following aortic dissection, 135f, 137f
  in atheromatous disease, 176f
  in coarctation of the aorta, 273, 273t, 289f,
    292f
  in intramural hematoma, 121f, 122f, 124f
Emboli
  to brain, 169
  pedunculation of thrombus or debris
    associated with, 170, 171f
Embryogenesis, 17, 18f
Endocarditis
  bioprosthetic valve, 252f
  mechanical valve, 253f
  case study of, 257–258
Endoleaks, 244
Endovascular therapy, 237–248
  for abdominal aortic aneurysms, 223, 226f,
    227
  devices for, 242, 242f
    sizing of, 242–243, 243f
  future of, 247f–249f, 247–248
  hybrid endovascular and open repair and, 245,
    245f–247f, 247
  imaging and, 240–242, 241f, 242f
  indications for, 237–239, 238f–240f, 238t
  pitfalls of, 244f, 244t, 244–245, 245f
  principles and techniques of, 239
  procedural techniques for, 243–244
  for thoracic aortic aneurysms, 200, 200f
  for traumatic disruption of the aorta, 319,
    330f
End-to-end anastomoses, for coarctation of the
    aorta, 281f
Esophageal arteries, variant anatomy of, 22

F

False aneurysms, 55
  case study of, 205, 205f
  in coarctation of the aorta, at site of surgical
    correction, 282f
Family history, 33
Fenestration, for acute aortic dissection, 79
Fluoroscopy
  in atherosclerotic intimal calcification,
    158f
  in coarctation of the aorta, 281f
  in intramural hematoma, 144f
Functions, aortic, 13t–14t
Fusiform aortic aneurysms, 195

G

Genetic testing, in Marfan syndrome, 299–300
Ghent diagnostic criteria, for Marfan syndrome,
  299, 301t–302t
Giant cell aortitis, 347, 348f, 348t
Giant cell arteritis, Takayasu's disease versus,
  342t

Gore TAG thoracic endoprosthesis, 242, 242f, 243

H

Hematomas, intramural. *See* Intramural hematomas.
Hemodynamics, in bicuspid aortic valve, 267f
Hilar overlay sign, in coarctation of the aorta, 275f
Histology, aortic, 6–8, 7f, 7t
    of adventitia, 7–8
    of intima, 6–7
    of media, 7
History taking, 33
Hypertension, aortic pulse wave and, 11, 11f

I

Infectious aneurysms, 337–340
    bacterial, 337
        clinical presentation and management of, 337
        case studies of, 338–340
    syphilitic, 337–338
        clinical presentation and management of, 338, 338f
Intercostal arteries, variant anatomy of, 22
Intima
    histology of, 6–8, 7f, 7t
    tear of. *See* Acute aortic dissection; Dissection.
Intimal calcification, 34, 34f
    atherosclerotic, 155–157, 156f–158f
    as marker of intimal location, 159, 159f
Intimal displacement, 34, 35f
Intramural hematomas, 113–129
    anatomic findings of, 114, 114f, 114t
    case studies of, 120–129, 143, 144f, 145f
    complications of, 115, 116t, 119, 119t, 120f
    definition of, 113
    diagnosis of, 116
    imaging of
        angiography for, 118
        computed tomography for, 117, 118f
        magnetic resonance imaging for, 117–118
        transesophageal echocardiography for, 117, 117f, 118f
    incidence of, 114
    long-term survival in, 119, 119f
    management of, 118–119, 119f
    mortality of, 115f, 115–116, 116t
    natural history of, 114–115
    pathogenesis of, 113, 114f
    predisposing factors for, 114
    surgical findings in, 126f
Intravascular ultrasound, endovascular therapy and, 242, 242f
Isthmus
    anatomy of, 5f, 5–6
    disease involvement of, 5–6
    imaging considerations for, 5

K

Kommerell's diverticulum, 19, 20f, 23f, 27f, 28f

L

Loeys-Dietz syndrome type 1, 299f

M

Magnetic resonance angiography, 21f
    in aortic atherosclerosis, 163f
Magnetic resonance aortography, 49–51, 50f
    in acute aortic dissection, 76t
    black blood imaging and, 50, 50f
    blood pool depiction on, 50–51, 51f
    bright blood imaging and, 50f
    comparison with other imaging modalities, 52t
    gadolinium-enhanced, 50, 51f
        abdominal aortic aneurysm on, 51f
        in coarctation of the aorta, 277f, 278, 295f
        in Takayasu's disease, 51f
        of thoracoabdominal aneurysm, 51f
    post-processing and, 51
    reformatting and, 51
    spin echo images and, 49–50
    in Takayasu's disease, 343, 343f
    time-of-flight, 50
Magnetic resonance imaging
    in abdominal aortic aneurysm, 220t, 222f
    in acute aortic dissection, 76t
    of aortic root, 3
    in atheromatous disease, 176f
    in coarctation of the aorta, 277, 277f, 278f
    comparison with other imaging modalities, 52t
    gadolinium-enhanced
        in acute coronary syndrome, 152f
        in coarctation of the aorta, 292f
        in thoracic aortic aneurysms, 206f
    in intramural hematoma, 117–118
    reformatted, in abdominal aortic aneurysm, 223f
    spin echo
        in acute coronary syndrome, 152f
        in aortic atherosclerosis, 163f
    in Takayasu's disease, 343
    in tumors of the aorta, 334f
Marfan syndrome, 297–313
    annuloaortic ectasia and, 196–197, 197f
    cardiovascular abnormalities in, 299
    case studies of, 307–314
    diagnosis of, 299t, 299–302, 300f, 301f, 302f
        aortic root surveillance for, 302
        genetic testing for, 300–302
        Ghent diagnostic criteria and, 300, 301t–302t
    genetic factors in, 297–298, 298t
    historical background of, 297
    management of, 303–306
        medical, 303
        surgical, 303–306, 303f–306f, 305t
    phenotypes in, 298
Mechanical valve endocarditis, 253f
    case study of, 257–258
Media, histology of, 7
Medial necrosis, cystic, 197
Medical history, 33
Middle aorta syndrome, 159
Mural thrombus, abdominal aortic aneurysms and, 218

Murmur, aortic insufficiency, 33
Mycotic aneurysms, 337

P

Pericardial rub, 33
Pericardial tamponade
    atrial septal defect associated with, management of, 79
    signs of, 33
Peripheral arteries
    function of, 13t–14t
    structure of, 13t–14t
Photomicrography, in giant cell arteritis, 348f
Physical examination, 33–34
Physiology, aortic, 8f, 8t, 8–15, 9f
    aortic pulse wave and, 9–10, 10f
        hypertension and, 11, 11f
    arterial pressure and arterial flow and, pressure waveform and, 15, 15f
    blood pressure and, 8–9, 9f, 10f
        arterial, age relationship of, 9, 10f
        pressure waveform and, 12, 12f, 12t, 14f, 15f
    pulse pressure contour and, 1f, 11, 12f
    reflected pressure waves and, 10t, 10–11, 11f
Plaques, aortic, 169
    thickness of, 170
Pleural effusion, left, 34
Positron emission tomography, in Takayasu's disease, 343
Pressure:volume relationships, 8
Prosthetic patch repair, for coarctation of the aorta, 281f
Proximal aorta
    function of, 13t–14t
    structure of, 13t–14t
Pseudoaneurysms, 55
    case study of, 205, 205f
    in coarctation of the aorta, at site of surgical correction, 282f
Pseudocoarctation of the aorta, 271, 272f
Pulmonary capillary wedge pressure tracing, contrast-enhanced, in Marfan syndrome, 312f
Pulseless disease. *See* Takayasu's disease.
Pump function, of aorta, 13t

R

Radiography. *See* Abdominal radiography; Chest radiography.
Rheumatoid arthritis, aortitis and, 347

S

Saccular aortic aneurysms, 195
    case studies of, 206, 206f, 349–350
    of descending thoracic aorta, 199–200
Seronegative aortopathy-associated aortitis, 348
Sinotubular junction
    anatomy of, 3, 3f
    disease involvement of, 3
    imaging considerations for, 3
Sinus of Valsalva aneurysms, 196, 251, 252f
    case study of, 253–254

Sinus of Valsalva fistulas, 251, 252f
case study of, 256–257
Spinal arteries, variant anatomy of, 22, 22f
Stenting
for acute aortic dissection, 79, 79f
for coarctation of the aorta, 280f, 280–281, 281f
reconstructed computed tomography after, 239f
for traumatic disruption of the aorta, 319, 330f
Strain plot, in acute aortic dissection, 110f
Structure, aortic, 13t–14t
Subclavian arteries
left
anatomy of, 19
embolization of, 208, 208f
right, aberrant, 19, 20f, 26f–28f
Subclavian patch aortoplasty, for coarctation of the aorta, 281f
Subcostal arteries, variant anatomy of, 22
Surgical inspection, 52
Syphilitic aneurysms, 337–338
clinical presentation and management of, 338, 338f
Systemic lupus erythematosus, aortitis and, 347, 348f
Systems review, 33

T

Takayasu's disease, 51f, 341–346
angiographic classification of, 341, 342t, 343, 343f
case studies of, 344–346
clinical presentation of, 341–343
giant cell arteritis versus, 342t
imaging of, 343, 343f, 344f, 344t
long-term morbidity and surgical mortality in, 343–344
treatment of, 343
Thoracic aorta
anatomy of, 5f, 5–6
disease involvement of, 5–6
imaging considerations for, 5
Thoracic aortic aneurysms, 195–213
of aortic arch, 198–199, 199f
of aortic root, 196–197
annuloaortic ectasia and, 196–197, 197f
sinus of Valsalva aneurysms as, 196, 251, 252f, 253–254, 256–257
of ascending aorta, 197–198, 198f
case studies of, 201–213
of descending thoracic aorta, 199f, 199–200
saccular, 199–200
endovascular repair of, 200, 200f

Thoracic aortic aneurysms (Continued)
etiology of, 196
extensive, 200f, 200–201, 201f
Thoracic endovascular aortic repair, 200, 200f
Thoracoabdominal aorta, 50f
Thoracoabdominal aortic aneurysms, 51f, 195, 200f, 200–201, 201f
case study of, 206, 207f
Thrombi
mural, abdominal aortic aneurysms and, 218
pedunculation of, 170, 171f
Thromboembolism, aortic, 171
Tracheal tug, 34
Transesophageal echocardiography, 38, 39f, 40f, 41t
in acute aortic dissection, 59f, 71, 72, 73f, 74f, 75t, 76t, 81f, 84f, 86f, 88f, 89f, 92f, 94f, 96f, 98f, 99f, 109f, 111f, 146f
in aortic atheromatous disease, 160f, 161f, 165f, 169, 170f
following aortic dissection, 136f, 138f, 139f
in aortic root aneurysm, 252g
in aortic root fistula, 252g
in aortic ulcers and penetrating ulcers, 183f, 184f, 187f, 189f, 191f
in atheromatous disease, 175f, 177f
in atherosclerotic intimal calcification, 158f
in bicuspid aortic valve, 264f, 265f
in coarctation of the aorta, 274f, 276, 277f, 290f, 293f–295f
comparison with other imaging modalities, 52
in intramural hematoma, 117, 117f, 118f, 121f, 122f, 124f, 128f, 145f
in Marfan syndrome, 309f, 311f, 312f
in mechanical valve endocarditis, 258f
in sinus of Valsalva aneurysm, 254f
in Staphylococcus aureus aneurysms, 340f
in Takayasu's disease, 346f
in thoracic aortic aneurysms, 204f, 205f
in traumatic disruption of the aorta, 318–319, 319f–321f, 319t, 320t, 323f, 328f
Transthoracic echocardiography, 35–37, 37f
in acute aortic dissection, 71, 72, 72f, 82f, 91f, 98f, 101f, 103f, 106, 146f
in aortic root to right atrium-right ventricle fistula, 255f
in aortic ulcers and penetrating ulcers, 189f
in atheromatous disease, 179f
in bicuspid aortic valve, 262f, 263f, 268f
in coarctation of the aorta, 273, 276, 276f, 277f, 283f, 284f, 287f, 293f, 295f
comparison with other imaging modalities, 52t
in Marfan syndrome, 308f, 311f, 313f, 314f
in sinus of Valsalva fistula, 257f

Transthoracic echocardiography (Continued)
in thoracic aortic aneurysms, 202f
in tumors of the aorta, 334f
Traumatic disruption of the aorta, 315–330
case studies of, 321–330
clinical findings prompting consideration of, 316
complete, 315
diagnosis of, 316–319
aortography in, 317–318, 318f, 319f
chest radiography in, 316
computed tomography in, 316–317, 317f
transesophageal echocardiography in, 318–319, 319f, 319t, 320f, 320t
mechanisms of disruption and, 315
partial, 315
sites and morphology of, 316, 316f
surgical findings in, 325f
treatment of, 319
Tubular aortic aneurysms, 195
Tumors, aortic, 333–335
case studies of, 333–335
surgical treatment of, 335f

U

Ulcers and penetrating ulcers, aortic, 181–193
case studies of, 184–193
imaging of, 181–182, 183f
management of, 182, 183f
endograft insertion for, 188f
surgical specimens of, 183f, 190f, 191f
Ultrasonography
of abdominal aorta, 37, 38f
in abdominal aortic aneurysm, 219f
advantages and disadvantages of, 220t
in acute aortic dissection, 104f, 105f
in atherosclerotic intimal calcification, 158f
comparison with other imaging modalities, 52t
in dissection, 148f
endovascular therapy and, 242, 242f
in intramural hematoma, 144f

V

Ventriculography
contrast, in aortic root to right atrium-right ventricle fistula, 256f
in Marfan syndrome, 312f

W

Windkessel, 8, 8f